CLINICAL CASES
Orthopaedic Surgery

Eugene C. Toy, MD
Vice Chair of Academic Affairs, Department of Obstetrics and Gynecology
The John S. Dunn, Senior Academic Chair and Program Director
The Methodist Hospital Ob/Gyn Residency Program
Houston, Texas
Clerkship Director, Clinical Professor
Department of Obstetrics and Gynecology
The University of Texas—Houston Medical School
Houston, Texas

Andrew J. Rosenbaum, MD
Resident of Orthopaedic Surgery
Division of Orthopaedic Surgery
Albany Medical Center
Albany, New York

Timothy T. Roberts, MD
Resident of Orthopaedic Surgery
Division of Orthopaedic Surgery
Albany Medical Center
Albany, New York

Joshua S. Dines, MD
Orthopaedic Surgeon
Sports Medicine and Shoulder Service
Hospital for Special Surgery
New York, New York
Assistant Professor of Orthopaedic Surgery
Weill Cornell Medical College
New York, New York

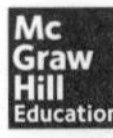

McGraw Hill Education (India) Private Limited
NEW DELHI

McGraw Hill Education Offices
New Delhi New York St Louis San Francisco Auckland Bogotá Caracas
Kuala Lumpur Lisbon London Madrid Mexico City Milan Montreal
San Juan Santiago Singapore Sydney Tokyo Toronto

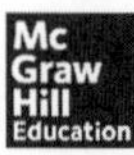 McGraw Hill Education (India) Private Limited

Clinical Cases: Orthopaedic Surgery

McGraw Hill Education (India) Edition 2013

RZZYCDRORBQRR

Reprinted in India by arrangement with The McGraw Hill Companies, Inc., New York

Sales territories: India, Pakistan, Nepal, Bangladesh, Sri Lanka and Bhutan

Library of Congress Cataloging-in-Publication Data

Toy, Eugene C.
Clinical Case: Orthopaedic surgery / Eugene Toy … [et al.]. — 1st ed.
p. ; cm
Orthopaedic surgery
Includes bibliographical references and index.
ISBN 978-0-07-179030-7 (pbk. : alk. paper) — ISBN 0-07-179030-6 (pbk. : alk. paper)
I Toy, Eugene C. II. Title: Orthopaedic surgery.
[DNLM: 1. Orthopaedic Procedures—methods—Case Reports. 2. Orthopaedic Procedures—methods—Problems and Exercises. 3. Musculoskeletal System—injuries—Case Reports. 4. Musculoskeletal System—injuries—Problems and Exercises. WE 18.2]
617.4'7—dc23 2012038036

ISBN-13: 978-93-5134-337-0
ISBN-10: 93-5134-337-5

Published by McGraw Hill Education (India) Private Limited, P-24, Green Park Extension, New Delhi 110 016, and printed at Rajkamal Electric Press, Kundli-131028, Haryana

DEDICATION

To runners everywhere, from the casual jogger to the serious and competitive marathoner—may the wind be at our backs, horizon before us, and may we never need the medical care in this book.

—ECT

To Kristin, my sister Caroline, and my parents: thank you for your support, encouragement, and love. To Dr. Eric Hume, my mentor and role model. And to my uncle David Dines, an inspiration and someone I can only hope to emulate as an orthopaedic surgeon.

—AJR

To Guy and Meisie, whose guidance, generosity, and genes inspired my orthopaedic dreams. And to the talented faculty of Albany Med, who are patiently making them real.

—TTR

To the residents, fellows, and colleagues with whom I work: Thank you for inspiring me to always continue learning and teaching. And, to Kathryn, Humphrey, and my parents for your unwavering support.

— JSD

CONTENTS

Contributors / vii
Acknowledgments / xvii
Introduction / xix

Section I
How to Approach Clinical Problems 1
Part 1. Approach to the Orthopaedic Patient 2
Part 2. Approach to Clinical Problem Solving 9
Part 3. Approach to Reading 14

Section II
Clinical Cases 21
Forty-Five Case Scenarios 23

Section III
Listing of Cases 417
Listing by Case Number 419
Listing by Case Topic (Alphabetical) 420

Index / 423

CONTRIBUTORS

Thomas J. Barrett, MD
Resident, Orthopaedic Surgery
Division of Orthopaedic Surgery
Albany Medical Center
Albany, New York
Open Tibia Fracture

Asheesh Bedi, MD
Assistant Professor and Orthopaedic Surgeon
Sports Medicine and Shoulder Surgery
Department of Orthopaedic Surgery
University of Michigan Health System
Ann Arbor, Michigan
Patellar Tendon Rupture
Lateral Epicondylitis (Tennis Elbow)

Marschall B. Berkes, MD
Resident, Orthopaedic Surgery
Department of Orthopaedic Surgery
Hospital for Special Surgery
New York, New York
Proximal Humerus Fracture
Meniscal Tears

David S. Brown, MD, PhD
Resident, Orthopaedic Surgery
Division of Orthopaedic Surgery
Albany Medical Center
Albany, New York
Shoulder Arthroplasty

Michael B. Cross, MD
Orthopaedic Surgeon
Hospital for Special Surgery
Adult Reconstruction and Joint Replacement Division
New York, New York
Hip Osteoarthritis

Matthew E. Cunningham, MD, PhD
Assistant Professor, Orthopaedic Surgery
Weill Cornell Medical College
Cornell University
Assistant Attending, Orthopaedic Surgery
Hospital for Special Surgery
New York, New York
Adolescent Idiopathic Scoliosis

Cory M. Czajka, MD
Resident, Orthopaedic Surgery
Division of Orthopaedic Surgery
Albany Medical Center
Albany, New York
Septic Knee

Joshua S. Dines, MD
Orthopaedic Surgeon
Sports Medicine and Shoulder Service
Hospital for Special Surgery
New York, New York
Assistant Professor of Orthopaedic Surgery
Weill Cornell Medical College
New York, New York
Proximal Humerus Fracture
Meniscal Tears
Ulnar Collateral Ligament Injury of the Elbow

David Y. Ding, MD
Resident, Orthopaedic Surgery
Department of Orthopaedic Surgery
New York University Hospital for Joint Diseases
New York, New York
Distal Radius (Colles) Fracture

John A. DiPreta, MD
Associate Clinical Professor
Division of Orthopaedic Surgery
Albany Medical College
Capital Region Orthopaedic Group
Albany, New York
Achilles Tendon Rupture
Lisfranc Injury

Christopher C. Dodson, MD
Assistant Professor of Orthopaedic Surgery
Thomas Jefferson Medical College
Attending Surgeon
Rothman Institute
Philadelphia, Pennsylvania
Cubital Tunnel Syndrome

Paul-Michel F. Dossous, MD, MPH
Resident, Orthopaedic Surgery
Division of Orthopaedic Surgery
Albany Medical Center
Albany, New York
Osteomyelitis

Matthew A. Dow, MD
Resident, Orthopaedic Surgery
Division of Orthopaedic Surgery
Albany Medical Center
Albany, New York
Developmental Dysplasia of the Hip

Scott J. Ellis, MD
Assistant Attending, Orthopaedic Surgery
Department of Foot and Ankle Surgery
Hospital for Special Surgery
New York, New York
Adult Acquired Flatfoot Deformity

Elizabeth R. Sibilsky Enselman, Med, ATC
Clinical Research Coordinator
Department of Orthopaedic Surgery
The University of Michigan
Ann Arbor, Michigan
Patellar Tendon Rupture
Lateral Epicondylitis

Michael Faloon, MD, MS
John Cobb Spine and Scoliosis Fellow
Hospital of Special Surgery
Senior Clinical Associate, Orthopaedic Surgery
Weill Cornell Medical College
New York, New York
Adolescent Idiopathic Scoliosis

Michael A. Flaherty, MD
Fellow, Orthopaedic Sports Medicine
University of Massachusetts Medical Center
Worcester, Massachusetts
Rotator Cuff Repair

Michael P. Gaspar, MD
Resident, Orthopaedic Surgery
Division of Orthopaedic Surgery
Albany Medical Center
Albany, New York
Carpal Tunnel Syndrome

Andrew Gerdeman, MD
Clinical Professor, Orthopaedics
Division of Orthopaedic Surgery
Albany Medical Center
Capital Region Orthopaedic Group
Albany, New York
Anterior Cruciate Ligament Reconstruction

Daniel W. Green, MD, FACS
Associate Professor, Orthopaedic Surgery
Weill Cornell Medical College
Associate Attending, Orthopaedic Surgeon
Hospital for Special Surgery
New York, New York
Pediatric Both Bone Forearm Fracture

Matthew H. Griffith, MD
Department of Orthopaedic Surgery
Reston Hospital Center
Reston, Virginia
Trigger Finger

Christopher C. Harrod, MD
Spine Fellow
Department of Orthopaedic Surgery and Neurosurgery
Thomas Jefferson University Hospital
Rothman Institute
Philadelphia, Pennsylvania
Lumbar Burst Fracture

Vishal Hegde
Class of 2013
Weill Cornell Medical College
New York, New York
Osteoporosis

Khalid Hesham, MD
Resident, Orthopaedic Surgery
Division of Orthopaedic Surgery
Albany Medical Center
Albany, New York
Rickets

Joel A. Horning, MD
Fellow, Orthopaedic Sports Medicine
University of Texas Health Science Center at San Antonio
San Antonio, Texas
Anterior Cruciate Ligament Reconstruction

Shazaan Hushmendy, BS
Class of 2013
Albany Medical College
Albany, New York
Supracondylar Fracture
Cauda Equina Syndrome

Kristofer J. Jones, MD
Chief Resident, Orthopaedic Surgery
Department of Orthopaedic Surgery
Hospital for Special Surgery
New York, New York
Ulnar Collateral Ligament Injury of the Elbow

Lana Kang, MD
Assistant Professor
Weill Cornell Medical College and
New York Presbyterian Hospital
New York, New York
Attending Surgeon
Hospital for Special Surgery
New York, New York
Consultant, Orthopaedic Surgeon
James J. Peters Veterans Affairs Medical Center
Bronx, New York
Dupuytren Disease

Christopher K. Kepler, MD, MBA
Fellow, Spine Surgery
Thomas Jefferson University
Philadelphia, Pennsylvania
Lumbar Burst Fracture

Hanna N. Ladenhauf, MD
Resident, Pediatric and Adolescent Surgery
Department of Pediatric and Adolescent Surgery
Paracelsus Medical University Hospital
Salzburg, Austria
Pediatric Both Bone Forearm Fracture

Joseph M. Lane, MD
Professor, Orthopaedic Surgery
Weill Cornell Medical College
Chief, Metabolic Bone Disease Service
Hospital for Special Surgery
New York, New York
Osteoporosis

James P. Lawrence, MD, MBA, FAAOS
Assistant Professor, Surgery
Division of Orthopaedic Surgery
Albany Medical Center
Orthopaedic Spine Surgeon
Capital Region Spine
Albany, New York
Cervical Radiculopathy
Cauda Equina Syndrome

Xiaowei A. Li
Class of 2014
Weill Cornell Medical Center
Cornell University
New York, New York
Hip Osteoarthritis

Dean Lorich, MD
Associate Professor, Orthopaedic Surgery
Weill Cornell Medical Center
Chief, Orthopaedics
New York-Presbyterian Hospital
Associate Director, Orthopaedic Trauma Service
Hospital for Special Surgery
New York, New York
Proximal Humerus Fracture

Jason A. Luciano, MD, MBA
Resident, General Surgery
Department of Surgery
University of Pittsburgh Medical Center
Pittsburgh, Pennsylvania
Acute Compartment Syndrome

Patrick G. Marinello, MD
Resident, Orthopaedic Surgery
Department of Orthopaedic Surgery
Cleveland Clinic Foundation
Cleveland, Ohio
Achilles Tendon Rupture

Owen McGonigle, MD
Resident, Orthopaedic Surgery
Department of Orthopaedics
Tufts Medical Center
Boston, Massachusetts
Intertrochanteric Hip Fracture

Andrew S. Morse, MD
Resident, Orthopaedic Surgery
Division of Orthopaedic Surgery
Albany Medical Center
Albany, New York
Carpal Tunnel Syndrome

Michael T. Mulligan, MD
Assistant Professor, Orthopaedic Surgery
Division of Orthopaedic Surgery
Albany Medical Center
Albany, New York
Carpal Tunnel Syndrome

Denis Nam, MD
Resident, Orthopaedic Surgery
Department of Orthopaedic Surgery
Hospital for Special Surgery
New York, New York
Periprosthetic Hip Fracture

Meredith Osterman, MD
Resident, Orthopaedic Surgery
Department of Orthopaedic Surgery
Thomas Jefferson University Hospital
Philadelphia, Pennsylvania
Cubital Tunnel Syndrome

Dean Papaliodis, MD
Resident, Orthopaedic Surgery
Division of Orthopaedic Surgery
Albany Medical Center
Albany, New York
Clavicle Fracture
Achilles Tendon Rupture

Anish G. R. Potty, MD, MRCS
Fellow, Orthopaedic Surgery
Hospital for Special Surgery
New York, New York
Osteoporosis

Steven Rayappa, MD, MS
Resident, Orthopaedic Surgery
Division of Orthopaedic Surgery
Albany Medical Center
Albany, New York
Femoral Neck Fracture

Timothy T. Roberts, MD
Resident, Orthopaedic Surgery
Division of Orthopaedic Surgery
Albany Medical Center
Albany, New York
The Approach to the Orthopaedic Patient
Femoral Neck Fracture
Tibial Plateau Fracture
Ankle Fracture
Supracondylar Humerus Fracture
Osteomyelitis
Slipped Capital Femoral Epiphysis
Cervical Radiculopathy
Cauda Equina Syndrome
Lumbar Burst Fracture
Total Knee Arthroplasty
Rickets

Andrew J. Rosenbaum, MD
Resident, Orthopaedic Surgery
Division of Orthopaedic Surgery
Albany Medical Center
Albany, New York
Posterior Hip Dislocation
Open Tibia Fracture
Pediatric Both Bone Forearm Fracture
Developmental Dysplasia of the Hip
Rotator Cuff Injury
Anterior Cruciate Ligament Reconstruction
Lisfranc Injury
Osteosarcoma

Michael T. Rozell, MD
Resident, Orthopaedic Surgery
Department of Orthopaedic Surgery
SUNY Upstate Medical University
Syracuse, New York
Lisfranc Injury

Anas Saleh, MD
Metabolic Bone Disease Unit
Hospital for Special Surgery
New York, New York
Osteoporosis

John Saunders, MD
Resident, Orthopaedic Surgery
Albany Medical Center
Albany, New York
Ankle Fracture

Mark A. Schrumpf, MD
Resident, Orthopaedic Surgery
Department of Orthopaedic Surgery
Hospital for Special Surgery
New York, New York
Ulnar Collateral Ligament Injury of the Elbow

Nirav J. Shah, MD
Resident, Orthopaedic Surgery
Division of Orthopaedic Surgery
Albany Medical Center
Albany, New York
Total Knee Arthroplasty

Gillian L. S. Soles, MD
University of California
Davis Medical Center
Sacramento, California
Calcaneus Fracture

Samuel A. Taylor, MD
Resident, Orthopaedic Surgery
Hospital for Special Surgery
New York, New York
Proximal Humerus Fracture
Meniscal Tears

Justin Tsai, MD
Resident, Orthopaedic Surgery
Department of Orthopaedic Surgery and
Rehabilitation Medicine
SUNY Downstate Medical Center
Brooklyn, New York
Anterior Shoulder Dislocation

Michael Van Hal, MD
Resident, Orthopaedic Surgery
Department of Orthopaedic Surgery
University of Pittsburgh Medical Center
Pittsburgh, Pennsylvania
Cervical Radiculopathy

Zachary S. Wallace, MD
Resident, Internal Medicine
Department of Medicine
Massachusetts General Hospital
Boston, Massachusetts
Gout
Rheumatoid Arthritis

Brad J. Yoo, MD
Assistant Professor, Orthopaedic Trauma Service
Department of Orthopaedics
University of California
David Medical Center
Sacramento, California
Calcaneus Fracture

George Zanaros, MD
Orthopaedic Surgeon
Division of Orthopaedic Surgery
Albany Medical Center
Capital Region Orthopaedic Group
Albany, New York
Clavicle Fracture

Joseph P. Zimmerman, MD
Resident, Orthopaedic Surgery
Division of Orthopaedic Surgery
Albany Medical Center
Albany, New York
Child Abuse

ACKNOWLEDGMENTS

The clerkship curriculum that evolved into the ideas for this series was inspired by two talented and forthright students, Philbert Yao and Chuck Rosipal, who have since graduated from medical school. It has been a tremendous joy to work with the excellent orthopaedic surgery residents and faculty members at Albany Medical Center and Hospital for Special Surgery. They have been some of the most diligent, astute, and wonderfully responsive group with whom I have collaborated. I am greatly indebted to my editor, Catherine Johnson, whose exuberance, experience, and vision helped to shape this series. I appreciate McGraw-Hill's believing in the concept of teaching through clinical cases, and I would like to especially acknowledge John Williams, the director of editing. I am also thankful to Tania Andrabi for her excellent production expertise.

Without my dear colleagues Drs. Konrad Harms, Priti Schachel, and Gizelle Brooks-Carter, this book could not have been written. At Methodist Hospital, I appreciate Dr. Marc Boom, Dr. Judy Paukert, and Dr. Alan Kaplan. I also appreciate Debby Chambers, an excellent administrator, who is extremely supportive to the mission of education. Most of all, I appreciate my ever-loving wife Terri and my four wonderful children, Andy, Michael, Allison, and Christina, for their patience and understanding.

Eugene C. Toy, MD

ACKNOWLEDGMENTS

INTRODUCTION

Mastering the cognitive knowledge within a field such as orthopaedic surgery is a formidable task. It is even more difficult to draw on that knowledge, procure and filter through the clinical and laboratory data, develop a differential diagnosis, and finally form a rational treatment plan. To gain these skills, the student often learns best at the bedside, guided and instructed by experienced teachers, and inspired toward self-directed, diligent reading. Clearly, there is no replacement for education at the bedside or operating room. Unfortunately, clinical situations usually do not encompass the breadth of the specialty. Perhaps the best alternative is a carefully crafted patient case designed to stimulate the clinical approach and decision making. In an attempt to achieve that goal, we have constructed a collection of clinical vignettes to teach diagnostic or therapeutic approaches relevant to pediatrics. Most importantly, the explanations for the cases emphasize the mechanisms and underlying principles, rather than merely rote questions and answers.

This book is organized for versatility: It allows the student "in a rush" to go quickly through the scenarios and check the corresponding answers, while allowing the student who wants more thought-provoking explanations to go at a more measured pace. The answers are arranged from simple to complex: a summary of the pertinent points, the bare answers, an analysis of the case, an approach to the topic, a comprehension test at the end for reinforcement and emphasis, and a list of resources for further reading. The clinical vignettes are purposely placed in random order to simulate the way that real patients present to the practitioner. A listing of cases is included in Section III to aid the student who desires to test his or her knowledge of a specific area or who wants to review a topic, including basic definitions. Finally, we intentionally did not primarily use a multiple-choice question format in our clinical case scenarios because clues (or distractions) are not available in the real world. Nevertheless, several multiple-choice comprehension questions are included at the end of each case discussion to reinforce concepts or introduce related topics.

HOW TO GET THE MOST OUT OF THIS BOOK

Each case is designed to simulate a patient encounter with open-ended questions. At times, the patient's complaint is different from the most concerning issue, and sometimes extraneous information is given. The answers are organized into four different parts:

PART I

1. **Summary:** The salient aspects of the case are identified, filtering out the extraneous information. Students should formulate their summary from the case before looking at the answers. A comparison to the summation in the answer will help to improve their ability to focus on the important data while appropriately discarding the irrelevant information—a fundamental skill in clinical problem solving.

2. A **Straightforward Answer** is given to each open-ended question.
3. The **Analysis of the Case** is composed of two parts:
   a. **Objectives of the Case:** A listing of the two or three main principles that are crucial for a practitioner to manage the patient. Again, the students are challenged to make educated "guesses" about the objectives of the case upon initial review of the case scenario, which helps to sharpen their clinical and analytical skills.
   b. **Considerations:** A discussion of the relevant points and brief approach to the specific patient.

PART II

Approach to the Disease Process consists of two distinct parts:

a. **Definitions:** Terminology pertinent to the disease process.
b. **Clinical Approach:** A discussion of the approach to the clinical problem in general, including tables, figures, and algorithms.

PART III

Comprehension Questions: Each case contains several multiple-choice questions, which reinforce the material or introduce new and related concepts. Questions about material not found in the text have explanations in the answers.

PART IV

Clinical Pearls: Several clinically important points are reiterated as a summation of the text. This allows for easy review, such as before an examination.

SECTION I

How to Approach Clinical Problems

Part 1 Approach to the Orthopaedic Patient

Part 2 Approach to Clinical Problem Solving

Part 3 Approach to Reading

Part 1. Approach to the Orthopaedic Patient

The transition from textbook learning to the application of information in a specific clinical situation is one of the most challenging tasks in medicine. It requires retention of information, organization of the facts, and recall of a myriad of data in precise application to the patient. The purpose of this book is to facilitate this process. The first step is gathering information, also known as establishing the database. This includes taking the history; performing the physical examination; obtaining selective imaging, such as plain x-rays; and ordering laboratory studies. Of these, the historical examination is the most important and useful. Sensitivity and respect should always be exercised during interactions with patients.

HISTORY

1. **Basic information:**

   a. *Age and sex:* It may seem obvious, but the age and sex of the orthopaedic patient is of tremendous diagnostic, therapeutic, and prognostic importance. For example, a first-time shoulder dislocation in a male less than 20 years of age is bound to recur at a rate of greater than 80%, whereas a first shoulder dislocation in a female greater than 40 years of age will only recur approximately 10% of the time.

   b. *Chief complaint:* What has brought the patient to your office? Urgent care clinic? Trauma bay? Has the patient suffered an acute traumatic injury, or has the patient been referred to you for chronic symptoms of several months in duration? Perhaps the most common complaint to orthopaedic physicians is pain. At a minimum, the acuity, severity, location, temporality, presence of associated symptoms, and relieving and exacerbating factors for any complaint of pain should be noted.

      - **Acute trauma:** In acute, high-energy traumatic situations, it is essential to carefully follow Advanced Trauma Life Support (ATLS) protocol to optimize patient survival and minimize morbidity. In many hospitals, traumatic scenarios are managed by emergency department physicians and trauma surgical teams. Orthopaedic surgeons play a vital, if supportive, role in acute life support management. After ensuring stability of the patient's airway, breathing, cardiovascular system, cerebral perfusion, and environment, the orthopaedist must work to stabilize major fractures, reduce dislocations, attenuate bleeding, provisionally irrigate contaminated lesions, and assess neurovascular deficits.

      - **Mechanism of injury:** In traumatic situations, whether low-energy falls from standing height or high-energy motor vehicular collisions (MVC), orthopaedic physicians must make special note of the mechanism of injury. Both the patient's positioning during injury and the direction of forces acting on the patient play a key role in the classification, treatment, and prognosis of many different types of orthopaedic injuries. In fact, several fracture classification systems are based on the very mechanism of injury, including high-energy, high-mortality pelvic fractures and comparatively lower energy "everyday" ankle fractures. For patients injured in MVCs, note whether the patient was wearing a seat belt. Likewise, was the motorcyclist wearing a helmet? Does the patient recall the accident, or did he or she lose consciousness? In the elderly especially, a hip fracture may represent more than just a broken bone. Such patients often fall as a result of syncope or presyncope, secondary to underlying cardiac and/or neurologic conditions. The fall may be the first presentation of uncontrolled atrial fibrillation or Alzheimer dementia.

- **Chronic symptomatology:** In patients with chronic symptomatology, the physician must work to carefully characterize the patient's symptoms with regard to acuity, severity, location, temporality, presence of associated symptoms, and relieving and exacerbating factors. At this point, the clinician may begin to generate a list of differential diagnoses that further inquiry, examination, and testing will narrow.
- **Concomitant injuries:** Does the patient have any other complaints? Does the patient complain of neck pain after crashing the car? Is the patient intoxicated? Patients under the influence of drugs or alcohol, or simply as secondary to a sympathetic response to the injury, may not immediately recognize a painful injury. This is especially true in patients with multiple distracting injuries. When evaluating the cervical spine, it is essential to rule out distracting injuries, as a painful broken femur may distract the patient from a vague neck ache, the result of an unstable ligamentous injury.

c. *Past medical history:* First, any history of systemic illnesses such as diabetes, cardiovascular disease, peripheral vascular disease, and crystalloid, rheumatoid, and seronegative arthritis must be investigated. Primarily musculoskeletal conditions such as osteoporosis and osteoarthritis and histories of fracture, sprains, strains, tears, and infections should also be elicited.

d. *Past surgical history:* Does the patient have a history of fracture fixation, joint replacement, spinal decompression, or other procedures, recent or distant, that may influence his or her management? A detailed knowledge of previous orthopaedic treatments is paramount for planning new interventions. For example, an acute periprosthetic femoral shaft fracture around a previous hip replacement is treated differently from hip fracture in a native (normal) joint. Although the patient without a history of joint replacement may benefit from an intramedullary rod, the canal is partially occupied by the prosthesis in the patient with the history of joint replacement, making intramedullary fixation impossible without an extensive revision of components. For any patient undergoing surgery on or around a previous orthopaedic implant, it is important to obtain documentation of the type of implant used, its size, manufacturer, and both when and by whom it was placed.

e. *Family history:* Inquire about a history a familial degenerative, metabolic bone, or connective tissue disorders. In patients with arthritis, for example, be certain to ask about a familial history of rheumatoid and autoimmune diseases, as these conditions may have a familial predilection. Such information may help target your differential diagnosis.

f. *Social history:* Does the patient abuse tobacco? Does the patient drink alcohol? If so, how much and for how long? Does the patient use illicit substances? Nicotine is a significant inhibitor of both wound and bone healing; in a study of open tibial shaft fractures, injuries took almost 70% longer to heal in smokers versus nonsmokers. Nicotine also has been shown to increase the rate of nonunion, or failed healing of bone. Inquire about the patient's vocation, hobbies, physical activities, and hand dominance. A high-performance college athlete, for example, may benefit more from an elective anterior cruciate ligament (ACL) repair than a 53-year-old concert pianist who spends most of her time sitting. The same concert pianist may require surgical reduction and fixation of a nondominant comminuted distal radius fracture versus the same fracture in an 86-year-old nonambulator for whom cast fixation is adequate.

g. *Allergies:* Inquire about previous reactions to medications, and be certain to distinguish between true hypersensitivity and adverse responses. A distant memory of "stomach upset" from penicillin is not necessarily reason to compromise on an effective, first-line antibiotic.

h. *Medications:* As usual, careful documentation of medications both past and present is important. Note dosages, durations of treatment, and indications when unclear. Pay special attention to history of steroids, bisphosphonate, anticoagulant, and antibiotic use, as these medications frequently influence perioperative management.

i. *Review of systems:* A general review of symptomatology is important in assessing the orthopaedic patient. Has the patient with knee pain been experiencing fevers and chills, suggestive of a septic joint? Has the patient concerned with insidious back pain been experiencing unintended weight loss and night sweats, representative, perhaps, of a vertebral body metastasis from an unknown primary tumor? Such diagnoses may be missed if a review of systems is not performed.

PHYSICAL EXAM

1. **Vital signs:** Note the patient's temperature, blood pressure, heart rate, respiratory rate, and peripheral oxygen saturation. Height, weight, and body mass index should also be considered.

2. **General appearance:** Note whether the patient is cachectic versus well-nourished, anxious versus calm, alert versus obtunded, comfortable versus distressed. Also note the patient's ambulatory status, gait, posture, and stance. Some clinicians argue that the physical exam "begins in the waiting room" as they observe patients make their way to the examination room.

3. **A basic approach to the musculoskeletal examination of the extremities:** Based on 5 elements: inspection, palpation, range of motion, neurovascular evaluation, and special tests.

   a. *Inspection:* The examination of any extremity should begin with inspection of the limb for gross deformities, open fractures, skin defects, rashes, blisters, burns, lacerations, or any other traumatic sequelae. Carefully survey the skin for tenting in the setting of displaced fractures, as protruding bone fragments can quickly erode through the skin, creating a delayed open fracture. Inspect for symmetry, atrophy, or gross defects such as dislocations, angulations, and rotational deformities. Note that a small skin "poke hole" injury from a femoral shaft fracture represents a deceptively large soft tissue injury, as the femur fragments must violate several inches of thick muscle, fascia, and skin to pierce the surface.

b. *Palpation:* Palpate long bones for regions of tenderness, step-off, crepitus, and swelling. Palpate joints for tenderness, crepitus, and effusions.

c. *Range of motion:* Evaluate range of motion, first passively, with the examiner moving the patient's limb through a range of motion, then actively, with the patient moving his or her own limb through a complete range of motion. Always compare the affected extremity to the contralateral side.

d. *Neurovascular evaluation:* Sensation and vascularity should be assessed. Check for palpable pulses distally and for capillary refill at the finger or toe pads. Reflex testing may be performed when appropriate. When relevant, strength should be graded on a scale of 0 to 5:

0. No visible or palpable contraction
1. Any flicker of motion or visible and/or palpable muscle contraction
2. Full range of movement out of the plane of gravity
3. Full range of motion against gravity only
4. Full range of motion against some resistance, but weaker than expected
5. Normal strength

e. *Special testing:* Special tests, or tests specific to a certain joint, bony region, or pathology, may next be performed. Details for special physical exam tests are discussed later within pertinent clinical cases.

4. **A basic approach to the examination of the spine:** The spine has a complex arrangement of integrated bony, muscular, ligamentous, nervous, vascular, and other structures; understanding its anatomy is paramount to performing an effective examination. Although there is considerable overlap between a basic extremity and basic spine examination, the difference in the spine exam is the neurologic focus on nerve root distributions of function. For example, a finding of thumb and index finger weakness and numbness may represent ipsilateral C6 or C7 nerve root compression to a "tunnel-visioned" examiner who is focused on the spine. To a hand surgeon, however, such a finding may be the result of an undiagnosed carpel tunnel syndrome. The key to a good examination and evaluation is being able to recognize the differential diagnosis for a particular finding and narrow its potential etiologies accordingly.

a. *Inspection:* Inspect the spine for gross deformities, curvatures, skin defects, and other additional pathology. In settings of trauma, observe the skull, both anteriorly and posteriorly for evidence of blunt trauma, which may represent hyperextension and hyperflexion cervical injuries, respectively. From behind the patient, look for asymmetric scapulae, deviation from a plumb line (a median vertical line dropped from C7 by suspending a weight on a string), and observe for rib humps when the patient is in a forward-bend position. In newborns and infants, observe for defects such as dimples or tufts of hair, which are suggestive of underlying congenital abnormalities such as spinal bifida.

b. *Palpation:* Similarly, palpate the spine for abnormal curvatures, areas of step-off or prominences, or regions of tenderness. In patients with complaints of pain, make sure to determine whether the tenderness is localized over bony spinous processes or over paraspinal musculature. The former is suggestive of bone pathology such as fracture or tumor. This is especially important when clearing the cervical spine (C-spine) in traumatic scenarios. Although the focus here is orthopaedic pathology, one should assess for other organic causes of back pain such as renal pathology, suggested by costovertebral tenderness. Sacroiliac tenderness, elicited with pelvic compression or a FABER maneuver (positioning the hip in **f**lexion, **ab**duction, external **r**otation and pushing on the knee may induce pain with sacroiliac pathology), is suggestive of seronegative spondylopathies, whereas rheumatoid arthritis may cause tenderness of the intervertebral joints.

c. *Range of motion:* Outside of an acute trauma scenarios, the patient should be taken through an active range of motion including forward flexion, extension, lateral (sideways) bending, and rotation. Decreased range of motion with an absence of significant pain may be indicative of generalized degenerative process. A substantially decreased range of motion may be indicative of ankylosing spondylitis. Passive or physician-guided ranging of motion should be avoided in the cervical spine, as this may lead to iatrogenic injury.

d. *Neurovascular evaluation:* For patients with concerns of spine pathology, a complete and thorough neurologic exam must be performed and carefully documented. Strength, graded 0 to 5, and sensation, graded 0 to 2 (0=insensate, 1=impaired, 2=normal), should be evaluated in the major myo-dermatomal distributions of the bilateral upper and lower extremity. Tables I–1 and I–2 show common muscular, sensory, and reflexive distributions of the major nerve roots supplying the brachial and lumbar plexuses, respectively. For patients with acute traumatic injuries to the spine, it is essential that motor and sensory function be examined bilaterally throughout the body and carefully documented at the time of initial presentation. For patients undergoing workup for radicular pain, chronic back pain, or similar degenerative processes, physical exam findings should closely correlate with radiographic findings if one hopes to have successful surgical outcomes. Clinical correlation is paramount, as magnetic resonance imaging (MRI) of the spine has a notoriously high false-positive rate in elderly individuals.

e. *Special testing:* Details for specific physical exam tests are discussed later within pertinent clinical cases.

5. **Clearing the cervical spine:** In the setting of high-energy trauma or in patients who have suffered blunt trauma to the head or neck, the cervical spine must be immobilized provisionally to prevent potentially catastrophic neurologic injury. Even if a patient does not initially complain of head, neck, or radicular pain, intoxication and other injuries may distract from the sometimes subtle pains of

Table I–1 • MOTOR, SENSORY, AND REFLEX DISTRIBUTIONS OF THE MAJOR CERVICAL NERVE ROOTS TO THE BRACHIAL PLEXUS

Nerve Root	Motor	Sensory	Reflex
C5	Deltoid	Lateral shoulder	Biceps
C6	Biceps, wrist extensors	Radial forearm, thumb, and index finger	Brachioradialis
C7	Triceps, wrist flexors	Middle finger	Triceps
C8	Finger flexors	Ring and small fingers	
T1	Hand intrinsics	Ulnar forearm	

unstable cervical bony or ligamentous injury. For this reason, protocols exist to guide physicians in "clearing" the C-spine (ie, safely discontinuing provisional immobilization when there is no evidence to suggest an occult cervical spine injury). In general, the elements necessary for clearing the C-spine include an absence of posterior neck tenderness, an absence of focal neurologic deficits, a normal level of alertness, an absence of intoxication, an absence of distracting injuries, and the ability of the patient to perform an active range of painless neck motion.

RADIOGRAPHIC EVALUATION

1. **X-ray:** Also known as plain films or radiographs. At a minimum, 2 images are acquired, taken in planes perpendicular to one another. These are usually anterior-posterior (AP) and lateral views. For traumatic injuries, x-rays of the joint above and below an area of interest should be obtained. Additionally, many types of specialty views are obtained, depending on the region of interest. A common example is the Mortise view of the ankle—an AP view with 15 degrees of internal rotation—which shows a smooth, uniform space between the tibia/fibula and the underlying talus. In ankle fractures, widening or disruption of this normally uniform space may clearly demonstrate injuries.

Table I–2 • MOTOR, SENSORY, AND REFLEX DISTRIBUTIONS OF THE MAJOR LUMBOSACRAL NERVE ROOTS TO THE LUMBAR PLEXUS

Nerve Root	Motor	Sensory	Reflex
L2	Hip flexors	Anterior thigh	
L3	Quadriceps	Anterior knees	Patella (L3-4)
L4	Ankle dorsiflexors	Medial leg	
L5	Extensor hallices longus, hip abductors	Lateral leg	
Sacral	Ankle plantar flexors (S1)	Lateral foot (S1)	Achilles (S1-2), Anal wink (S2-4), Bulbocavernosus (S3-4)

2. **Computed tomography (CT):** CT is essentially a series of x-rays, reassembled by a computer into 3-dimensional images or "slices." CT plays an integral role in assessing complex anatomy such as acetabular and spine fractures and comminuted fractures and is often more sensitive than plain x-ray in diagnosis of nondisplaced or healing fractures. CT also plays a role in preoperative planning.

3. **Magnetic resonance imaging:** MRI is an indispensible tool for evaluating soft tissue structures such as ligaments, tendons, menisci, and nerves. When set to a T2-weighted signal, physiologic processes resulting in edema and tissue inflammation, such as infection, autoimmune processes, bone or soft tissue injury, and spinal cord or disc pathology, can be clearly visualized. MRI avoids ionizing radiation and is considered safe to use in the absence of ferromagnetic implants such as certain types orthopaedic hardware or cardiac pacemakers.

4. **Ultrasound:** Useful for detecting effusions, guiding needles for aspiration, evaluating for soft tissue abscesses or hematomas. Like MRI, ultrasound avoids ionizing radiation; it is frequently used in pediatric imaging.

5. **Nuclear medicine scans:** Bone scans, typically performed after administration of intravenous radioisotope technetium-99m, are a helpful tool for detecting bone pathology such as osteomyelitis, tumor, or healing fracture. After injection, the radioisotope localizes to regions of increased bony metabolic activity and is observable on specialized image detectors. Similarly, radioisotope-tagged white blood cells may be used in a similar fashion. Known as a tagged white blood cell scan, this modality is especially sensitive for detecting osteomyelitis.

6. **Dual-emission x-ray absorptiometry (DXA) scan:** DXA scanning is a radiographic method of measuring bone mineral density used in the diagnosis and management of osteoporosis.

LABORATORY TESTS

1. **Preoperative laboratory testing:** Patients suffering from high-energy traumatic injuries and patients undergoing elective orthopaedic procedures should undergo basic preoperative laboratory testing. This generally includes a complete blood count, basic metabolic panel, blood type and screening, and the basic coagulation tests, prothrombin time and partial thromboplastin time.

2. **Inflammatory laboratory studies:** Patients in whom infection is suspected should receive testing for an erythrocyte sedimentation rate (ESR) and C-reactive protein (CRP). These are 2 nonspecific inflammatory markers that may be used to assist with the diagnosis of, and to assess the efficacy of therapy in, chronic bone or joint infections. In patients undergoing workup for autoimmune disease, basic laboratory studies should minimally include ESR, CRP, rheumatoid factor, anticitrullinated protein, antinuclear antibody, and possibly HLA-B27 testing. Referral to a rheumatologic specialist is generally recommended.

3. **Synovial fluid analyses:** Frequently, orthopaedists are confronted with erythematous, swollen, and painful joints that must be aspirated to confirm a diagnosis. Synovial fluid should be sent for Gram stain, culture of aerobic and anaerobic organisms, crystal analysis, and synovial fluid cell counts, including white blood cell counts. The presence of bacteria on Gram stain is typically an indication for surgical irrigation and debridement of the joint, as bacteria in a closed joint can rapidly and irreversibly damage cartilage and other synovial structures. Crystal analysis may help with the diagnosis of gout (uric acid crystals) or pseudogout (calcium pyrophosphate crystals). Crystalloid arthropathy are typically managed nonoperatively.
4. **Urine pregnancy test (β-human chorionic gonadotropin):** In women of child-bearing age, it is important to eliminate the possibility of pregnancy when considering surgery or when exposing patients to ionizing radiation from x-rays, CT, or radioisotope scans.

Part 2. Approach to Clinical Problem Solving

There are typically 4 distinct steps that an orthopaedic surgeon takes to solve most clinical problems systematically:

1. Making the diagnosis
2. Assessing the severity of the disease or injury
3. Rendering a treatment based on the severity of the disease or injury
4. Following the patient's response to the treatment

MAKING THE DIAGNOSIS

The diagnosis is made by careful evaluation of the database, analysis of the information, assessment of the risk factors, and development of the list of possibilities (the differential diagnosis). The process includes knowing which pieces of information are meaningful and which may be thrown out. Experience and knowledge help to guide the physician to "key in" on the most important possibilities. A good clinician also knows how to ask the same question in several different ways and to use different terminology when appropriate. For example, patients at times may outright deny having any "current medical problems" but will deliver a laundry list of insulins, beta-blockers, or anti-depressants when asked about their current medications. Reaching a diagnosis may be achieved by systematically reading about each possible cause and disease. The patient's presentation is then matched up against each of these possibilities, and each potential diagnosis is either placed high up on the list as a potential etiology or moved lower down because of the disease's prevalence, the patient's presentation, or other clues. A patient's risk factors may influence the probability of a diagnosis.

Although orthopaedic trauma diagnoses are seemingly straightforward fracture identifications, concomitant symptoms such as weakness or paralysis, paresthesias, or pulselessness may complicate the diagnosis of a "simple" fracture. An intimate appreciation for both anatomy and physiology is required to generate the differential diagnosis, even in the setting of acute trauma—could the patient with a proximal tibia/fibula fracture and an inability to extend his great toe be experiencing paralysis from common peroneal nerve entrapment; from decreased effort, secondary to extreme anxiety and discomfort; from neurovascular compromise, secondary to an acute compartment syndrome; or from a yet undiscovered concomitant lumbar spine injury?

For the patient in the office complaining of several days of shoulder or knee pain, a long list of possible diagnoses can be pared down to 2 to 3 most likely diagnoses based on physical exam, selective imaging, and laboratory tests. For example, a woman who complains of left knee pain and has a history of a meniscal tear may have degenerative joint disease; another patient who has left knee pain and recent fevers and chills may have a septic joint infection. Furthermore, a patient complaining of left knee pain and a history of chronic steroid use for her Crohn disease may not have true knee pathology at all, but rather referred pain from avascular necrosis of the ipsilateral hip.

ASSESSING THE SEVERITY OF THE DISEASE

After ascertaining the diagnosis, the next step is to characterize the severity of the disease process; in other words, describe "how bad" a disease is. Most commonly, with traumatic injuries such as fractures and dislocations, this is done using a variety of classification schemes.

To students and residents unfamiliar with fracture classification systems, it may seem overly "academic" to call the broken ankle a "Lauge-Hansen S/ER-IV" or the broken hip an "AO 31-B2." However, classification systems play an important role in communicating the location, mechanism, and severity of an injury while simultaneously guiding its treatment. Classification schemes allow injuries to be standardized for research purposes and allow physicians to deliver more accurate prognoses to patients. The attending physician, hearing that the on-call resident has reduced and splinted an S/ER IV ankle fracture, can instantly picture this severe injury and can tell the resident to admit the patient for operative fixation the following morning.

Chronic orthopaedic conditions should be stratified in the same way. Degenerative joint disease of the hip may be mild in nature and effectively treated with nonsteroidal anti-inflammatory drugs (NSAIDs) and activity modification; or it may be severe, with the patient all but demanding a steroid injection or even a joint replacement.

TREATMENT BASED ON SEVERITY OF THE DISEASE OR INJURY

Both the treatment and prognosis for virtually any given orthopaedic diagnosis relates directly to its severity. For example, a closed tibial shaft fracture may be treated in a cast if its alignment after reduction falls within certain radiographic parameters. That same fracture, should it shift even a few millimeters, may need an intramedullary rod down its center, or a plate placed on its side, to hold the tenuous reduction. Had the skin over the fracture been damaged during the injury, it would have required urgent operative irrigation and debridement with concomitant intramedullary rodding or placement into an external fixator. Had there been a segment of bone lost during the injury, the patient may have required several staged procedures with vascularized bone grafting, soft tissue flapping, or even bone lengthening through an Ilizarov apparatus.

Orthopaedics is a broad field, with treatments ranging from quick splint application in the office to extensive and invasive procedures such as pelvic fracture reductions and internal fixation. An overview of some basic orthopaedic treatments and some of their most common indications follows. Details regarding orthopaedic treatment indications, techniques, and outcomes are discussed in the cases that follow.

Nonoperative Treatments

An orthopaedic reduction means simply to manipulate the bone or joint in such a way that anatomic positioning is restored. The principles of immobilization are simple: Hold the bones or tissues in, or as close to, their anatomic state to optimize healing and to minimize stresses on surrounding tissues. In their most simplistic form, most reduction maneuvers involve application of both axial traction and force in the direction opposite to that of the mechanism of injury. For a dorsally angulated distal radius fracture, for instance, reduction is performed by pulling axial traction and by applying volar-directed force to return the angulated carpus to its correct position. In general, immobilization should stabilize the joint above and below a fracture. One should always attempt to restore length, rotation, and angulation.

1. **Casting and splinting:** Defined as the application of plaster, fiberglass, or similar materials to immobilize a particular region of the body. Casts are generally applied circumferentially around an affected body part, providing more rigid and more durable immobilization. Splints may span and partially cover a region, but they allow tissues to swell and are easily removed. Several common casting techniques are detailed below; splints are applied similarly to these methods.
   a. *Short arm cast:* Applied from below the elbow to just proximal to the metacarpal-phalange joints at the midpalmar crease. These are generally indicated for reducible distal radius fractures. Short arm casts may be extended to a thumb spica cast wherein the thumb is immobilized up to the interphalangeal joint.
   b. *Long arm cast:* Similar distally to a short arm cast, but extends to the proximal third of the humerus with the elbow in approximately 90 degrees of flexion. Generally indicated in pediatric forearm fractures because, unlike short arm casts, it prevents rotation of the forearm by locking the wrist in the same plane as the arm. Long arm casts can also be extended to thumb spica casts and are thereby used to treat nondisplaced scaphoid fractures.
   c. *Short leg casts:* Extends from the tibial tubercle to just proximal to the metatarsal-phalange joints. Typically indicated in the treatment of stable ankle fractures. In general, it is important to dorsiflex the ankle to neutral, or 90 degrees with respect to the tibia, as prolonged plantar flexion may result in an equinus contracture of the Achilles tendon.

d. *Long leg cast:* Similar to a short leg cast, but extends to the proximal thigh. Typically indicated in the treatment of nonoperative tibial shaft fractures. Like long arm casts, this cast effectively blocks rotation of the extremity. The knee should be immobilized in 5 to 20 degrees of flexion.

e. *Hand splinting:* For immobilization of almost all metacarpal and phalanx fractures. The metacarpal-phalange joints should be immobilized between 70 and 90 degrees of flexion to prevent stiffening and contracture. Interphalangeal joints are immobilized in extension. Together, this is referred to as the "intrinsic plus" position because it mimics the hand position achieved with contraction of the hand intrinsic muscles.

2. **Bracing:**

   a. *Knee immobilizer:* A prefabricated brace extending from the mid-thigh to the mid-leg that holds the knee in near-complete extension. Typically used to stabilize knee dislocations, patella repairs, minimally displaced tibia plateau fractures, and postoperative arthroscopy patients.

   b. *Sarmiento (functional) bracing:* Typically consists of 2 pieces of half-cylindrical shells that strap together circumferentially around the site of a humeral shaft fracture. Often used as definitive treatment for humeral shaft fractures.

   c. *Bledsoe bracing:* Hinged braces that attach above and below a joint (typically the knee or elbow) to allow motion in a single plane. The desired degree of motion may be preset. For example, an elbow Bledsoe brace may be set from 0 to 90 degrees of flexion to protect from the extremes of flexion/extension as well as preventing varus/valgus forces in a postoperative distal humerus fracture.

3. **Traction:** Historically, many types of lower extremity fractures were treated with the patient in traction and on prolonged bedrest. Hip fractures and femoral shaft fractures, for example, are commonly displaced as a result of strong muscular deforming forces. Problems with hygiene, skin breakdown, and the difficulty of maintaining reductions made casting of these injuries nearly impossible. Therefore, such injuries were treated in traction, or with a constant, controlled axial force that pulls fractures into alignment. Because the skin can only tolerate limited prolonged pressure before breakdown occurs, traction pins were commonly employed. Placed through the distal femoral metaphysis or through the proximal tibia, large-diameter pins could transmit the traction forces necessary to counter deforming muscular contractions. Modern intramedullary rodding, prostheses, and generally improved surgical techniques have antiquated most indications for traction. However, traction is still used provisionally for patients awaiting definitive surgical fixation or for patients who are not medically fit to undergo major fixation procedures. Halo immobilization and Gardner-Well tong traction are another form of skeletal traction still in use today. With pins placed firmly into the skull, axial traction may be applied to the spine to assist in the reduction of injuries such as spinal facet dislocations, immobilization of unstable cervical spine injuries, and sometimes in pediatric patients to help correct scoliosis.

Operative Treatments

1. **Fracture fixation:**
   a. *Open reduction internal fixation (ORIF):* One of the mainstays of orthopaedic trauma surgery. Applies to virtually any situation in which a fracture site is directly opened and the bones reduced and fixated with a variety of implants such as screws, plates, wires, cement, and sutures.
   b. *Intramedullary nailing:* Similar to ORIF; however, the implant goes directly through the medullary canal, not on the surface of the bone. Furthermore, ORIF generally requires *direct* reduction of fracture fragments, whereas the fracture fragments in an intramedullary nailing procedure are typically indirectly reduced. Patients are sometimes surprised to hear that their scars will be nowhere near the site of their actual fracture.
   c. *External fixation:* External fixation is a method of temporarily stabilizing fractures and/or joints in the setting of hemodynamic instability, significant swelling, significant soft tissue injury, or other contraindications to primary fixation. Pins are typically placed in the cortices above and below a fracture site and then connected to an external frame that holds the alignment until definitive fixation may take place. These are commonly employed in multitrauma scenarios in which a patient with multiple long bone fractures and other organic injuries needs quick, temporary stabilization. Of course, if the reduction is well-aligned and the fixator remains in place long enough, external fixation may be the definitive treatment.
   d. *Percutaneous pinning:* A method of fixing fractures using thin wires placed through the skin under x-ray fluoroscopic guidance. Commonly used in settings such as hand fractures or supracondylar pediatric humerus fractures. Casts or splints are used in conjunction with pin placement to support the immobilized bone. After adequate callus formation, pins are typically pulled out through the skin without the need for further fixation.
2. **Arthroplasty:** Arthroplasty means the reconstruction of a joint. Common orthopaedic arthroplasty procedures involve the knee, hip, and shoulder, although implants are available for many other joints in the body. Arthroplasty is typically performed on an elective basis and is used as elective treatment for patients with severe degenerative joint disease and some cases of inflammatory arthritis. Elderly patients with displaced femoral neck fractures may undergo primary arthroplasty as definitive treatment for their fracture because attempted repair of the fragments has a very high incidence of failure.
3. **Arthroscopy:** Arthroscopy simply refers to the minimally invasive technique of using a camera to evaluate and treat intraarticular pathology. Common arthroscopic procedures include diagnostic explorations, meniscal debridements, removal of loose bodies, ligamentous repairs such as ACL reconstructions, and tendinous/joint capsule reconstructions. Thanks to the minimally invasive approach, procedures are often performed on an outpatient basis.

FOLLOWING THE RESPONSE TO TREATMENT

The final step in the approach to disease is to follow the patient's response to therapy. The "measure" of response should be monitored and documented. Some responses are clinical, such as improvement, or lack thereof, in a patient's subjective joint pain, activity level, range of motion, and strength. The physician must be skilled at eliciting this subjective data in an unbiased and standardized manner. Fractures, whether treated operatively or nonoperatively, are typically followed with serial x-rays. Intervals between imaging often vary with regard to the nature of the injury: A lateral malleolar ankle fracture treated in a cast is likely to remain stable and may require only biweekly imaging until there is clear evidence of bony healing. By contrast, a comminuted distal radius fracture treated in a cast has a much greater propensity to collapse and may need close monitoring if it is to be treated nonoperatively. Patients with conditions such as chronic osteomyelitis may require 6 to 8 weeks of intravenous antibiotic treatment, during which serial ESR and CRP studies help the clinician determine the duration and efficacy of treatment.

Part 3. Approach to Reading

The clinical problem-oriented approach to reading is different from the classic "systematic" research of a disease. Outside of isolated traumatic injuries, patients rarely present with a clear diagnosis; hence the clinician-in-training must become skilled in applying textbook information to the clinical setting. Furthermore, the reader retains more information when reading with a purpose. In other words, one should read with the goal of answering specific questions. Likewise, the clinician-in-training should have a plan for the acquisition and use of the information. The process is similar to having a mental "flow chart," with each step sifting through diagnostic possibilities, risk factors, therapies, and potential complications. There are several fundamental questions that facilitate clinical thinking:

- What is the most likely diagnosis?
- What should be the next step?
- What is the most likely mechanism for this injury or condition?
- What are the risk factors for this injury or condition?
- How is the diagnosis confirmed?
- What is the best therapy?
- What complications are associated with this injury or condition and its treatment?

WHAT IS THE MOST LIKELY DIAGNOSIS?

The method of establishing the diagnosis has been covered in the previous section. One way of attacking this problem is to develop standard "approaches" to common clinical situations. It is helpful to recognize the most common presentation of a given disease. For example, the most common cause of knee effusion is degenerative joint disease.

The clinical scenario would be something such as:

A 50-year-old overweight female is referred to your office with complaints of right knee pain and swelling.

With no other information to go on, the student would note that this patient has a painful knee effusion. Using "most common cause" information, the clinician would make an educated guess that the patient has degenerative joint disease.

However, what if the scenario also included the following phrase?

The right knee is mildly erythematous and warm to the touch.

Now the most likely diagnosis is an inflammatory arthritis. Degenerative joint disease rarely presents with inflammatory signs such as localized redness or warmth.

WHAT SHOULD BE THE NEXT STEP?

This question is difficult because the next step has many possibilities; the answer may be to obtain more diagnostic information, to stage the illness, or to introduce therapy. The next step is often a more challenging question than "What is the most likely diagnosis?" because there may be insufficient information to make a diagnosis, and thus the next step may be to pursue additional diagnostic testing. Another possibility is that there *is* enough information for a probable diagnosis, and thus the next step is to stage the disease or to administer treatment. Hence from clinical data, a judgment must be rendered regarding where one falls on the "make a diagnosis → stage the disease → treat based on stage → follow the response" continuum. Frequently, students and training clinicians are taught to "regurgitate" information that someone has written about a particular disease, but they are not yet skilled at determining the next step. This talent is learned optimally at the bedside, in a supportive environment, with freedom to make educated guesses, and with constructive feedback. The sample scenario that follows describes one's thought process through a case of lower back pain:

- **Make the diagnosis:** "Based on the information available, I believe that this 48-year-old male has a right-sided acutely herniated nucleus pulposus at L4-5. This is based on right-sided lateral leg and shin paresthesias, an isolated EHL weakness of 4/5, and a positive straight leg raise test."
- **Stage the disease:** "I don't believe that this is severe disease, since he does not have progressive symptoms, bowel/bladder dysfunction, saddle anesthesia, profound or bilateral weakness, or constitutional symptoms suggestive of infection or malignancy."
- **Treat based on stage:** "Therefore, my next step is to treat him with NSAIDs, acetaminophen, activity modification, and a muscle relaxant."
- **Follow the response:** "I want to follow the treatment by assessing his pain and clinical exam. I will reassess him in 1 week."

In a similar patient, when the clinical presentation is more immediately concerning—for example if the patient were experiencing urinary retention and profound weakness in his bilateral lower extremities—the next step would likely be diagnostic in nature, such as an MRI of the lumbosacral spine to evaluate for cauda equina syndrome. Finally, if given an MRI showing a large centrally-herniated lumbar disc, the next step would be emergency surgical decompression.

WHAT IS THE MOST LIKELY MECHANISM FOR THIS INJURY OR CONDITION?

This question goes further than making the diagnosis, requiring the clinician to understand the underlying mechanism behind the process. For example, a clinical scenario may describe a 61-year-old female who becomes hypoxic during an intramedullary rodding procedure for a femur fracture. The surgeon must first recognize fat embolism syndrome, which may occur intraoperatively during the intramedullary reaming of long bones. Then, the surgeon must understand the process by which the reamer disseminates the intramedullary fat into the bloodstream, leading to the mechanical obstruction of pulmonary blood flow and the triggering of a secondary inflammatory response in which platelets and erythrocytes aggregate and cause a localized toxic injury to the pulmonary vascular endothelium. Students and junior clinicians are advised to learn the mechanisms by which common injuries are created. Ankle fractures, for example, are often classified by the direction of the force acting on the ankle and the position of the foot during injury. If the foot is supinated during a low-energy external rotation injury, one is more likely to injure the lateral malleolus or disrupt the lateral ankle ligaments. Conversely, if the foot is pronated during the same external rotation injury, one is more likely to suffer injury to the medial malleolus or deltoid ligaments.

WHAT ARE THE RISK FACTORS FOR THIS INJURY OR CONDITION?

Understanding the risk factors for certain conditions helps the practitioner establish a diagnosis and determine how to interpret tests. For example, understanding the risk for osteonecrosis after a 4-part fracture of the proximal humerus may direct the surgeon to perform a primary shoulder hemiarthroplasty instead of fixing the fracture with plates, sutures, and screws. In an older individual with a history of osteoporosis, multiple medical comorbidities, and tobacco use, surgeons may opt to perform a primary partial replacement instead of attempting fixation. In younger individuals with the same injury, open reduction and internal fixation may be attempted, as younger patients will typically have better bone stock and blood supply than their older counterparts. Additionally, younger individuals have higher physical demands than are typically tolerated by current shoulder prostheses.

HOW IS THE DIAGNOSIS CONFIRMED?

Although confirming the diagnosis of a traumatic fracture may be as simple as acquiring an x-ray of the affected bone, many injuries and diseases relevant to orthopaedics have complicated workups and diagnoses that physicians-in-training must be familiar with. In a young patient with complaints of snuffbox tenderness after a fall onto an outstretched arm, obtaining x-rays of the wrist with scaphoid views is typically the next step in diagnosis. However, what if the x-rays are negative, despite the telltale history and physical exam findings? Occult fractures of the scaphoid are treated in spica casts with follow-up x-rays at 1 to 2 weeks from injury to identify evidence of healing fracture. If symptoms persist despite negative films, an MRI or bone scan may be performed to confirm the diagnosis of an occult fracture. Clinicians-in-training should strive to know the indications for—and limits of—diagnostic tests, not just in the setting of traumatic injuries, but for many types of common bone and joint conditions.

WHAT IS THE BEST THERAPY?

To answer this question, the clinician needs to reach the correct diagnosis and assess the severity of the condition, and then he or she must weigh the situation to reach the appropriate intervention. For the student and even junior-most residents, knowing exact steps of a surgical procedure is not as important as understanding the operative and nonoperative treatment options, identifying the best possible treatment, and recognizing its potential complications. It is essential for the training surgeon to be able to concisely and clearly verbalize the diagnosis and communicate his or her rationale for a proposed therapy. A common error is for students and residents to "jump" to a surgical treatment, almost like a random guess, and to therefore receive only "right or wrong" feedback when all of the logical steps in the management process are not completely understood. A guess at a proposed treatment may well be correct, but for the wrong reason; conversely, the student's "shot-down" answer may actually be a very reasonable one, with only a small misstep in thinking along the way. Injuries or conditions and their proposed treatments should be presented in a stepwise, logical fashion so that feedback may be received at each decision point.

WHAT COMPLICATIONS ARE ASSOCIATED WITH THIS INJURY OR CONDITION AND ITS TREATMENT?

Clinicians must be cognizant of the complications of a disease, so that they will understand how to follow and monitor the patient. Sometimes, the training physician will have to make the diagnosis from clinical clues and then apply his or her knowledge of the consequences of the pathologic process. For example, a woman who presents with a comminuted both bone forearm fracture after a fall from a balcony is at significant risk for developing a compartment syndrome in the short term, as well as developing forearm synostosis or complications from Volkmann ischemia in the long term. Furthermore, the gold standard treatment—open reduction internal fixation of the radius and ulna with plates and screws—has several associated complications of its own, including posttraumatic synostosis, infection, and neurovascular injury. Physicians must be mindful of the potential complications arising from certain conditions or injuries—for example, which types of fractures are at significant risk for developing, say, a compartment syndrome and thus need to be monitored every few hours versus those that may be admitted and addressed the following morning. A basic knowledge of complications after both operative and nonoperative therapies for a variety of orthopaedic conditions is paramount. Of course, whenever possible, potential complications should be discussed with patients *before* intervention.

CLINICAL PEARLS

- There is no substitute for a meticulous history and physical examination.
- There are 4 steps to the clinical approach to the patient: making the diagnosis, assessing its severity, treating based on severity, and following the response.
- Remember to distinguish between **pain,** a subjective complaint, and **tenderness,** an objective finding on physical exam.
- In virtually all trauma situations, the physician must never assess passive range of motion for the cervical spine; active, or patient-driven, range of motion for the cervical spine may be permitted in certain situations.
- Herniated discs may present with a variety of nonspecific physical exam findings such as tenderness to palpation over spinous processes, paravertebral musculature, the sciatic notch, and the sciatic nerve.
- Be mindful of Waddell signs when examining a potentially malingering patient. These include pain out of proportion (to light touch), a lack of contralateral hip extensor effort when attempting a straight leg raise, nonanatomic distributions of symptoms, and exaggerated responses or overreactions.
- To clinically clear the cervical spine after trauma, the patient must be sober, without focal neurologic deficit, midline tenderness, or distracting injury; have a normal level or alertness; and be able to actively range his or her neck through a complete range of painless motion.
- Casts, whether applied to an arm or a leg, should end short of the metacarpophalangeal and metatarsophalangeal joints, respectively. In general, the patient should be able to move his or her fingers and/or toes within the cast.
- When placing traction pins in the distal femur, one should start medially to gain the most control over the pin near the superficial femoral artery. When placing a proximal tibial traction pin, one should start laterally to best control the pin around the common peroneal nerve.
- Both nailing and rodding are interchangeable terms describing an intramedullary fixation technique. A technical difference does exist in that nails are tapered at their end, whereas rods are cylindrical.

REFERENCES

Bates B. A *Guide to Physical Examination and History Taking*. 5th ed. Philadelphia, PA: J. B. Lippincott Company; 1991.

Brown DE, Neumann RD (eds). *Orthopaedic Secrets*. 3rd ed. Philadelphia, PA: Hanley & Belfus/Elsevier; 2004.

Egol KE, Koval KJ, Zukerman JD (eds). *Handbook of Fractures*. 4th ed. Philadelphia, PA: Lippincott Williams & Wilkins; 2010.

Flynn JM (ed). *Orthopaedic Knowledge Update: Ten*. Rosemont, IL: American Academy of Orthopaedic Surgeons; 2011.

Rhee JM, Yoon T, Riew D. Cervical radiculopathy. *J Am Acad Orthpaed Surg*. 2007;15:486-494.

Thompson JC. *Netter's Concise Atlas of Orthopaedic Anatomy*. Philadelphia, PA: Saunders Elsevier; 2002.

Toy EC, Liu TH, Campbell AR. *Case Files: Surgery*. 2nd ed. New York: McGraw-Hill Medical; 2007.

SECTION II

Clinical Cases

CASE 1

A 20-year-old, right-hand-dominant male athlete, the star wide receiver on his collegiate football team, had just caught the game-winning touchdown. As his teammates gathered around him to celebrate, they noticed that he was clutching his right shoulder and appeared to be in a great deal of pain. Soon after, in the emergency department (ED), he refused to let anyone move his right arm from its current position of slight abduction and external rotation. The team physician notes that the front of his shoulder appears "full" and that the acromion is prominent in comparison with the contralateral side. He has a strong radial pulse, and sensation to light touch is intact throughout the whole extremity. He refuses a motor exam. An anteroposterior (AP) radiograph of the shoulder is obtained by the ED and is seen in Figure 1–1.

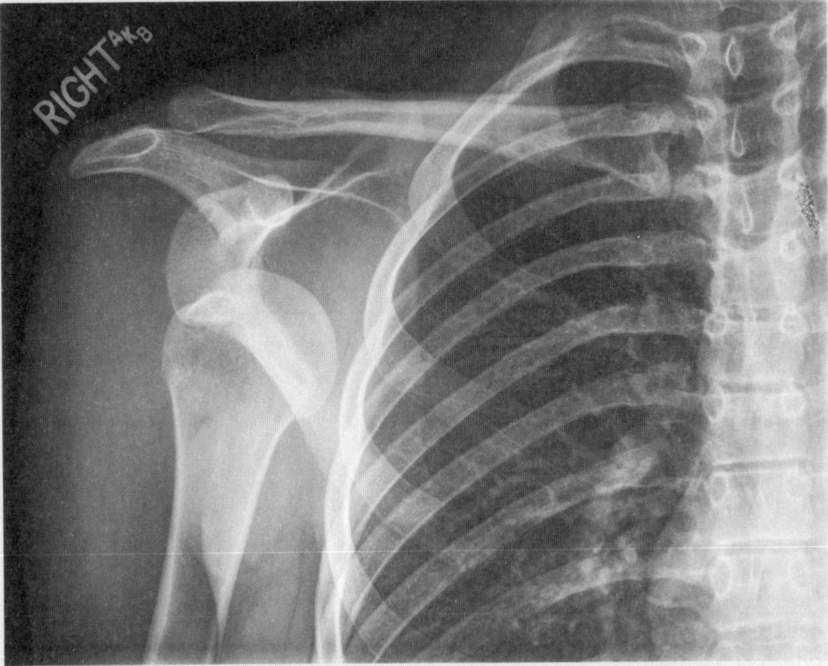

Figure 1–1. AP radiograph of the shoulder.

- What is the most likely diagnosis?
- What abnormalities are seen in the radiograph?
- What other abnormal findings are likely to be noted in this patient?
- What is the best treatment for this patient?

ANSWERS TO CASE 1: Anterior Shoulder Dislocation

Summary: A 20-year-old athlete sustained trauma to the right shoulder resulting in obvious deformity and pain, with an AP radiograph of the right shoulder demonstrating a dislocation and osseous defect of the posterolateral aspect of the humeral head.

- **Most likely diagnosis:** Anteroinferior glenohumeral dislocation
- **Radiographic abnormality:** These plain films depict a right glenohumeral dislocation and a **Hill-Sachs lesion,** which is an indentation fracture of the posterolateral humeral head caused by impaction on the anterior glenoid rim after anterior glenohumeral dislocation.
- **Associated physical exam findings:** Deltoid spasm/dysfunction, positive apprehension and/or crank test, 3+ sulcus sign, rotator cuff tear (especially in older patients), clicking/catching during movement, positive load-shift test, Bankart lesion, and other bony abnormalities of the humerus and/or glenoid rim.
- **Best treatment:** Prompt closed reduction, if acutely dislocated; nonoperative immobilization in external rotation versus operative Bankart repair (open or arthroscopic), possible bone fragment incorporation, and possible glenoid augmentation, if indicated.

ANALYSIS

Objectives

1. Identify the anatomic structures that serve as stabilizers of the glenohumeral joint.
2. Be familiar with the epidemiology, clinical presentation, and initial management of anterior shoulder dislocations.
3. Understand the clinical indications for operative stabilization procedures.

Considerations

The 20-year-old football player has just sustained his third traumatic anterior shoulder dislocation requiring urgent reduction. Although patients with a history of repeated dislocations may recognize what has happened, a thorough history, exam, and workup should be performed. **Special attention must be directed to the patient's neurovascular exam—both before and after reduction—as the dislocation may cause neurovascular damage.** This is more commonly observed in the elderly. The decision of whether to obtain radiographs of the dislocated shoulder or proceed directly to closed reduction is often governed by the unique circumstances of each case. Individuals with a history of dislocations and high pain tolerance may tolerate immediate reductions. Others may need sedation. After the joint is reduced and the reduction confirmed radiographically, the next step should be to investigate the patient's history of recurrent shoulder dislocations. Factors such as time between events, management of the initial dislocation, and circumstances surrounding each dislocation are especially important. This information will guide both the short-term and long-term management of the patient. The patient described in the vignette would typically be a candidate for further workup and operative stabilization if clinically warranted.

APPROACH TO: Anterior Shoulder Dislocation

DEFINITIONS

SHOULDER LAXITY: A clinical exam finding referring to the ability of the humeral head to translate on the glenoid. Laxity varies significantly between individuals and is only considered pathologic if it is accompanied with additional symptomatology such as pain.

SHOULDER INSTABILITY: A pathologic state associated with painful, excessive translation of the shoulder. Instability, unlike asymptomatic laxity, should be considered for treatment.

BANKART LESION: The most common sequelae of an anterior shoulder dislocation (up to 85% of cases). Bankart lesions are described as detachment of the antero-inferior labrum from the glenoid rim, accompanied by detachment of the inferior glenohumeral ligament from its glenoid origin. Described as a bony Bankart lesion when the glenoid rim itself fractures in lieu of a labral detachment.

HILL-SACHS LESION: An osteochondral depression in the posterior humeral head caused by impaction of the head on the anterior glenoid during anterior dislocation. If severe, Hill-Sachs lesions may contribute to recurrent instability.

CLINICAL APPROACH

Epidemiology

The glenohumeral joint is the most mobile and most commonly dislocated joint in the human body. Dislocations in the anterior direction are by far the most frequently occurring, representing up to 90% of all shoulder dislocations. Posterior dislocations are significantly less common and may be more insidious in presentation. Rarer still are inferior dislocations (known as **luxatio erecta**) and superior dislocations.

The age distribution of anterior dislocations is bimodal in nature. An early peak occurs among men in their second decade of life. Young males are also more likely to have recurrent dislocations: Rates of as high as 90% have been reported in athletes who suffer a dislocation before the age of 20 years. The latter peak represents women in their sixth and seventh decades. Although this population group is less likely to suffer a recurrent dislocation, they experience higher rates of associated injuries such as rotator cuff tears, vascular injuries, and nerve damage.

Anatomy of the Glenohumeral Joint

The glenohumeral joint is a complex array of structures that act together to provide the greatest range of motion of any joint in the human body. These structures can be loosely divided into *static* and *dynamic* stabilizers. **Static stabilizers** passively support the humeral head in the glenoid; they include the congruence between the humeral head and **glenoid fossa, the labrum, glenohumeral ligaments, and the joint capsule. Dynamic stabilizers** describe the **rotator muscles and periscapular musculature.**

Static Stabilizers: The glenoid fossa itself engages only a minor proportion of the humeral head, analogous to a golf ball on a tee. The fibrocartilaginous labrum (attached circumferentially to the glenoid rim) helps deepen the glenoid concavity by up to 50%. The anterior inferior attachment of the labrum to the glenoid is tight, whereas the superior attachment is looser and attaches to the long head of the biceps near its origin. Perhaps the most important static stabilizers are the glenohumeral ligaments, particularly the anterior band of the inferior glenohumeral ligament.

A **Bankart lesion** refers to a traumatic separation of the inferior glenohumeral ligament and labral complex from the glenoid rim. Disruption of this complex is a well-recognized cause of recurrent anterior instability. A **bony Bankart lesion** refers to avulsion of a portion of the glenoid rim attached to the anteroinferior labral complex during a traumatic anterior dislocation. The glenohumeral ligaments, along with their attachments and specific functions, are listed in Table 1–1. Together, these ligaments act to stabilize the shoulder in different arrays of flexion/extension, abduction/adduction, and internal/external rotation. The joint capsule, aside from providing structural support to the glenohumeral joint, additionally acts to maintain a negative intraarticular pressure that helps "suck" the humeral head down into the glenoid fossa.

Table 1–1 • ANATOMY AND FUNCTION OF THE GLENOHUMERAL LIGAMENTS

	Origin	Insertion	Function
Superior glenohumeral ligament	Superoanterior glenoid rim	Lesser tuberosity	Stabilizes shoulder against inferior translation in adduction
Middle glenohumeral ligament	Slightly below that of the superior glenohumeral ligament	Medial to lesser tuberosity	Stabilizes shoulder against anterior/posterior translation in 45 degrees of abduction
Inferior glenohumeral ligament (anterior band)	Anterior labrum	Humeral neck	Stabilizes shoulder against anterior translation in abduction and external rotation
Inferior glenohumeral ligament (posterior band)	Posterior labrum	Humeral neck	Stabilizes shoulder against posterior translation in internal rotation/flexion

Dynamic Stabilizers: Dynamic stabilizers of the glenohumeral joint are the muscles of the shoulder that contract in a highly coordinated fashion to produce smooth, stable movement throughout normal ranges of motion. Specifically, these include the rotator cuff muscles (subscapularis, supraspinatus, infraspinatus, and teres minor) as well as the latissimus dorsi, trapezius, pectoralis major, and the long head of the biceps.

Clinical Presentation

The most common clinical presentation of an anterior shoulder dislocation is after an acute traumatic event. Typically, the injury involves one falling on a shoulder that is in **extension, external rotation,** and **abduction** (common in athletes like the patient in Case 1). An additional mechanism of injury includes dislocations from direct force to the posterior shoulder, which can also result in anterior dislocation. In older patients or patients with a history of recurrent dislocations, the glenohumeral joint can be extremely unstable and may dislocate with minimal trauma or even during sleep.

Physical Exam: Patients with acutely dislocated shoulders usually have obvious physical deformity on visual inspection. Shoulders will appear "full" anteriorly and may have a visual or palpable depression of the posterior shoulder. Active and passive range of motion is limited by significant pain.

When presented with a patient who has had multiple episodes of dislocation, there are several bedside maneuvers classically associated with the diagnosis of **anterior instability.** In the apprehension test, the patient is placed in the supine position and asked to place their arm in a comfortable position. The arm is then gradually externally rotated and abducted by the examiner. A positive test is one in which the patient exhibits apprehension or guards against this shift in position due to the subjective feeling of instability—in other words, the patient anticipates a potential for dislocation and resists further external rotation and abduction. Interestingly, actual pain is usually typically elicited with this maneuver. The relocation test is performed concurrently with a positive apprehension test: When the patient begins to exhibit guarding, a posteriorly applied force should relieve the sensation of impending dislocation.

The *load and shift test* can be used to assess both anterior and posterior instability. The examiner applies an axial load on the elbow to drive the humeral head into the glenoid fossa and simultaneously applies an anterior and posterior force on the humeral head with the remaining hand. Translation of the humeral head 0 to 1 cm in either direction is considered mild, whereas translation of greater than 2 cm or translation beyond the glenoid rim is considered severe.

Finally, the presence of generalized ligamentous laxity should be evaluated. Signs of metacarpophalangeal hyperextension or elbow recurvatum are suggestive of underlying pathologic conditions such as Ehlers-Danlos syndrome and therefore require an appropriate workup if present.

Radiographic Evaluation: A trauma series of a suspected anteriorly dislocated shoulder should be obtained whenever possible. Obtaining an axillary view in the acute setting is often difficult as a result of extreme pain, even after copious narcotic administration. In such instances, a **Velpeau axillary radiograph** may be obtained by having the patient lean backward over an x-ray cassette and angling the caudally directed beam downward from above the shoulder.

A pathognomonic radiologic finding for anterior glenohumeral dislocation is the *Hill-Sachs lesion*, which describes an osteochondral indentation fracture of the posterolateral humeral head. It is caused by the impaction of relatively soft humeral head against the hard glenoid rim after a dislocation and can deepen with recurrent events. These defects can be easily missed on AP radiographs. The Stryker notch view is especially useful in detecting such lesions and is obtained by having the supine patient place the palm of the hand of the affected extremity on the crown of the head and directing the beam toward the coracoid process.

Magnetic resonance imaging remains the gold standard imaging technique for evaluating soft tissue injuries associated with anterior dislocation and should be obtained when planning an operative stabilization procedure outside.

TREATMENT

Closed Reduction

Closed reduction should be attempted as soon as the patient has been appropriately evaluated and images obtained. Multiple techniques for reduction have been described in the literature. Sedation and/or analgesia serve both to reduce the patient's discomfort during the reduction as well as to relax the pericapsular musculature, thus allowing for easier reduction. The *Stimson technique* involves attaching weights to the affected extremity with the patient in the prone position. The gentle traction overcomes muscular spasm over a period of time and allows for reduction to occur. The **Hippocratic maneuver** and **traction-countertraction** techniques achieve reduction by combining traction with internal and external rotation movements. The most significant difference between these techniques is the method of countertraction: In the Hippocratic maneuver, the practitioner places his or her foot in the patient's axilla to stabilize the body while he or she is pulling the affected arm. In the traction-countertraction method, an assistant provides countertraction by pulling on a sheet wrapped around the patient's body from under the axilla. Postreduction films should always be obtained. If reduction proves extremely difficult and does not occur after multiple attempts, soft tissues are likely interposed between the humeral head and glenoid. In such instances, closed reduction is futile, and urgent operative open reduction should proceed.

After closed reduction, the shoulder is typically immobilized using a sling or shoulder immobilizer. Some recent literature, however, has failed to clearly demonstrate benefits of immobilization. More commonly agreed on is a gradual rehabilitation, focused on increasing range of motion. Older patients generally are immobilized for shorter periods of time.

Operative Treatment

Absolute indications for operative treatment include failed closed reduction secondary to soft tissue interposition and significant glenoid bone loss. Biomechanical studies have shown that stability decreases exponentially with bone defects of 6 to 7 mm or greater in size.

Relative indications for operative treatment include those with a history of recurrent dislocations, as well as the initial shoulder dislocation in the young, highly active patient. The question of operative versus nonoperative management of the latter subgroup of patients has been the source of multiple investigations. Studies show an up to 90% recurrence rate in patients younger than 30 years of age managed nonoperatively after their first dislocation.

The most commonly performed stabilization procedure is repair of the anteroinferior labral/inferior glenohumeral ligament complex, known as the Bankart repair (open or arthroscopic). Other procedures include glenoid cavity deepening, tendon transfers, and capsular shifts. Patients with **t**raumatic dislocations who exhibit **uni**lateral instability and in whom **B**ankart lesions are present should be considered for **s**urgical intervention—such scenarios are sometimes referenced by the mnemonic **TUBS** (**t**raumatic, **u**nidirectional, **B**ankart, **s**urgery). Conversely, the mnemonic **AMBRI** is sometimes used to describe populations for whom rehabilitation is the preferred initial treatment. AMBRI describes patients with a history of **a**traumatic dislocations with **m**ultidirectional instability, involvement of **b**ilateral shoulders who should be initially treated by **r**ehabilitation; however, if surgery is needed, an **i**nferior capsular shift should be considered. Simply put, TUBS and AMBRI are mnemonics to describe the presentation and treatment of patients at either end of the instability spectrum.

OTHER TYPES OF GLENOHUMERAL DISLOCATION

Posterior glenohumeral dislocations represent up to 15% of all shoulder dislocations. In general, they are less symptomatic in the acute phase and are sometimes found incidentally in the elderly during workup for unrelated pathology. They may also be seen as the sequelae of strong involuntary muscle contractions such as those caused by seizures or electric shock, when the strong pericapsular muscles responsible for internal rotation (latissimus dorsi, pectoralis major, and subscapularis) overpower the relatively weaker external rotators. A **reverse Hill-Sachs** lesion may be seen on the anteromedial aspect of the humeral head following posterior dislocation.

Inferior glenohumeral dislocations (luxatio erecta) are exceedingly rare and classically present with a startling, pathognomonic clinical presentation. Luxatio erecta occurs when the arm is forced into a frozen hyperabducted state—sometimes referred to as the "Superman" position because of its likeness to the superhero's famous flight stance. With the humeral head forced inferiorly, deltoid and other muscular attachments pull the arm into extreme abduction. Neurovascular compromise almost always accompanies this type of dislocation.

COMPREHENSION QUESTIONS

1.1 A 33-year-old rugby player is seen for follow-up after a first-time anterior shoulder dislocation 6 weeks ago while being tackled. The shoulder has remained reduced. On exam, he has a good range of painless active and passive motion. Which of the following is considered a dynamic stabilizer of the glenohumeral joint?

A. Glenoid fossa

B. Anteroinferior labral complex

C. Coracohumeral ligament

D. Subscapularis muscle

E. Anterior band of the inferior glenohumeral ligament

1.2 Which of the following describes a technique for diagnosis of anterior shoulder instability in the patient in Question 1.1?

A. Pivot shift

B. Velpeau axillary

C. Load and shift

D. Stimson maneuver

E. Hippocratic maneuver

1.3 Early radiographs of the patient in Question 1.1 determined the patient to have a small Hill-Sachs lesion. Which of the following radiographs is best suited for visualizing this lesion?

A. West Point

B. Stryker notch

C. Scapular Y

D. AP

E. Axillary

1.4 A 22-year-old amateur wrestler is seen in the ER after a first-time anterior shoulder dislocation. As a result of understaffing, he waits 3 hours for conscious sedation. Appropriate reduction is eventually achieved after 2 manipulation attempts. He is neurovascularly intact and is discharged in a shoulder immobilizer. Which of the following has been shown to be the greatest predictor of future dislocation after a first-time anterior shoulder dislocation?

A. Prolonged reduction

B. Chronic pain with motion after reduction

C. Age at time of first dislocation

D. Tobacco use greater than 1 pack per day

E. Heavy labor occupations

ANSWERS

1.1 **D.** The periscapular musculature stabilizes the glenohumeral joint during and throughout its full range of motion, thus acting as dynamic restraints. The other answers listed are static restraints.

1.2 **C.** The load and shift test is a bedside examination technique that can aid in the diagnosis of anterior shoulder disability. Because it can be performed in various degrees of arm abduction, it can sometimes aid in identifying the specific deficient structure contributing to anterior shoulder instability.

1.3 **B.** The Stryker notch view provides an excellent view of the posterolateral humeral head. Hill-Sachs lesions can be easily visualized with other views, however, especially if the defect is large (as seen in Figure 1–1).

1.4 **C.** Age has been shown to be the most consistent predictor of instability: in young patients < 20 years of age, recurrent rates are reportedly as high as 80% to 90%; in those >40 years of age, rates drop precipitously to approximately 10% to 15%.

CLINICAL PEARLS

- Anterior dislocations of the glenohumeral joint are the most common, representing up to 90% of all shoulder dislocations.
- When a true axillary radiograph cannot be obtained, a Velpeau axillary radiograph should be preformed to evaluate a dislocated glenohumeral joint.
- Urgent closed reduction is critical in the setting of a dislocated shoulder, with a thorough and well-documented neurovascular exam performed.
- Both Bankart and Hill-Sachs lesions are seen concurrently with shoulder dislocations and can contribute to recurrent instability.

REFERENCES

Brown DE, Neumann RD, eds. Shoulder instability. In: *Orthopedic Secrets*. 3rd ed. Philadelphia, PA: Hanley & Belfus; 2004:107-111.

Dodson CC, Cordasco FA. Anterior glenohumeral joint dislocations. *Orthop Clin North Am*. 2008;39:507-518.

Lintner SA, Speer KP. Traumatic anterior glenohumeral instability: the role of arthroscopy. *J Am Acad Orthop Surg*. 1997;5:233-239.

Piasecki DP, et al. Glenoid bone deficiency in recurrent anterior shoulder instability: diagnosis and management. *J Am Acad Orthop Surg*. 2009;17:482-493.

Provencher MT, Ghodadra N, Romea AA. Arthroscopic management of anterior instability: pearls, pitfalls, and lessons learned. *Orthop Clin North Am*. 2010;41:235-337.

Sahajpal DT, Zuckerman JD. Chronic glenohumeral dislocation. *J Am Acad Orthop Surg*. 2008;16:385-398.

CASE 2

A 32-year-old right-hand-dominant female was standing on a stool in her kitchen, lost balance, and fell onto her outstretched right hand. She arrives at an urgent care clinic and is complaining of pain and deformity about her wrist. She did not sustain any other injuries and has no significant past medical history. Physical exam reveals her right wrist to have intact skin, and it is swollen and ecchymotic. She has significant tenderness to palpation about the wrist, which has a mild, dorsally angulated deformity. There is no snuffbox tenderness. She readily flexes her distal interphalangeal joints and abducts her fingers. She weakly extends the thumb and fingers. There is brisk capillary refill throughout, and sensation is intact in the median, radial, and ulnar nervous distributions. Anteroposterior (AP) and lateral wrist films are obtained and can be seen in Figure 2–1.

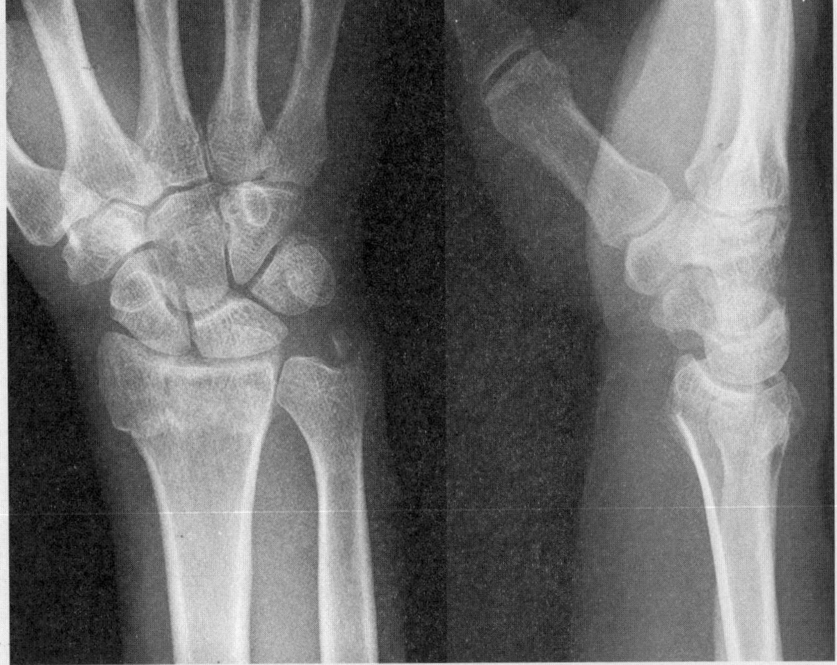

Figure 2–1. AP and lateral plain radiographs of a right wrist in a skeletally mature individual.

- ▶ What is the most likely diagnosis?
- ▶ What additional injuries are you most concerned about?
- ▶ What is the most appropriate initial treatment for this patient?

ANSWERS TO CASE 2:
Distal Radius (Colles) Fracture

Summary: A 32-year-old, right-hand-dominant female sustained a wrist injury after falling on an outstretched hand. She has pain and a dorsally angulated deformity about the distal radius. Wrist x-rays show an intraarticular distal radius fracture with concomitant ulnar styloid fracture.

- **Most likely diagnosis:** This is an intraarticular distal radius fracture that involves the distal radioulnar joint (DRUJ) with a concomitant ulna styloid fracture. This may be classified as a Frykman type VI distal radius fracture.
- **Additional injuries to be concerned:** Scaphoid fractures, radial head fractures (Essex Lopresti), elbow dislocation, proximal humerus fractures, shoulder dislocations, and clavicle fractures.
- **Initial treatment:** All displaced fractures should undergo closed reduction. A hematoma block with or without sedation provides analgesia for closed reduction. The goals of reduction include anatomic repositioning of fragments for healing, limiting postinjury swelling and pain, and relieving compression on median nerve and other surrounding neurovascular structures.

ANALYSIS

Objectives

1. Understand the anatomy of the distal forearm and proximal wrist.
2. Be familiar with basic treatment options for distal radius fractures with regard to both nonoperative and operative management.
3. Recognize potential complications arising from initial injuries and their treatments.

Considerations

This 32-year-old patient sustained an injury to her dominant hand from a fall. Because the patient will be focused on her wrist, it is important to remember to evaluate the entire extremity, focusing on areas of potential injury such as the snuffbox, elbow and radial head, shoulder, and clavicle. If warranted by mechanism, full trauma workup should be initiated. A careful history should elucidate whether the patient suffered a simple mechanical fall or whether there were underlying etiologies behind her accident, such as syncope or gait instability. Examination of the skin is important to ensure that there is not an open fracture that would necessitate urgent operative debridement and washout. Next, a careful neurovascular exam needs to be performed. Extension of the thumb by the extensor pollicus longus should be evaluated because the tendon can be trapped or lacerated as it passes the Lister tubercle. Particular attention should be paid to the median nerve. Carpal tunnel compression symptoms are common secondary to forced hyperextension of the wrist, as well as local hematoma formation, impingement by fracture fragments, and increased compartment pressures.

Finally, after a complete and thorough exam is performed and documented, the fracture should be immobilized, regardless of whether it meets requirements for operative fixation. This is typically performed by cast or splint immobilization.

APPROACH TO: Distal Radius Fracture

DEFINITIONS

COLLES FRACTURE: An eponym originally describing extraarticular fractures of the distal radius. More commonly used today as a lay term for any dorsally angulated distal radius fracture.

SMITH FRACTURE: An eponym for volarly angulated distal radius fractures, most commonly incurred after a fall or blow to the dorsum of the wrist. This is sometimes referred to as a reverse Colles fracture.

CHAUFFEUR FRACTURE: An avulsion fracture of the radial styloid, historically as the result from hand-cranked automobiles in which engine backfire forced the crank back into the chauffeur's hand. Also known as a "backfire" or Hutchinson fracture. Today these result from falls onto outstretched hands, with axial compressive force driving the scaphoid into the radial styloid as the wrist is both ulnarly deviated and dorsiflexed.

BARTON FRACTURE: A shear fracture of the volar or dorsal lip of the distal radius, resulting in dislocation or subluxation of the wrist, most commonly in the volar direction.

CLINICAL APPROACH

Anatomy and Mechanisms of Injury

The distal radius consists of the metaphysic, or metaphyseal region, as well its articulating surfaces, which include the scaphoid facet, lunate facet, and the sigmoid notch. The metaphysics flares distally, and its cortical bone becomes thin, especially at its dorsal and radial aspects. **Thin bone at this region is prone to comminution, and therefore, many distal radius fractures eventually collapse dorsoradially, despite initial anatomic reductions.**

Radiographic Evaluation

Several distal radius and ulna measurements are helpful in evaluating the severity of injury and can later be used to assess reduction. Although these values are well-established, they can vary greatly between individuals. If doubt exists regarding the adequacy of alignment, contralateral comparison views should be obtained. Figures 2–2 and 2–3 are AP and lateral radiographs of normal wrists, respectively, showing measurements of the following alignment parameters:

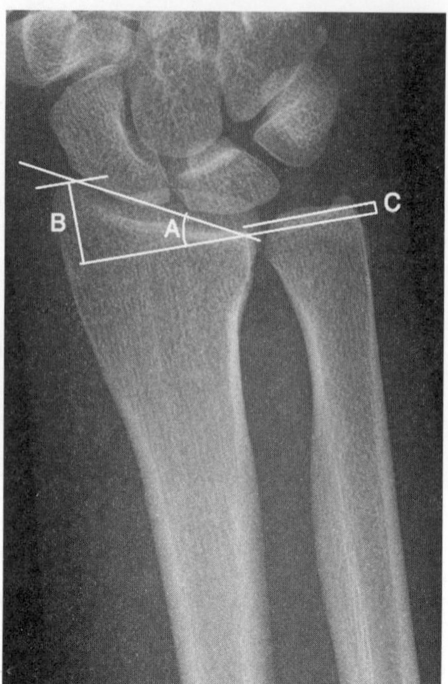

Figure 2–2. An AP plain radiograph of a normal wrist showing the radiographic measurements: radial inclination (A), radial length (B), and ulna variance (C).

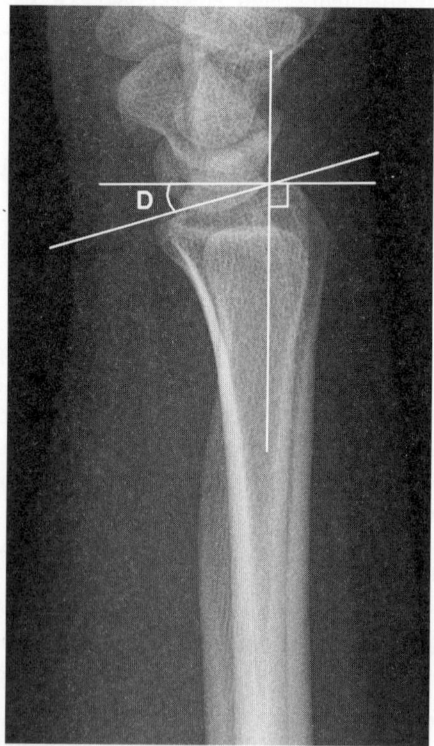

Figure 2–3. A lateral plain radiograph of a normal wrist with measurement of palmar tilt (D).

1. **Radial inclination (normally 23 degrees).** Measured on an AP wrist film as the angle between a line drawn from the radial styloid to the medial corner of radius and a line drawn perpendicular to long axis of radius.

2. **Radial length (normally 12 mm).** Measured on an AP wrist film as distance in millimeters between the tip of the radial styloid and most distal point of the ulnar head of the radius.

3. **Ulnar variance (normally ± 0-2 mm).** On AP: distance between medial corner of the articular surface of the radius and most distal point of articular surface of the ulnar head.

4. **Dorsal/palmar tilt (normally 11 degrees).** On true lateral: angle between line perpendicular to the long axis of radius and line from most distal points of volar and dorsal lips of radius. Palmar tilt is the most important parameter to restore, as it has the greatest bearing on functional outcome.

Classification

Several distal radius fracture classification schemes exist, including informal descriptive classifications to formal systems based on mechanism (Fernandez classification) or extent of articular involvement (Frykman classification). Often, fractures of the distal radius are described with regard to whether the fracture is open or closed, intra- or extraarticular with regard to the radiocarpal joint and/or the DRUJ, whether the fracture is comminuted or simple, the direction of displacement if present, and whether there is an associated ulna styloid fracture.

TREATMENT

Nonoperative Treatment

Closed reduction and cast immobilization is the mainstay of treatment. All displaced distal radius fractures should have attempted closed reduction, regardless of severity. If swelling is significant or if superficial skin injury is present, fractures may be initially splinted with delayed casting. Nondisplaced fractures may be cast in situ, typically with a short arm cast. If the fracture remains stable with the acceptable radiologic parameters discussed previously, then fractures may be treated definitively with a cast. Acceptable parameters for active, healthy patients include restoration of palmar tilt, a neutral tilt or up to 10 degrees of dorsal angulation, restoration of radial length within 2 to 3 mm of the contralateral wrist, the absence of intraarticular stepoff >1 to 2 mm, and less than a 5-degree loss of radial inclination.

Close follow-up with serial radiographs is necessary, as some fractures have a tendency to collapse. As mentioned, even the most anatomic of reductions may collapse in the setting of dorsal comminution and other types of metaphyseal comminution or bone loss. For low-demand, elderly patients in whom the risks of surgery outweigh the benefits, fractures may be treated definitively with a cast, splint, or brace.

Operative Treatment

Several modes of operative treatment exist, including plate fixation, percutaneous pinning, and even external fixation. The current mainstay of treatment is an open-reduction internal fixation with plate and screws that may be placed either dorsally or volarly. **Surgical indications include metaphyseal instability, especially with comminuted dorsal-medial cortices; intraarticular fractures with articular step off >1 to 2 mm or significant comminution; open fractures; DRUJ instability; or secondary loss of reduction with loss of radial inclination of >5 degrees, loss of radial length of >2 to 3 mm, or dorsal angulation >10 degrees. Additional relative indications include bilateral fractures, an impaired contralateral extremity, and associated carpal fractures.**

OUTCOMES AND COMPLICATIONS

Several factors are associated with elevated risk of re-displacement after closed reduction of a distal radius fracture. These include patient age >80 years, significant displacement before initial reduction, significant metaphyseal comminution, and immediate displacement after reduction requiring multiple attempted reductions.

Malunion is a significant complication after nonoperative treatment. Malunion can lead to negative effects on radiocarpal mechanics, loss of motion, and pain at the DRUJ. Acute carpal tunnel syndrome that does not resolve soon after reduction may lead to median nerve damage.

Posttraumatic osteoarthritis is a common sequelae of all intraarticular fractures and correlates strongly with inadequate articular reduction. Anatomic restoration of the articular surface is paramount for long-term functional success.

Complex regional pain syndrome (CPRS) may develop. Cardinal features of CPRS include abnormal or neuropathic pain, temperature changes, abnormal localized diaphoresis, joint stiffness/atrophy/swelling, and bone changes. **Tendon rupture and tenosynovitis can occur, most frequently involving the extensor pollicus longus (EPL) tendon.** A higher risk of EPL rupture is associated with dorsal plating versus volar plating when surgical fixation is performed, because prominent dorsal plates may lead to repetitive wear on the tendon, leading to eventual rupture. EPL rupture may also occur in the absence of internal fixation, because callus formation from even minimally displaced fractures and vascular disruption may lead to gradual tendinous attrition and eventual rupture.

COMPREHENSION QUESTIONS

2.1 A 27-year-old right-hand-dominant man sustains a right distal radius fracture after a trip and fall. He is treated with closed reduction. Which radiographic parameter has the greatest bearing on functional outcome?

A. Radial height

B. Radial inclination

C. Ulnar variance

D. Palmar tilt

E. Bauman angle

2.2 A 50-year-old engineer suffers a comminuted distal radius fracture that fails an initial attempt at cast immobilization. He undergoes elective open-reduction internal fixation of the fracture with a dorsal plating technique. Which tendon is most likely to rupture after dorsal plate fixation of a distal radius fracture?

A. Flexor carpi radialis

B. Extensor pollicus longus

C. Abductor pollicus longus

D. Extensor pollicus brevis

E. Extensor digitorum

2.3 A 52-year-old female fell from her bicycle while trying to light a cigarette while navigating a busy intersection. She suffers a right-sided, dominant distal radius fracture. The fracture is closed and simple, extends into the radiocarpal joint, and is almost 100% displaced dorsally. On additional radiographs, she has a small, nondisplaced fracture of her ipsilateral radial head. Which of the following, if present, is associated with the highest risk of displacement after closed reduction and cast immobilization?

A. Intraarticular involvement

B. Age >50 years old

C. The severity of prereduction dorsal displacement

D. Ipsilateral fracture of the radial head

E. Tobacco history

ANSWERS

2.1 **D.** Although radial height, radial inclination, and ulnar variance are important reduction parameters for the successful nonoperative treatment of distal radius fractures, palmar tilt has been shown to have the greatest bearing on long-term functional outcomes. Bauman angle is found in the pediatric elbow and is most commonly used to assess supracondylar fractures. Bauman angle is measured between the axis of the humeral shaft and the physis of the lateral condyle.

2.2 **B.** The extensor pollicus longus has been shown to be more prone to rupture with dorsal plating than the flexor carpi radialis, abductor pollicus longus, extensor pollicus brevis, and the extensor digitorum. EPL rupture is thought to occur secondary to repetitive wear of the tendon on a prominent plate. Although several different methods are described, irreparable EPL ruptures may be treated with transfer of the redundant extensor indicis proprius to the thumb to regain thumb extension.

2.3 **C.** Of the several factors associated with re-displacement after closed reduction of distal radius fractures, the severity of initial displacement is likely the most significant. Additional risk factors include patient age >80 years (not 50 years), significant metaphyseal comminution (she had a simple, 2-part fracture), and immediate displacement after reduction requiring multiple attempted reductions (not mentioned in the vignette). Intraarticular involvement, positive tobacco history, and even concomitant fractures have not been clearly associated with a high risk of failed closed reduction.

CLINICAL PEARLS

- Distal radius fractures are amongst the most common fractures treated in the United States at more than 650,000 cases per year.
- Patients with distal radius fractures may have incurred more than a simple wrist injury, especially in high-energy trauma scenarios. It is therefore essential to assess similarly injured structures such as the scaphoid, radial head, shoulder, and clavicle.
- The incidence of distal radius fractures as the result of simple falls mirrors that of hip fractures. Both may be evidence of osteopenia or osteoporosis, and patients at risk should be worked up accordingly.

REFERENCES

Buchholz RW, Court-Brown CM, Heckman JD, Tornetta P, eds. Distal radius and ulna fractures. In: *Rockwood and Green's Fractures in Adults*. 7th ed. 2 vol. Philadelphia: Lippincott Williams & Wilkins; 2010:829-880.

Egol KE, Koval KJ, Zukerman JD, eds. Distal radius. In: *Handbook of Fractures*. 4th ed. Philadelphia: Lippincott Williams & Wilkins; 2010:269-280.

CASE 3

A 33-year-old male patient is brought to the emergency department (ED) by ambulance after a high-speed motor vehicle collision (MVC) that occurred approximately 2 hours ago. He was the unrestrained passenger in a car that was traveling approximately 65 miles per hour (mph) when it rear-ended a pick-up truck. There was a prolonged extrication at the scene. On arrival to the ED, the patient is writhing in pain on the gurney, complaining of right hip pain. His vital signs are within normal limits, and a trauma workup reveals deformity to the patient's right lower extremity, but no other injuries. On examination, the patient's right hip is slightly flexed, adducted, and internally rotated. Although he cannot extend his hip, he is able to extend his great toe, as well as dorsiflex and plantarflex his foot. His right lower extremity is warm and well perfused with brisk pulses; sensation to light touch is also grossly intact. The patient denies any prior medical or surgical history. An anteroposterior (AP) plain radiograph of the pelvis is shown (Figure 3–1).

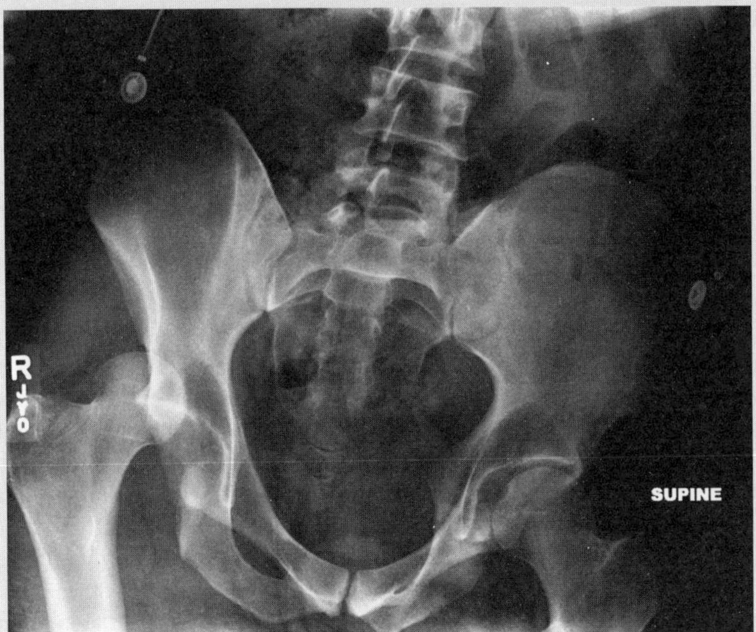

Figure 3–1. AP radiograph of the pelvis showing a posterior dislocation of the right hip.

- What is your most likely diagnosis?
- What is the mechanism of this injury?
- What is your next step in therapy?

ANSWERS TO CASE 3:
Posterior Hip Dislocation

Summary: A 33-year-old male patient is brought to the ED 2 hours after a high-speed MVC and prolonged extrication complaining of right hip pain. On exam, his right lower extremity is slightly flexed, adducted, and internally rotated. It is neurovascularly intact. An AP radiograph of his pelvis identifies a right hip dislocation.

- **Most likely diagnosis:** Posterior dislocation of the right hip
- **Mechanism of injury:** Axial load on a flexed hip (a dashboard injury)
- **Next step in therapy:** Emergent closed reduction within 6 hours to decrease the risk of femoral head osteonecrosis and sciatic nerve injury

ANALYSIS

Objectives

1. Know the diagnostic approach to hip dislocations.
2. Understand that a native hip dislocation is an orthopaedic emergency.
3. Be familiar with the technique used to reduce a dislocated hip.
4. Know the postreduction workup and management.
5. Know the complications associated with hip dislocations.

Considerations

This 33-year-old male patient presents to the ED with a right hip dislocation 2 hours after a high-speed MVC. **The first priority is a trauma workup, applying advanced trauma life support (ATLS) principles.** This patient has no other injuries, and therefore, the next step must be to evaluate the imaging obtained to rule out an associated femoral neck fracture, followed by emergent reduction. It is imperative that the orthopaedist perform a complete and well-documented physical examination, noting any neurovascular compromise or other injuries to the right lower extremity before reduction. Successful reduction is dependent on the ability of ED physicians to perform conscious sedation with good muscle relaxation. If they are unable to do this, the patient may require reduction in the operating room under general anesthesia. A repeat AP pelvis radiograph should be obtained to confirm reduction, followed by a computed tomography (CT) scan through the acetabulum. This will evaluate for a concentric reduction and the presence of any intra-articular fragments and associated fractures of the femoral head and acetabulum. **After reduction, the patient's hip should be ranged and assessed for stability and a repeat neurovascular exam performed.** The patient must be counseled on the risk of osteonecrosis of his hip, the high association of this injury with other injuries (ipsilateral knee injuries are common), and hip precautions.

APPROACH TO: Hip Dislocation

DEFINITIONS

OSTEONECROSIS (AVASCULAR NECROSIS): Process by which bone tissue dies due to either a temporary or permanent disruption to the bone's blood supply. It is associated with excessive steroid use, sickle cell disease, alcoholism, deep diving (caisson disease), Gaucher disease, lupus, and rheumatoid arthritis. It can also be posttraumatic, such as after a hip dislocation, or idiopathic in nature.

HIP PRECAUTIONS: Restrictions designed to prevent posterior dislocation of the hip. They are applied after total hip arthroplasty performed via a posterior approach as well as after native posterior hip dislocations. The precautions prohibit patients from crossing their legs, bending their hip past a 90-degree angle, and twisting their hip inward.

ALLIS MANEUVER: One of several described methods by which to reduce a dislocated hip. The patient is placed in the supine position, and the pelvis is stabilized by an assistant applying pressure. The physician then applies in-line longitudinal traction to the femur followed by gentle flexion of the hip to 90 degrees. Internal and external rotation of the hip ensues, with continued traction until reduction is achieved. Reduction is often signified by an audible and palpable clunk.

CLINICAL APPROACH

Etiology and Mechanism of Injury

Posterior hip dislocations are caused by high-energy mechanisms and comprise greater than 90% of all native hip dislocations (Figure 3–2). They are referred to as *dashboard injuries* because of their high association with motor vehicle accidents in which the patient is subjected to an axial load on a flexed hip occurring when the knee is driven violently into the dashboard. Other causes include falls and athletic injuries. **In all of these instances, the hip is positioned in a flexed, adducted, and internally rotated position (Figure 3–2). Anterior dislocations, which are uncommon and comprise fewer than 10% of hip dislocations,** occur via an external rotation and abduction force and are not discussed.

Anatomy

The inherent stability of the hip joint is provided by its ligamentous, bony, and muscular architecture, as well as the labrum. **Its main blood supply is via the medial femoral circumflex artery,** with other contributions from the lateral femoral circumflex artery, artery of the ligamentum teres (obturator), and the inferior and superior gluteal arteries. The sciatic nerve lies close to the hip joint, exiting anterior to the piriformis in the greater sciatic notch.

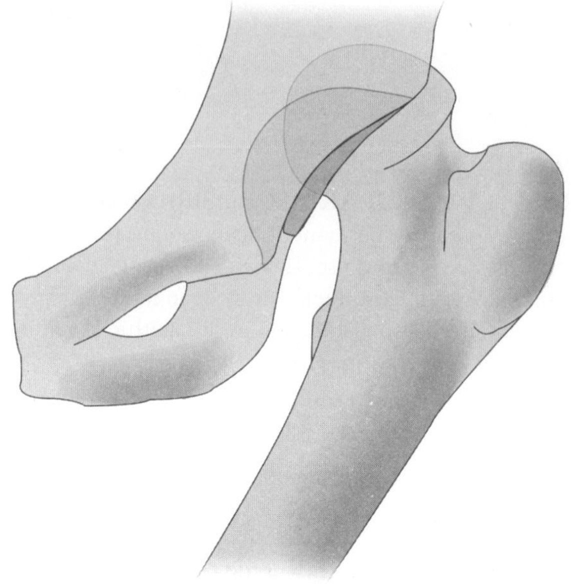

A

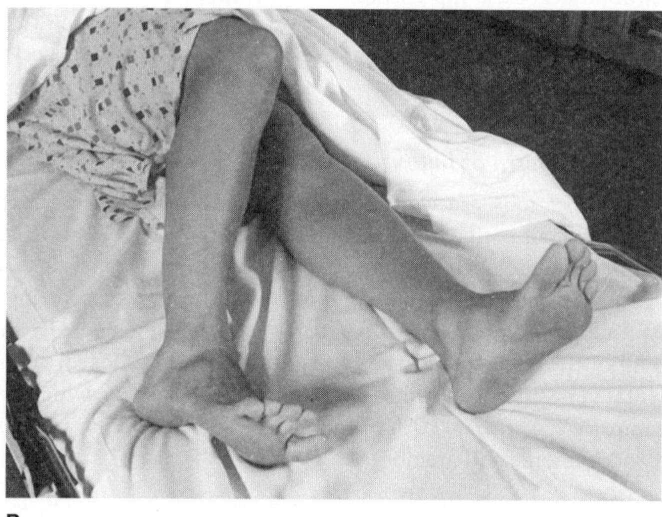

B

Figure 3–2. Posterior dislocation of the hip. (**A**) Posterior dislocation of the hip. (**B**) The clinical appearance of a posterior dislocation of the right hip. (Reproduced, with permission, from Tintinalli J, et al. *Tintinalli's Emergency Medicine: A Comprehensive Study Guide.* 7th ed. New York, NY: McGraw-Hill; 2010:Fig. 270–12.)

Table 3–1 • THE THOMPSON AND EPSTEIN CLASSIFICATION FOR HIP DISLOCATION

Type	Description
I	Dislocation with or without minor fracture
II	Posterior fracture-dislocation with a single, significant posterior acetabular rim fragment
III	Posterior fracture-dislocation with posterior rim comminution with or without a major fragment
IV	Posterior fracture-dislocation involving the acetabular floor
V	Dislocation associated with a femoral head fracture

Initial Management, Diagnosis, and Classification

Given their high-energy mechanisms, ATLS protocol must be followed in the initial management of the patient presenting with a hip dislocation. After this, a complete physical exam is performed, and in the setting of a posterior hip dislocation, the position of the patient's affected extremity is often telltale. The limb will be flexed, adducted, and internally rotated. Neurologic and vascular status must be documented. An AP pelvic radiograph should be obtained and will confirm the diagnosis. With posterior dislocations, the femoral head appears smaller than its contralateral side, joint congruency is lost, and the lesser trochanter difficult to visualize as a result of the internal rotation of the femur. The femoral neck of the affected side must be adequately visualized and evaluated for fracture, as this would change the treatment plan and require operative intervention.

The Thompson and Epstein classification for hip dislocation is one of the most widely used, based on radiographic characteristics, and is described in Table 3–1.

Treatment and Postreduction Management

A hip dislocation is an orthopaedic emergency, and closed reduction attempts must be performed as soon as possible to reduce the period of avascularity to the hip. It must be reiterated, however, that adequate imaging be obtained before any reduction attempts to rule out an ipsilateral femoral neck fracture. Reduction can be performed in the ED if conscious sedation and muscle relaxation can be achieved. If adequate sedation and relaxation is unattainable in the ED, the hip must be reduced in the operating room under general anesthesia.

There are many described reduction techniques for posterior dislocations, including the Allis and Bigelow maneuvers and the East Baltimore lift. In the Allis maneuver, which requires the patient to be supine on the table, the patient's pelvis is stabilized by an assistant applying pressure. The physician then applies in-line longitudinal traction to the femur followed by gentle flexion of the hip to 90 degrees. Internal and external rotation of the hip ensues with continued traction until reduction is accomplished. Reduction is often signified by an audible and palpable clunk.

A repeat AP pelvic radiograph must be obtained to confirm a successful reduction. Once this is confirmed, the hip should be ranged gently to assess stability and a CT scan performed to evaluate for a concentric reduction, the presence of intraarticular fragments, and the presence of femoral head and acetabular fractures.

Posterior acetabular wall fractures with >40% wall disruption lead to an unstable hip, whereas it remains stable when <20% of the wall is disrupted. An irreducible hip dislocation, which is caused by bony or soft-tissue interposition within the joint, requires emergent open surgical intervention to reduce the pressure on the hip's articular cartilage and subsequent risk for avascular necrosis. A nonconcentric reduction may also require open operative intervention or skeletal traction for the same reasons seen with irreducible hips.

If the hip is found to be clinically and radiographically stable after reduction, an abduction pillow or knee immobilizer must be used to prevent inadvertent movements by the patient that could compromise reduction and cause recurrent dislocation. Strict hip precautions should be enforced at all times and prohibit patients from crossing their legs, bending their hip past a 90-degree angle, and twisting their hip inward.

There is no one specific approach to rehabilitation after a hip dislocation, and the patient's weight-bearing status and need for postreduction traction or bed rest are controversial and surgeon dependent.

Complications

The risk of developing posttraumatic osteonecrosis of the femoral head is what makes hip dislocations an orthopaedic emergency. **The critical time to reduction, which in theory will restore blood flow to the femoral head, has not been definitively determined. However, it is thought that a greatly increased risk of avascular necrosis occurs with a delay in reduction of greater than 6 to 12 hours.** It is important to note that those who incur hip dislocations via higher energy mechanisms are more likely to develop osteonecrosis as a result of greater initial damage to the surrounding blood supply. Osteonecrosis commonly occurs within 2 years. Other complications include development of posttraumatic arthritis, sciatic nerve palsy, and recurring dislocations. Furthermore, many patients presenting with hip dislocations have other significant systemic injuries as well as ipsilateral knee and bony injuries.

COMPREHENSION QUESTIONS

3.1 A 45-year-old driver is involved in a motor vehicle collision and sustains a posterior dislocation of the left hip. What is the most likely concomitant injury?

A. Lumbar burst fracture

B. Right knee meniscus tear

C. Left knee anterior cruciate ligament tear

D. Subdural hematoma

3.2 A 28-year-old man is about to be discharged from the hospital after a motor vehicle collision in which he sustained a right hip dislocation. Before leaving, he asks to review what positions he can and cannot place his hip. You explain to him that posterior hip precautions prohibit:

A. Leg crossing
B. Flexing the hip to greater than 90 degrees
C. Twisting the hip inward
D. Hip extension
E. A, B, and C

3.3 A 41-year-old woman sustains a left posterior hip dislocation. After a successful attempt at closed reduction in the emergency room using conscious sedation, what is the next step in management?

A. CT scan of the hip and pelvis
B. Hip spica cast application
C. Further evaluation of hip stability via an exam under anesthesia in the operating room
D. Femoral skeletal traction pin

ANSWERS

3.1 **C.** The traumatic hip dislocation in this case is due to a dashboard injury in which the forces are first transmitted through the knee en route to the hip. Thus the possibility of a concurrent ipsilateral knee injury should be explored through careful clinical examination and possibly magnetic resonance imaging.

3.2 **E.** Choices A, B, and C are posterior hip precautions. Hip extension is not and can be performed by those who have had a posterior dislocation or have undergone hip replacement via a posterior approach. However, it is considered an anterior hip precaution and therefore should not be done in those who undergo hip replacement via an anterior approach or who have dislocated anteriorly.

3.3 **A.** The next step in management after reduction of a posterior hip dislocation is obtaining a CT scan to evaluate for damage (ie, fracture or impaction deformity) to the femoral head and acetabulum. Furthermore, a CT scan will identify an incongruent reduction and free intraarticular joint fragments. Such findings may require additional intervention.

CLINICAL PEARLS

- Posterior hip dislocations are caused by high-energy mechanisms and comprise greater than 90% of all native hip dislocations.
- In the setting of a posterior dislocation, the hip is positioned in a flexed, adducted, and internally rotated position.
- A hip dislocation is an orthopaedic emergency, and closed reduction attempts should be performed as soon as possible to reduce the period of avascularity to the hip.
- An AP pelvic radiograph must be obtained to confirm reduction, and a CT of the hip should be done to evaluate joint congruency, presence of intraarticular fragments, and presence of femoral head and acetabular fractures.
- Posterior hip precautions prohibit patients from crossing their legs, bending their hip past a 90-degree angle, and twisting their hip inward.
- Complications associated with hip dislocations include osteonecrosis, posttraumatic arthritis, sciatic nerve palsy, and recurring dislocations.

REFERENCE

Foulk DM, Mullis BH. Hip dislocation: evaluation and management. *J Am Acad Orthopaed Surg*. 2010;18(4):199-209.

CASE 4

A 76-year-old Caucasian female is brought to the emergency department (ED) with complaints of left groin pain after stumbling and falling in the hallway of her home. Previously she ambulated without assistance, but she states that now she cannot bear weight on her left leg. Although she did not lose consciousness, she recalls feeling "a little light-headed" before she fell. She has no other complaints or pains. She takes several medications for a history of cardiac arrhythmias, including warfarin. On physical exam, the patient is laying comfortably in the stretcher with her left leg held in slight external rotation. She reports pain with gentle passive rotation of her hip. There is a slight ecchymosis over her left greater trochanter. She readily dorsi- and plantarflexes her left ankle and flexes and extends her toes; her sensation is intact throughout her leg. Gentle palpation of all other joints is negative for tenderness or notable deformity. Her temperature is 98°F, blood pressure 134/88 mmHg, and heart rate is 155 beats/min. An electrocardiogram shows a rapid, erratic ventricular rate without discernible p waves. Initial laboratory tests show a hemoglobin and hematocrit of 11.5 g/dL and 35.0%, respectively, and an international normalized ratio (INR) of 3.4. A radiograph is obtained and can be seen in Figure 4–1.

- ▶ What is the most likely diagnosis?
- ▶ What is the best treatment for this patient?
- ▶ What are other additional immediate concerns for this patient?

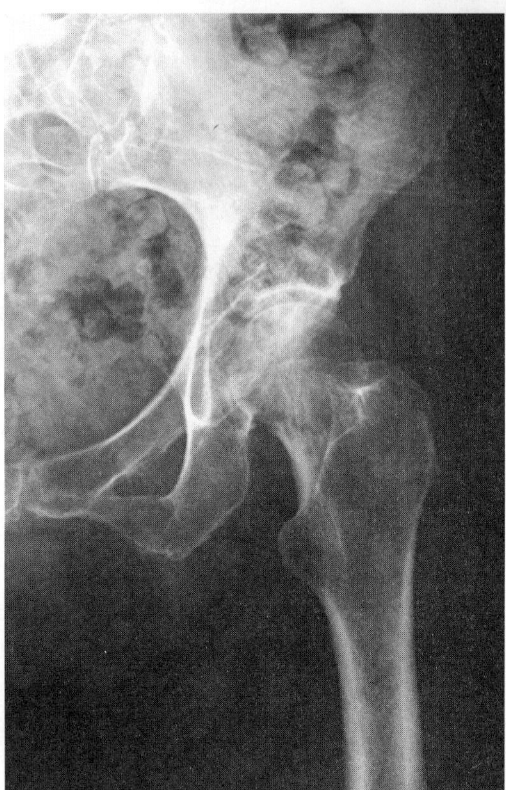

Figure 4–1. AP radiograph of the left hip.

ANSWERS TO CASE 4:

Femoral Neck Fracture

Summary: A 76-year-old woman complains of left hip pain after suffering a presyncopal fall onto her left hip. She suffers a nondisplaced femoral neck fracture.

- **Most likely diagnosis:** Anteroposterior (AP) radiograph of the left hip showing a fracture that extends obliquely across the femoral neck. The femoral head is not significantly displaced from the femur, but impacted into the neck and rotated away from the midline. This results in a valgus deformity.
- **Treatment options:** Although treatment options always include nonoperative management—historically treated with prolonged bed rest and traction—fractures of the femoral neck are best treated surgically. Basic methods include fixation with screws and hip arthroplasty.
- **Additional concerns:** The patient's elevated INR puts her at risk for significant perioperative bleeding, especially if she requires hip prosthesis placement. Furthermore, her history of unsteady gate and dizziness requires a thorough

workup for presyncope. Her cardiac comorbidities, age, and additional aspects of her history place her at risk for multiple perioperative complications. Anesthesia, internal medicine, and/or cardiology are often consulted for assistance with perioperative risk management.

ANALYSIS

Objectives

1. Distinguish different types of femoral neck fractures and their classifications.
2. Determine the appropriate treatment options for various types of femoral neck fractures with regard to patient age, comorbidities, and prior activity level.
3. Understand the mechanics and anatomy of the hip with special regard to its blood supply.
4. Be familiar with the complications associated with femoral neck fractures.

Considerations

This mechanism of injury—a low-energy, direct fall onto the great trochanter—is perhaps the most common cause of hip fracture in elderly patients. The affected extremity may be **shortened and externally rotated** with displaced fractures; however, in neck fractures that are nondisplaced, physical signs may be subtle and limited to pain with weight bearing or with movement, especially rotation, of the hip. Femoral neck fractures are not usually associated with neurovascular injury unless accompanied by other injuries; these should be of greater suspicion in younger patients who have sustained hip fractures from high-energy mechanisms.

This patient exhibits many risk factors for an insufficiency fracture of the hip, including her postmenopausal age, female sex, white race, and history of tobacco use. Despite these risk factors, however, the patient maintained a fairly active lifestyle, ambulating and participating in many daily activities; such activity levels help guide expectations and treatments.

Additionally, this patient has atrial fibrillation that is not rate-controlled on presentation. Her anticoagulation status, secondary to warfarin use, precludes all but the most drastic of surgical interventions. The patient's elevated INR must be reversed before invasive procedures are performed. An unstable cardiac history of arrhythmias or valve replacements necessitates careful evaluation and optimization before surgery, balancing the importance of anticoagulation with perioperative bleeding. Fortunately, this patient's nondisplaced neck fracture need not be fixed in an emergent manner; however, some types of nondisplaced hip fractures, as discussed below, demand a more prompt, emergency fixation to preserve blood supply to vulnerable bone. During her hospitalization, this patient should have her presyncopal symptoms and coagulation addressed by her medical team.

Preoperative risks must be addressed quickly and minimized when possible, as many studies show improved patient outcomes with early (<4 days in some studies) versus delayed surgical interventions. Advantages include reduced hospital stays, risks of pulmonary complications, venous thromboembolism, and pressure ulceration.

APPROACH TO:
Femoral Neck Fracture

DEFINITIONS

AVASCULAR (OSTEO)NECROSIS (AVN): Bone death secondary to inadequate blood supply. May be idiopathic; secondary to biological, chemical, or physical insults; or, in femoral neck fractures, the result of traumatic loss of vascular supply.

CALCAR FEMORALE: Dense, vertically oriented bone originating in the posteromedial portion of the femoral shaft under the lesser trochanter. It radiates laterally toward the posterior aspect of the greater trochanter, reinforcing the femoral neck posteroinferiorly.

INTRACAPSULAR FEMORAL NECK: This term refers to the area of the femoral neck that is located within the joint capsule. Anteriorly, the capsule attaches to the intertrochanteric line. Posteriorly, it attaches 1 to 1.5 cm proximal to the intertrochanteric line at the base of the neck.

EXTRACAPSULAR FEMORAL NECK: This term refers to the more distal area of the femoral neck, which is located outside the joint capsule. This predominantly metaphyseal region has excellent blood supply and therefore has a comparatively low risk of nonunion/AVN.

CROSS-TABLE LATERAL X-RAYS: A radiographic view that allows perpendicular assessment of the femoral neck without need for manipulation of the affected extremity. It is obtained by flexing the contralateral hip out of the x-ray plane and obtaining x-rays perpendicular to the femoral neck.

HEMIARTHROPLASTY: A surgical procedure that replaces the femoral portion of the hip joint; the femoral head and neck are removed and replaced with a prosthesis containing a femoral head component that swivels in the remnant acetabulum.

CLINICAL APPROACH

Anatomy

The hip joint is a ball-and-socket joint consisting of the femoral head articulating with the acetabulum. The femoral neck is characterized by a 120 to 135-degree angle formed between the femoral neck and femoral shaft in the coronal plane and 15 to 25 degrees of anteversion, or forward rotation, in the sagittal plane. The predominantly cortical bone in the femoral neck has a highly organized arrangement, with trabeculae oriented in the direction of major stress forces across the hip joint.

In adults, blood supply to the femoral neck and head is primarily through the medial circumflex femoral artery, a branch of the deep femoral (or profunda femoris) artery. Additional supplies are from the lateral femoral circumflex artery and the foveal artery, which travels through the ligamentum teres directly into the femoral head. Both circumflex femoral vessels form an extracapsular anastomotic ring at the base of the femoral neck and then penetrate the capsule to become intracapsular, thereby ascending to supply the head. Unlike the shaft of the femur, the intracapsular portion of its neck is devoid of periosteum; all healing must therefore occur through endosteal means, which necessitates an intact blood supply. It is critical to restore anatomic alignment in displaced fractures and to stabilize nondisplaced fractures to prevent future compromise to blood supply.

Mechanism of Injury

High-energy trauma, regardless of age, sex, or comorbidity, may cause femoral neck fractures. In the elderly or debilitated, however, femoral neck fracture most commonly occurs secondary to low-energy falls, either directly through forces on the greater trochanter, which transmits a force onto the femoral neck, or from forceful external rotation of the limb. Additional mechanisms include the repetitive loading forces experienced by athletes that gradually weaken portions of bone over time and manifest in stress fractures. Similar stress fractures may occur in patients with osteoporosis.

Evaluation and Diagnosis

In the setting of high-energy mechanisms, advanced traumatic life support protocols should be initiated to evaluate for any life-threatening injuries. With low-energy mechanisms such as a fall from standing, the patient should be evaluated for additional acute injuries such as head, cervical spine, or limb trauma. In patients without a history of acute trauma, other causes must be evaluated, including repetitive load cycling, particularly in physically active males and females with osteoporosis secondary to medical conditions including anorexia nervosa and renal or endocrine disorders.

The affected extremity should be evaluated for shortening, rotation, and neurovascular integrity. In some cases, physical signs may be very subtle. Gentle range of motion of the hip may elicit pain. Radiographic evaluation should use both an AP pelvis and a cross-table lateral image of the involved side. **When history and physical exam are clinically suggestive of fracture despite normal x-ray findings, magnetic resonance imaging or bone scan may reveal occult fractures.**

Classification

Femoral neck fractures are described using a variety of methods, including classification by anatomic location, by displacement of the fracture fragments, or by the vertical angulation of the fracture lines.

Anatomic Descriptors: Simple anatomic descriptors include the following:

Subcapital fracture: An intracapsular fracture located at the junction between the femoral head and neck.

Transcervical fracture: An intracapsular fracture extending across the mid-portion of the femoral neck.

Basicervical fracture: An extracapsular fracture located at the base of the femoral neck. Although this fracture is anatomically located within the femoral neck, it is often treated as an intertrochanteric fracture because of the biomechanical forces across this fracture.

Table 4–1 • GARDEN CLASSIFICATION OF FEMORAL NECK FRACTURES WITH RADIOGRAPHIC FEATURES		
	Fracture Definition	**Radiographic Features**
Type I	Valgus impacted, incomplete fracture	Trabecular lines of femoral head form valgus angle with acetabulum trabeculae (ie, apex points toward midline).
Type II	Complete, but nondisplaced fracture	Trabecular lines of femoral head are parallel to acetabulum trabeculae.
Type III	Complete fracture with partial displacement and varus angulation	Trabecular lines of femoral head form varus angle with acetabulum trabeculae (ie, apex points away from midline).
Type IV	Complete fracture with complete displacement	Femoral head is discontinuous with the femoral neck and remains located in acetabulum with its trabecular lines parallel to the acetabulum.

Garden Classification: Describes fractures based primarily on the degree of displacement noted in the AP radiograph. The risk of avascular necrosis and nonunion is predicted to be higher with increasing grade. The orientation of trabecular bone of the head with regard to that of the acetabulum is helpful in distinguishing these fracture types. Table 4–1 outlines the definitions and radiographic features of the Garden classification of femoral neck fractures.

Pauwel Classification: Fractures are categorized according to the angle that they form with the horizontal plane: **grade I, 0 to 30 degrees; II, 30 to 70 degrees; and III, >70 degrees.** At low angles, the forces of weightbearing are perpendicular to the fracture line and actually assist healing by compressing the pieces together to promote bone growth. As the angle increases, however, these forces become shear forces, exacerbating displacement of the pieces or failure of fixation. Pauwel type III fractures are thus associated with significant instability and high risks of nonunion and avascular necrosis. The stability of a fracture pattern no doubt influences the method of its treatment.

TREATMENT

Regardless of fracture type, the goals are almost universal: Minimize patient discomfort, restore hip function, and allow mobilization as early and safely as possible. Although most nondisplaced extremity fractures are treated with nonoperative immobilization, the difficulties of effective, comfortable, or practical immobilization of the hip are almost insurmountable. Furthermore, in the rare cases of nonoperative hip fracture treatment, subsequent displacement rates are as high as 40%. Nonoperative management is therefore reserved for only those absolutely medically unfit for surgery or severely demented and pain-free nonambulators.

Nondisplaced Fractures

Internal Fixation: Surgical fixation of nondisplaced fractures is most commonly achieved with cancellous lag screws percutaneously placed through the femoral neck. Typically, 3 screws are inserted in an **inverted-triangular configuration,** first using thin K-wires placed under x-ray fluoroscopy, which are then replaced by cannulated, or hollow, screws inserted over the wires. Care should be taken to **avoid starting the screws distal to the level of the lesser trochanter,** as the extreme tension forces on this side of the bone would be prone to stress riser forces and propagation of fracture.

General indications for percutaneous pinning include impacted and nondisplaced femoral neck fractures (ie, Gardner I or II fractures or those with low Pauwel angles [type I]). **In situ screw fixation is contraindicated, however, in patients with pathologic fractures or severe osteoarthritis or rheumatoid arthritis; such patients should be alternatively managed with prosthetic replacement.**

Displaced Fractures

Fracture Reduction and Fixation: There are a variety of surgical treatment options for displaced fractures, which vary significantly with regard to patient age, previous activity level, and comorbidities.

In young, otherwise healthy individuals, displaced transcervical or subcapital fractures pose a unique challenge. Here, prompt reduction of the femur is essential to restoring blood flow to support adequate healing. Femoral neck fractures in young individuals are generally considered an orthopaedic emergency, as risks of osteonecrosis may increase with increasing time until reduction. **Reductions, too, must be anatomic to maximally preserve the blood supply.**

Reduction in displaced neck fractures is typically achieved by externally rotating and flexing the hip under gentle traction to disengage fragments, then internally rotating to approximate the ends. Reduction must be evaluated by AP and cross-table lateral views. If prompt reduction is achieved, percutaneous pins, using the methods previously described, may be used to fix the unstable reduction. If reduction cannot be achieved using these closed methods, open reduction and internal fixation should be performed. Such constructs may be performed with sliding-screw or fixed-angle devices. If there is significant comminution, extensive damage, and stripped vasculature and soft tissue support, or significant comminution of the femoral neck, especially in the compression load-bearing calcar femorale region, the risks of AVN are high.

Arthroplasty: In elderly patients, patients with limited ambulatory status (those who previously ambulated with walkers or crutches or were wheelchair bound), and patients with underlying significant arthritis or osteoporosis, arthroplasty is generally the treatment of choice. By replacing the femoral head and neck, arthroplasty eliminates the risks of nonunion, avascular necrosis, and hardware failure that may be a consequence of internal fixation. Arthroplasty may be **total** (a replacement of both the acetabular cup and the femoral neck and head) or **hemi** (meaning the replacement of the femoral components placed into a native acetabulum). Hemiarthroplasty prostheses may be unipolar, involving a static implant that swivels in the acetabular cup, or, more commonly, bipolar, which provide an extraarticulating junction between the femoral head shell and inner ball. **Although total arthroplasty is the most extensive and invasive option, it may afford the highest level of function to elderly albeit healthy individuals who previously maintained active lifestyles.**

Complications

Femoral neck fractures impose a high mortality risk in the elderly population, reaching up to 30% at 1 year. Surgical treatment with internal fixation carries its own risks, most commonly:

Nonunion: Displaced femoral neck fractures generally take longer to heal, often 6 months or longer. The total rate of nonunion is reported to be 6%.

Hardware failure: This complication is most commonly reported concomitantly with nonunion and may require a conversion arthroplasty to fix.

Avascular necrosis: This tends to be a delayed complication, more commonly a complication of fractures displaced at presentation. AVN may not be evident until at least 2 years postoperatively. Conversion total arthroplasty is preferred over hemiarthroplasty, as the acetabulum often also exhibits degenerative changes due to collapse of the femoral head.

COMPREHENSION QUESTIONS

4.1 A 42-year-old man complains of right hip pain after being ejected from an all-terrain vehicle. He denies neurologic changes or other symptoms. His right leg does not appear to be shortened or externally rotated. Right hip radiographs demonstrate a complete, nondisplaced transcervical fracture. What is the most appropriate treatment for this patient?

A. Nonoperative observation with pain control, limited weightbearing, and close follow-up

B. Percutaneous pinning

C. Bipolar hemiarthroplasty

D. Total hip arthroplasty

4.2 A 66-year-old avid cross-country skier sustains a displaced femoral neck fracture after a fall down an icy embankment. What is the best treatment option for this patient?

A. Bipolar hemiarthroplasty

B. Open reduction internal fixation

C. Unipolar hemiarthroplasty

D. Nonoperative treatment with close follow-up

E. Total hip arthroplasty

4.3 A 72-year-old man sustains a completely displaced, subcapital femoral neck fracture after tripping over a step on a neighbors porch. Awake and lucid in the ED, he is most likely to assume which of the following positions for his fractured extremity?

A. Flexion and external rotation
B. Extension and external rotation
C. Flexion and neutral rotation and flexion
D. Extension and neutral rotation
E. Flexion and internal rotation

ANSWERS

4.1 **B.** The patient's young age and fracture severity are the major determinants of management. Of the surgical options listed, percutaneous pinning is the least invasive option in the setting of nondisplaced fractures. Regardless of displacement, closed reduction with internal fixation is the recommended choice of treatment in this age group. Arthroplasty is more commonly performed in the elderly population.

4.2 **E.** Given the presence of a displaced femoral neck fracture in an elderly patient, arthroplasty (options A, C, and E) is indicated. Given this patient's previously active lifestyle, total hip arthroplasty, option E, would best restore this patient to his previous level of function.

4.3 **A.** Patients with intracapsular pathology of the hip tend to hold their extremities in a position of external rotation and flexion. This patient has suffered subcapital fracture of the femoral neck, which is an intracapsular injury, thus resulting in hematoma formation and increased pressure within the hip socket. In a position of external rotation and flexion, the volume of the hip socket is greatest, and thus patients find relative comfort in this position. Additionally, children with septic arthritis of the hip will assume this position, as pain from pressurized inflammatory responses is similarly minimized.

CLINICAL PEARLS

- In the absence of absolute medical contraindications to surgery, the great majority of hip fractures are treated operatively.
- Despite significant improvements in the ability to surgically treat hip fractures and manage medical comorbidities, the mortality of hip fractures in patients $\geq$ 80 years of age is upward of 30% within 1 year from fracture.

REFERENCES

Buchholz RW, Court-Brown CM, Heckman JD, Tornetta P, eds. Femoral neck fractures. In: *Rockwood and Green's Fractures in Adults*. 7th ed. 2 vol. Philadelphia, PA: Lippincott Williams & Wilkins; 2010:1561-1596.

Egol KE, Koval KJ, Zukerman JD, eds. Femoral neck fractures. In: *Handbook of Fractures*. 4th ed. Philadelphia, PA: Lippincott Williams & Wilkins; 2010:378-387.

CASE 5

An 81-year-old white woman is brought to the emergency department (ED) with complaints of right hip pain after losing her balance while using the sink in her bathroom. Currently she is unable to bear weight on her right leg. She denies losing consciousness, feeling light-headed, or having chest discomfort or palpitations before the fall. She states her leg just "gave out." She did not hit her head. Before her injury, she ambulated with the assistance of a cane. The patient lives alone and was unable to move herself to a phone to call for help and was not found until almost 36 hours after the fall occurred. She has no other complaints of injury. Her past medical history is significant for hypertension, hypercholesterolemia, non–insulin-dependent diabetes mellitus, hypothyroidism, osteoporosis, and a history of a proximal humerus fracture 9 months prior. On exam, the patient is lying with her right leg slightly shortened and externally rotated. She experiences significant pain with gentle passive rotation and palpation over her hip. Her skin, as well as motor and sensory function, are intact throughout her right lower extremity. Palpation of all other joints is negative for tenderness or notable deformity. Her temperature is 98°F, blood pressure 100/60 mmHg, and heart rate is 105 beats/min. Electrocardiogram shows sinus tachycardia. An anteroposterior (AP) radiograph of the right hip is obtained (Figure 5–1).

- ▶ What is the most likely diagnosis?
- ▶ What are the treatment options available to this patient?
- ▶ What other potential medical issues must be considered based on this patient's history?

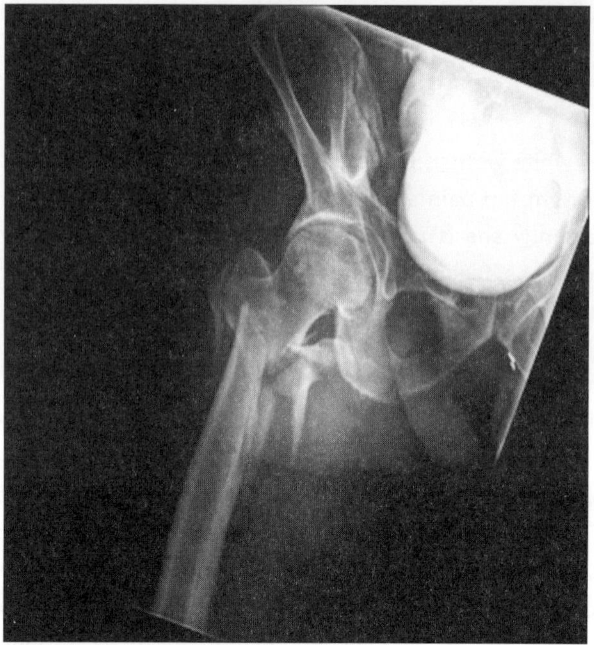

Figure 5–1. AP radiograph of the right hip.

ANSWERS TO CASE 5:

Intertrochanteric Hip Fracture

Summary: An 81-year-old woman complains of right hip pain after falling from standing and suffering a right intertrochanteric fracture.

- **Most likely diagnosis:** Right intertrochanteric fracture
- **Treatment options:** Intertrochanteric femur fractures are best treated surgically. The goal is stable internal fixation to allow early weightbearing and mobilization. Fixation implant choices include cephalomedullary hip screws, sliding hip screws, and, to a lesser extent, prosthetic replacements or external fixators. Like femoral neck fractures, nonoperative management is reserved only for patients whose medical comorbidities put them at excessive risk for surgery.
- **Additional medical concerns:** This patient was found collapsed, many hours after her fall. She has been without oral intake for this entire time. The patient must be evaluated for dehydration, electrolyte imbalances, nutritional deficits, pressure ulcers, potential rhabdomyolysis and associate acute kidney failure, and hemodynamic instability, as intertrochanteric fractures may be associated with a large amount of blood loss into the thigh.

ANALYSIS

Objectives

1. Identify and characterize intertrochanteric hip fractures with regard to their stability.
2. Be familiar with the basic treatment options available for fixation of intertrochanteric fractures.
3. Understand the significance of hip fractures on mortality rates.

Considerations

This patient suffered a low-energy fall from standing, with a direct impact onto her great trochanter. This represents the most common mechanism for intertrochanteric hip fractures, which are most commonly seen in elderly female patients.

On physical exam, it is important to look at the position of the affected extremity. With displaced fractures, the extremity may be shortened and externally rotated. In nondisplaced fractures, conversely, physical signs may be subtle or simply limited to pain with range of motion of the hip and an inability to bear weight. Intertrochanteric hip fractures are not commonly associated with neurovascular injury or open fractures; however, evaluation for such characteristics is essential. In younger patients with intertrochanteric fractures secondary to high-energy mechanisms, neurovascular and associated injuries are more common. Such patients, of course, should undergo a complete and thorough advanced traumatic life support workup before orthopaedic injuries are addressed.

Several studies have shown improved patient outcomes with prompt surgical intervention for hip fractures; however, medical comorbidities must first be evaluated. In this case, the patient should be treated for dehydration and potential electrolyte imbalances and worked up for a potential rhabdomyolysis. **Hip fractures are associated with increasing age (> 70 years), female sex, and low bone mass. Intertrochanteric fractures are the most common pattern, accounting for approximately 50% of all hip fractures, with femoral neck fractures being the second most frequent.** Other common osteoporosis-related fractures include fractures of the vertebral bodies, distal radius, and proximal humerus. Hip fractures may also be seen in younger patients after high-energy injuries such as motor vehicle accidents and falls from height.

APPROACH TO: Intertrochanteric Fracture

DEFINITIONS

INTERTROCHANTERIC: The region between the greater and lesser trochanters of the proximal femur. This area is extracapsular, is made up of predominantly cancellous bone, and has an abundant blood supply.

SLIDING HIP SCREW: An extramedullary device that consists of a lateral side plate and a femoral head lag screw. The lag screw is not fixed into the side plate, allowing a controlled collapse at the fracture site. This creates compression over the fracture site and may promote healing.

CEPHALOMEDULLARY NAIL: An intramedullary device that combines features of an intramedullary nail and a sliding hip screw. Cephalomedullary nails are frequently employed in unstable and reverse obliquity fracture patterns.

REVERSE OBLIQUITY: A type of unstable fracture pattern characterized by an oblique fracture line extending from the medial cortex proximally to the lateral cortex distally.

TIP-APEX DISTANCE: The sum of the distances from the tip of the lag screw to the apex of the femoral head on the AP and lateral radiographic views. The measurement is expressed in millimeters. A measurement of less than 25 mm has been shown to minimize the risk of screw cutout.

CLINICAL APPROACH

Anatomy

The femoral head is connected to the shaft by the femoral neck, which projects medially to the shaft at an angle of 120 to 130 degrees. The greater trochanter projects superiorly and laterally above the neck–shaft junction. The lesser trochanter is located at the inferior junction of the neck and shaft on the posteromedial side and is the site of insertion for the iliopsoas muscle. The 2 trochanters are connected posteriorly by a crest of thickened cancellous bone, known as the intertrochanteric crest. The piriformis and short external rotators insert along here. A strong plate of vertically oriented bone called the calcar femorale is located posteriorly between the lesser and greater trochanters. Intertrochanteric fractures may displace secondary to the pull of the musculotendinous attachments on their respective fragments: Greater trochanter fragments may be abducted and externally rotated by the gluteus medius and short external rotators, whereas the shaft will be displaced proximally, medially, and posteriorly by the adductors and hamstrings.

Mechanism of Injury

Low-energy falls from standing account for more than 90% of hip fractures in patients >50 years of age. Fractures secondary to high-energy mechanisms commonly affect men less than 40 years of age.

Evaluation and Diagnosis

Patients most commonly present with pain in the proximal thigh and inability to ambulate after a fall. The affected extremity should be evaluated for shortening, rotation, and neurovascular integrity. Pain with log rolling or axial loading of the hip has a high association with occult fracture. Radiographic evaluation should include an AP pelvis x-ray and AP and cross-table lateral x-rays of the affected side. A traction film or an internal rotation view may assist in the visualization of subtle fractures. If a fracture is observed to extend beyond into the subtrochanteric region—defined as the region 0 to 5 cm below the lesser trochanter—full-length femur films should be acquired, as such facture patterns often require larger, longer intramedullary devices that should be planned preoperatively. When there is sufficient clinical suggestion of fracture despite normal x-ray findings, magnetic resonance imaging may be useful in establishing the diagnosis.

Classification

The Evans classification system divides intertrochanteric fractures into stable and unstable fracture patterns. In stable fracture patterns, the posteromedial cortex is intact or has minimal comminution, and thus it may still function to buttress against fracture collapse. In unstable fracture patterns, the posteromedial cortex is often too comminuted to prevent collapse of the fracture fragments, and fractures may fall into varus and retroversion without appropriate fixation. Intertrochanteric fractures with subtrochanteric extension are similarly unstable secondary to their propensity to collapse. Reverse obliquity is a special type of unstable fracture pattern in which the fracture line extends from the proximal medial to the distal lateral intertrochanteric region. In reverse obliquity fractures, the distal fragment may displace medially secondary to both sheer forces and musculotendinous deforming forces if proper fixation is not obtained.

TREATMENT

Nonoperative Treatment

Nonoperative treatment should be considered only for patients who are nonambulatory without significant pain and those for whom surgical treatment carries an unacceptable risk of mortality. Nonsurgical management is associated with increased mortality rate, pneumonia infections, urinary tract infections, joint contractures, deep vein thrombosis, decubitus ulcers, and dementia.

Operative Treatment

Like femoral neck fractures, operative fixation is the standard of care for the vast majority of intertrochanteric fractures. Unlike nondisplaced femoral neck fractures, however, intertrochanteric fractures do not necessarily demand urgent operative intervention, because the abundant blood supply to the intertrochanteric region makes complications such as nonunion and avascular necrosis relatively rare. That stated, **fracture fixation should ideally occur within the first 24 to 48 hours after fracture, as this lowers the risks associated with prolonged hospitalization and immobilization.** The goal of surgery is to provide stable internal fixation to allow full weightbearing and early mobilization. The most common implants used include sliding hip screws and cephalomedullary nails.

Sliding Hip Screws: Before development of the cephalomedullary nail, the sliding hip screw was the most commonly used device for both stable and unstable fracture patterns. There are many sliding hip screw designs, but all consist of a side plate fixed to the lateral cortex of the femur and a lag screw placed into the femoral head. The lag screw should be inserted so that it is within 1 cm of subchondral bone and in a central position in the femoral head. Central placement should be assessed on both lateral and AP views. A tip-apex distance of less than 25 mm is ideal and associated with a decreased incidence of screw cutout. Recent literature has demonstrated that sliding hip screws have a higher rate of failure when used on unstable fracture patterns, especially reverse obliquity fractures. Sliding hip screws continue to have excellent outcomes in stable fracture patterns, however, with results that are at least equivalent to those of cephalomedullary nails. Theoretically, sliding hip screws allow a greater collapse and thus compression of fracture fragments as compared to cephalomedullary devices, a characteristic that is often desirable in the treatment of stable intertrochanteric fracture patterns.

Cephalomedullary Nails: This device combines features of a sliding hip screw with an intramedullary nail. Advantages include its ability to be inserted percutaneously with limited blood loss, limited fracture exposure, and decreased soft tissue damage. In addition, owing to its intramedullary location, these devices are subjected to lesser bending moments, resulting in its theoretical increased resistance to varus forces. There are several variations of the cephalomedullary nail, but all consist of an intramedullary nail and a femoral head component. The femoral head component generally consists of one or more screw or blade devices that fix within the center of the femoral head and neck and then interlock distally with the intramedullary nail component. Insertion of the intramedullary nail may be performed through the piriformis fossa or through the greater trochanter. Piriformis nails are typically straight, as the piriformis fossa falls directly in line with the medullary canal of normal femurs; trochanteric nails have a slight lateral curve that allows them to be passed through the greater trochanter and then directed down the medullary canal. Cephalomedullary nails are best suited for unstable intertrochanteric fractures, including those with subtrochanteric extension, reverse obliquity, and comminuted posteromedial cortices. When combined with a long intramedullary component, cephalomedullary nails may also be used in the treatment of subtrochanteric fractures (ie, fractures occurring 0-5 cm distal to the lesser trochanter).

Complications

Intertrochanteric fractures, like femoral neck fractures, are associated with a high mortality rate, even when prompt operative fixation is achieved. **After fracture, patients have an increased relative risk of mortality that is at least double that of their age-matched peers.** Mortality rates range from 8.4% to 36% within the first year after hip fracture.

Loss of fixation is a complication seen with intertrochanteric fractures. This most commonly results from varus collapse of the proximal fragment with superior cutout of the lag screw from the femoral head. The incidence of fixation failure is reported to be as high as 20% in unstable fracture patterns. **As stated, cutout may be significantly reduced when the tip-to-apex distance is <25 mm.**

Nonunion is rare, occurring in fewer than 2% of patients. It is most common in patients with unstable fracture patterns. Due to the highly vascular nature of intertrochanteric bone, however, nonunion and avascular necrosis are significantly less common after fixation in intertrochanteric fractures than in femoral neck fractures.

COMPREHENSION QUESTIONS

5.1 A patient with an intertrochanteric hip fracture undergoes open reduction and sliding hip screw application. Postoperative radiographs demonstrate that the lag screw is inferiorly and anteriorly positioned in the femoral head, with a tip-apex distance of 44 mm. This patient is at greatest risk for which of the following complications?

A. Lag screw cutout

B. Lag screw loosening

C. Nonunion

D. Periprosthetic fracture

E. Lag screw breakage

5.2 A 49-year-old woman with no significant past medical history is involved in a motor vehicle accident in which she sustains a reverse obliquity-type intertrochanteric femur fracture. What is the most appropriate treatment for her injury?

A. Total hip arthroplasty

B. Bipolar hemiarthroplasty

C. External fixation

D. Sliding hip screw

E. Cephalomedullary nail fixation

5.3 Which of the following most typically represents the patient demographic and scenario in which intertrochanteric femur fractures occur in the United States?

A. High-speed motor vehicle ejection accident in a 26-year-old man

B. Fall from standing in a 69-year-old woman

C. Fall from 3-story balcony in a 56-year-old man

D. Soccer-related internal rotation twisting injury in a 19-year-old woman

E. Twenty-year-old male pedestrian struck by a vehicle directly over the greater trochanter

ANSWERS

5.1 **A.** A tip-to-apex distance of less than 25 mm is associated with a decreased cutout rate of femoral head lag screws.

5.2 **E.** A reverse oblique intertrochanteric hip fracture is optimally treated with cephalomedullary nail fixation. Patients treated with a sliding hip screw for reverse-obliquity fractures have a much higher failure rate, nearly 56% in one study compared with 3% in the intramedullary nail group. Total hip arthroplasty, bipolar hemiarthroplasty, and external fixation are very rarely used treatment options for intertrochanteric fractures. Arthroplasty is never ideal for an otherwise healthy 49-year-old woman.

5.3 **B.** Although each of these mechanisms could result in an intertrochanteric femur fracture, elderly women with low-energy mechanisms most typically suffer these fractures. The average age of intertrochanteric fracture is 66 to 76 years, with published female-to-male ratios ranging from 2:1 to 8:1.

CLINICAL PEARLS

- Suspect a hip fracture in any patient presenting with a foreshortened leg, held in flexion and external rotation.
- Low-energy falls from standing account for greater than 90% of hip fractures in patients >50 years of age.
- The stability of intertrochanteric fractures depends chiefly on the integrity of the posteromedial cortex of the proximal femur, a thick area of vertically oriented cortical bone that buttresses against fracture collapse.

REFERENCES

Abrahamsen B, Van Staa T, Ariely R, Olson M, Cooper C. Excess mortality following hip fracture: a systematic epidemiological review. *Osteoporosis Int*. 2009;20(10):1633-1650.

Baumgaertner MR, Curtin SL, Lindskog DM, et al. The value of the tip-apex distance in predicting failure of fixation of peritrochanteric fractures of the hip. *J Bone Joint Surg Am*. 1995;77:1058-1064.

Ekman EF. The role of the orthopaedic surgeon in minimizing mortality and morbidity associated with fragility fractures. *J Am Acad Orthop Surg*. 2010;18:278-285.

Haidukewych GJ, Israel TA, Berry DJ. Reverse obliquity fractures of the intertrochanteric region of the femur. *J Bone Joint Surg Am*. 2001;83-A(5):643-650.

Kaplan K, Miyamoto R, Levine B, Egol K, Zuckerman J. Surgical management of hip fractures: an evidence-based review of the literature. II. Intertrochanteric fractures. *J Am Acad Orthop Surg*. 2008;16:665-673.

Morgan SJ. Fractures of the hip. In: Lieberman, ed: *AAOS Comprehensive Orthopaedic Review*. Rosemont, IL: American Academy of Orthopaedic Surgeons; 2009:597-609.

Russell T. Intertrochanteric fractures. In: Bucholz RW, Heckman JD, eds: *Rockwood and Green's Fractures in Adults*. 7th ed. Philadelphia, PA: Lippincott Williams & Wilkins; 2010:1597-1640.

CASE 6

A 61-year-old woman with a previous right total hip replacement presented with severe left hip osteoarthritis and underwent a left total hip replacement. The patient was doing well and walking pain-free, when at 4 months postoperatively, she tripped while stepping off a curb and landed directly onto her left side. She did not lose consciousness and only complained of left hip and groin pain and was not able to ambulate after the fall. She was taken to the emergency department for evaluation. Her past medical history is noncontributory, and her surgical history is as previously noted. Findings on physical exam include pain with axial loading and internal/external rotation of the left hip. Her skin is intact, and she has good sensation to light touch and motor function through the L4-S1 distribution. She does not have any tenderness to palpation around the knee or distally. She has 2+ dorsalis pedis and posterior tibial pulses. An anteroposterior (AP) radiograph of the left hip is obtained (Figure 6–1).

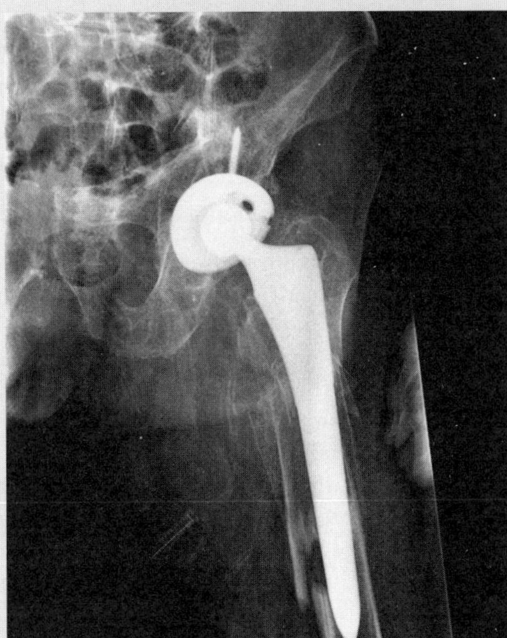

Figure 6–1. AP radiograph of the left hip demonstrating a periprosthetic femur fracture.

- What is the most likely diagnosis?
- What other aspects must be considered before determining the appropriate treatment for this patient?
- What is the most appropriate treatment for this patient?

ANSWERS TO CASE 6:
Periprosthetic Hip Fracture

Summary: A 61-year-old woman with a recent left total hip replacement sustained a fall and injury to her left hip. Plain films of the left hip show a periprosthetic femur fracture.

- **Most likely diagnosis:** Left periprosthetic femur fracture.
- **Additional considerations:** After identifying the fracture pattern and location, the 2 most important aspects to consider are the stability of the prosthetic femoral stem and the quality of the remaining bone stock.
- **Best treatment:** Revision of the femoral component to a cementless, porous coated long stem that bypasses the fracture by at least 2 cortical diameters. Fracture fixation is also required with cables, a plate, and/or strut graft.

ANALYSIS

Objectives

1. Understand what to look for on radiographs in the setting of a periprosthetic fracture, including fracture location, prosthesis fit, and bone stock.
2. Understand the Vancouver classification system of periprosthetic hip fractures and how it can be used to guide the appropriate method of treatment.
3. Be familiar with the basic treatment options for periprosthetic hip fractures.
4. Recognize potential complications arising from their treatment.

Considerations

This patient is a 61-year-old woman who sustained a fall and a left periprosthetic femur fracture. Although the patient presented complaining of left hip pain and sustained no other obvious injuries, it is important to rule out concomitant injuries, including head trauma or other musculoskeletal injuries. A thorough neurovascular examination of the left lower extremity, including sensory, and vascular assessments of the foot and ankle is mandatory. Movement of the hip, quadriceps, and hamstring may be limited as a result of pain, but a thorough assessment of the distal musculature should be performed. In addition, key questions regarding the patient's functional status before the fall may provide valuable insight: Was the patient able to ambulate without assistance? Did the patient have any thigh pain before the fall (which may indicate the presence of an already loose femoral component)?

Given the patient's inability to ambulate, she should be admitted to the hospital for definitive management of her fracture. An appropriate medical workup should be performed, including a chest x-ray, electrocardiogram, and laboratory tests before proceeding to the operating room. The medical team performing risk stratification of the surgery should understand that revision surgery will likely require a prolonged operative time and increased blood loss versus a primary, elective total hip arthroplasty. The orthopaedic team must preoperatively plan the surgical procedure and ensure that all implants and options that may be used are readily available. **Most important, the patient must understand that in revision hip surgery, both the rates of postoperative dislocation and infection are increased compared with primary hip surgery.**

APPROACH TO: Periprosthetic Hip Fracture

DEFINITIONS

PERIPROSTHETIC FRACTURE: A break in the bone surrounding a joint replacement prosthesis.

POROUS COATING: In total hip replacement, cementless implants commonly have a region where the surface is covered in microscopic pores, which enhances bone ingrowth for implant fixation.

SUBSIDENCE: In the setting of a total hip replacement, refers to the femoral stem migrating distally after initial implantation, indicating a high likelihood of a loose stem.

CLINICAL APPROACH

Etiologies

As the number of patients in the population living with a total hip arthroplasty continues to rise, the incidence of periprosthetic fractures also continues to increase. Patients with total hip replacements span a wide age range, with elderly patients being at increased risk for low energy falls, whereas younger, more active patients may be at risk for higher energy trauma. The Mayo Clinic Joint Replacement Database reported the largest series of periprosthetic hip fractures and noted an incidence of 1% (238 of 23,980) in primary hip arthroplasties and 4% (252 of 6349) in revision hip arthroplasties, although the overall incidence has been reported to be as high as 18%. Periprosthetic hip fractures can occur both intraoperatively and postoperatively, and it is key to accurately classify these fractures to determine the appropriate treatment plan. The most critical consideration is to determine the stability of the implant, as simple fixation of a fracture surrounding a loose femoral stem is likely to fail as a result of implant subsidence.

Risk factors for periprosthetic hip fractures are similar to those of the general population. In the elderly, low-energy falls, particularly in the setting of osteoporosis or inflammatory arthropathy, can lead to periprosthetic fractures. Another consideration pertains to the type of femoral component fixation and the use of either a proximally or fully-porous coated implant. Currently, the majority of femoral stems in primary total hip arthroplasty are implanted using cementless fixation, in which the femoral stem has a proximal porous coating, allowing bony ingrowth and fixation at the proximal aspect of the stem. This enables the stress from weightbearing to be transferred from the femoral head, through the proximal bone and calcar of the femur, and then distally through the native femoral shaft. With these wedge-fit tapered designs, proximal fractures may occur. With cylindrical fully-porous coated stems, distal "split" fractures can occur.

Clinical Presentation

Patients typically present with a low-energy mechanism of injury, such as a fall from standing, and have pain in the hip and femur, with or without the ability to ambulate. It is key to determine any other sites of injury, including head trauma, and whether or not the patient had any shortness of breath, lightheadedness, dizziness, or symptoms indicating a cardiac or neurologic cause of their injury. Any symptoms in the lower extremity before the injury should also be noted, along with signs of start-up thigh pain (pain initiated with ambulation on rising from a chair) that may indicate a loose femoral stem.

Prior surgical records and reports should be obtained to determine the prior surgical approach, implant type and size, and any perioperative complications including infection. The presence of prior infection should raise concerns of an active infection, and further testing should be performed to rule out infection such as hip aspiration, or cultures obtained intraoperatively. Of note, normal laboratory markers for occult infection such as the erythrocyte sedimentation rate and C-reactive protein can be falsely positive in the setting of a fracture and thus are of limited utility. As always, a thorough medical history should be obtained. A detailed examination of the affected lower extremity, including a complete neurovascular examination, and assessment of prior incisions and skin integrity should be performed. In addition, any leg length discrepancy should also be noted to assist with preoperative planning.

Diagnosis

The diagnosis of a periprosthetic hip fracture can typically be made using standard radiographs. Radiographs should include an AP of the pelvis, AP and lateral of the hip, and AP and lateral of the femur. Visualization of the entire femur is critical to assess the presence and distal extent of the fracture. To determine the stability of the implant, comparison to prior radiographs is useful to assess any increase in periprosthetic bone loss or implant subsidence that may suggest component loosening. With cementless femoral implants, the point at which the metal stem narrows proximally to become the femoral neck is typically aligned with the proximal, medial aspect of the native femur. If this point on the femoral stem migrates distally (or a fracture causes the medial aspect of the native femur to migrate proximally or displace), then the femoral stem is loose and needs to be revised. It is critical to assess both the acetabular and femoral components for both position and signs of loosening, as signs of acetabular loosening may warrant revision of the acetabular component during concomitant fixation of the femur fracture. Ultrasound, computed tomography, and magnetic resonance imaging are not routinely required.

TREATMENT

The treatment of a periprosthetic hip fracture is guided by the **Vancouver classification system** (Table 6–1). Type A fractures include fractures of the greater trochanter (A_G) and lesser trochanter (A_L). Greater trochanter fractures are stable when minimally displaced, but may require surgical treatment with a plate if displaced proximally. Lesser trochanter fractures can often be treated nonoperatively. However, if a significant portion of the calcar is involved, leading to destabilization of the stem, then revision of the femoral stem with fixation of the calcar/lesser trochanter with cables or supplementary plate fixation surrounding the greater trochanter is required.

Type B fractures occur around or just below the tip of the femoral stem. A B1 fracture occurs around a well-fixed stem and can be treated with plates and screws and possibly cortical strut allografts and cables. A B2 fracture occurs around or just below an unstable stem, and thus revision of the femoral stem is required. Typically, long porous-coated cementless stems are used to bypass the fracture and to achieve distal fixation. In addition, the fracture fragment is fixed using plates, cables, or cortical strut allografts. A B3 fracture is distinguished from a B2 fracture, as B3 fractures possess insufficient bone stock. Therefore, B3 fractures are also treated with femoral component revision and fracture fixation, but often require special techniques such as bone grafting or implantation of a proximal femoral replacement.

Type C fractures occur well below the femoral prosthesis and thus are treated with fixation of the fracture itself, without revision of the femoral or acetabular components.

Table 6–1 • THE VANCOUVER CLASSIFICATION SYSTEM OF PERIPROSTHETIC FEMUR FRACTURES

Vancouver Classification Type	Description	Treatment
A_L	Lesser trochanter fracture	Nonoperative if minimally displaced and femoral stem stable; revision of femoral stem and fixation of fracture if stem is loose
A_G	Greater trochanter fracture	Nonoperative if minimally displaced; fixation of fracture with cables or hook plate if displaced
B1	Fracture around or just below a well-fixed stem	Fixation of fracture with plates, screws, cables, and/or cortical strut allograft
B2	Fracture around or just below an unstable stem	Revision of the femoral stem with fixation of the fracture
B3	Fracture around or just below an unstable stem with poor remaining bone stock	Revision of the femoral stem with fixation of the fracture (often requires supplemental bone grafting or revision with proximal femoral replacement)
C	Fracture well distal to the tip of the stem, which does not affect the stability of the implant	Fixation of the fracture, without revision of the femoral stem

Complications

Complications after the treatment of periprosthetic hip fractures **include failure of the fracture to heal appropriately (nonunion), failure of femoral stem fixation (commonly owing to misdiagnosis of the initial stability of the stem), infection, dislocation, thromboembolic complications, and medical morbidity and mortality related to the surgical treatment itself.**

COMPREHENSION QUESTIONS

6.1 An 82-year-old man with a history of a prior left hip fracture treated with a bipolar hemiarthroplasty was in his usual state of health when he sustained another fall onto his left hip. He is neurovascularly intact and complains only of left hip pain. An AP left hip radiograph was taken and is shown in Figure 6–2. According to the Vancouver classification system, what type of periprosthetic fracture has this patient suffered?

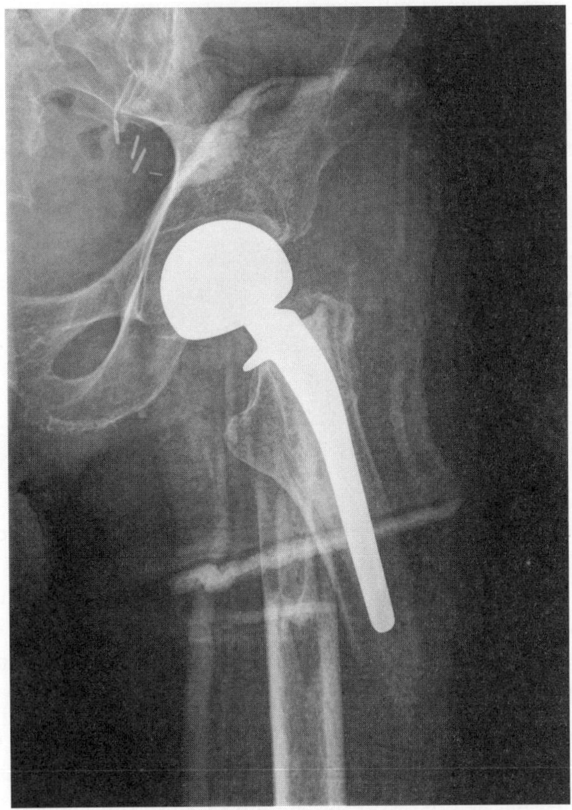

Figure 6–2. AP radiograph of the left hip demonstrating a periprosthetic femur fracture surrounding a bipolar hemiarthroplasty.

A. Type A_L
B. Type A_G
C. Type B1
D. Type B2
E. Type C

6.2 A 75-year-old woman who is 2 years removed from a right total hip arthroplasty sustains a fall and a nondisplaced greater trochanter fracture. The femoral stem appears stable on both anteroposterior and lateral radiographs of the hip and femur. Which of the following is the most appropriate treatment?

A. Open reduction and internal fixation of the fracture using a greater trochanter plate and cables

B. Resume all activities as tolerated, with no restrictions

C. Weightbearing as tolerated, but with no passive adduction past midline and no active abduction of the lower extremity

D. Nonweightbearing to the right lower extremity

6.3 A 79-year-old woman undergoes successful treatment of a Vancouver B2 periprosthetic femur fracture with a long porous-coated cementless stem, cables, and a cortical strut allograft. Which of the following complications is she at an increased risk for as compared with those patients who have undergone primary total hip arthroplasty?

A. Infection

B. Dislocation

C. Deep vein thrombosis

D. A and B

E. A, B, and C

ANSWERS

6.1 **C.** This patient sustained a periprosthetic left femur fracture. Because the stem appears stable proximally with no fracture extending proximally and no radiolucency surrounding the stem, this is likely a Vancouver B1 fracture. Vancouver B2 fractures would be similarly at the tip of the prosthesis, but would involve a loosened stem. Vancouver A fractures involve 1 of the 2 trochanters. Type C fractures occur distal to the prosthesis.

6.2 **C.** This patient sustained a nondisplaced greater trochanter fracture (A_G) and thus should initially be treated conservatively. The patient can continue to be weightbearing as tolerated, but should observe hip abduction precautions (movements that may cause the greater trochanter fracture to displace). The patient should receive sequential radiographs, and if the fracture demonstrates worsening displacement, then open reduction internal fixation of the fracture can be considered.

6.3 **E.** Revision hip surgery, particularly in the setting of a periprosthetic fracture, is extremely challenging. Unfortunately, the results are often less satisfactory than those seen with elective primary hip replacement. Postoperative complications occur more frequently in this setting and include infection, dislocation, and deep vein thrombosis, in addition to nerve palsy, cortical perforation, and fracture.

CLINICAL PEARLS

- The incidence of periprosthetic hip fractures continues to rise as a result of the increasing number of patients in the population with total hip arthroplasties.
- Radiographs of the entire femur must be obtained to assess the presence and entire extent of the fracture, along with stability of the femoral stem.
- Key aspects to consider regarding the classification and treatment of periprosthetic hip fractures are the stability of the femoral stem and the quality of the remaining bone stock.
- If the femoral stem is suspected to be unstable or loose, revision of the femoral stem should be performed, as fixation of a fracture in the setting of a loose femoral stem often leads to fracture nonunion and implant failure.

REFERENCES

Berry DJ. Epidemiology: hip and knee. *Orthop Clin North Am*. 1999;30:183-190.

Brady OH, Garbuz DS, Masri BA, et al. Classification of the hip. *Orthop Clin North Am*. 1999;30: 215-220.

Duncan CP, Masri BA. Fractures of the femur after hip replacement. *Instr Course Lect*. 1995;44: 293-304.

Pike J, Davidson D, Garbuz D. Principles of treatment for periprosthetic femoral shaft fractures around well-fixed total hip arthroplasty. *J Am Acad Orthop Surg*. 2009;17:677-688.

CASE 7

A 26-year-old African American male athlete reports to clinic after injuring his knee the night before while he was practicing squats and dead lifts for his upcoming weightlifting competition. He states he felt a "pop" as he began to stand during his second set of squats. He complains of intense pain and an inability to lift his leg or bear any weight on it. These symptoms began immediately after the pop. During the physical examination, the patient is found to have pain with palpation just below the patella. Although he is found to have good quadriceps tone, he is unable to perform a straight leg raise. All motor and sensory findings are otherwise normal. It is decided that radiographs should be obtained, which subsequently show patella alta. His past medical history and review of systems are otherwise unremarkable.

- ▶ What is the most likely diagnosis?
- ▶ What is the best treatment for this condition?

ANSWERS TO CASE 7:
Patellar Tendon Rupture

Summary: A 26-year-old African American male athlete who is a competitive weightlifter injured his left knee while performing dead lifts in the gym. He felt a pop in his knee and reported pain with considerable swelling to the anterior aspect. He has pain with palpation over the inferior pole of the patella and is unable to perform a straight leg raise, even though he has good quadriceps tone. All motor and sensory findings are otherwise normal. An x-ray identifies patella alta. His past medical history and review of systems are otherwise unremarkable.

- **Most likely diagnosis:** Patellar tendon rupture
- **Treatment:** Surgery for patellar tendon repair within 2 weeks. Before surgery, he is to ice and elevate his leg to help diminish the local swelling. The leg should be braced in extension to minimize further gapping and proximal retraction of the patella. After surgery, the leg will be protected in extension followed by gradual, progressive range-of-motion exercises.

ANALYSIS

Objectives

1. Learn the causes of patellar tendon rupture.
2. Understand the prevalence of the injury.
3. Be familiar with the populations that are most often affected.
4. Understand the therapy options.

Considerations

This is a 26-year-old African American male athlete who has presented with a story, physical exam, and radiographic findings consistent with a patellar tendon rupture. Although his story identifies repetitive microtrauma as the likely cause of his patellar tendon rupture, other predisposing factors must be investigated. In the setting of a competitive weightlifter, such as this gentleman, anabolic steroid use as a contributing factor should be contemplated. Because this is an acute rupture in a healthy young adult, surgical repair is indicated within 2 weeks from the date of injury. Surgical technique will vary based on the location of the rupture. Because most tears occur at the osseotendinous juncture between the tendon and inferior pole of the patella, bone tunnels and heavy suture will likely be required. It is also important to note that although no palpable gap was felt below the inferior patellar pole on physical exam, this would not be an uncommon finding.

APPROACH TO: Patellar Tendon Rupture

DEFINITIONS

TENDINITIS: A term describing tendon inflammation.

TENDINOSIS: A term referring to chronic inflammation of a tendon, in which damage occurs at the cellular level. It is thought to be caused by repetitive micro-trauma that increases the chance of a tendon rupture.

JUMPER'S KNEE: A phrase used to describe patellar tendon pathology, including tendonitis and tendinosis. These conditions typically occur in athletes involved in jumping sports such as basketball and volleyball and are therefore referred to as Jumper's knee.

BLUMENSAAT LINE: A line drawn along the roof of the intercondylar notch on a lateral radiograph with the knee in 30 degrees of flexion. This line should intersect the inferior border of the patella. In patella alta, which occurs in the setting of a patella tendon rupture, the distal pole of the patella is elevated above this line.

INSALL-SALVATI RATIO: Determined on a lateral radiograph and is the length of the patella tendon/length of the patella (the greatest diagonal length). The relationship should be 1.0. A ratio of 1.2 or more indicates patella alta, whereas a ratio of less than or equal to 0.8 indicates patella baja (seen in the setting of a quadriceps tendon rupture).

EXTENSOR MECHANISM OF THE KNEE: A network consisting of the quadriceps musculature, quadriceps tendon, patella, patellar tendon, tibial tubercle, and adjacent soft tissues that serves to extend or straighten the knee joint with the leg elevated and to stabilize the knee joint when the foot is planted on the ground.

CLINICAL APPROACH

Etiology

The patella's role in the extensor mechanism is to establish a **mechanical advantage** in knee extension by increasing the **moment arm** of the quadriceps muscle. **For the patellar tendon to rupture, an eccentric and violent quadriceps contraction must occur with the knee partially flexed.** Less frequently, penetrating trauma can cause a tear. Ruptures can be classified as complete or incomplete and as intrasubstance or as occurring at the insertion site of the tendon onto the inferior pole of the patella (an avulsion-type injury). Tendon avulsion from the tibial tuberosity is encountered less frequently.

It is uncommon for the patellar tendon to rupture in healthy tendon, and when it does, it is most commonly due to repetitive microtrauma. Although there is no clear age or sex predisposition for this injury, it is more commonly seen in those with an underlying disease that causes weakness in the tendon, predisposing it to rupture. Such diseases include rheumatoid arthritis, diabetes, lupus, gout, and chronic renal insufficiency. The tendon may also become weakened from anabolic steroid use or chronic use of corticosteroid medication injected directly into the tendon.

Physical Examination

The patient typically presents with a gross deformity of the knee, which includes an effusion and proximal retraction of the patella when compared with the contralateral, normal knee. Palpation may reveal an intrasubstance defect or one at its inferior pole. With an acute tear, the patient will have difficulty weightbearing, and the knee may buckle or feel as if it is going to "give out." When asked, the patient may recall an audible "pop" that had occurred at the time of injury and may be unable to perform a straight leg raise. However, one's ability to perform a straight leg raise does not completely rule out the presence of a patellar tendon rupture. In certain cases, the tendon can be ruptured while the adjacent medial and lateral retinacula of the knee remain intact, enabling the patient to perform some active extension. In such cases, the patient will, however, likely lack several degrees of terminal extension.

Radiographic Diagnosis

Anteroposterior (AP) and lateral radiographs are usually sufficient in confirming the diagnosis. The **Blumensaat line** and the **Insall-Salvati ratio** are derived from the lateral radiographs and aid in identifying both quadriceps and patellar tendon injury (Figure 7–1). At times, it may be useful to obtain a lateral radiograph of the

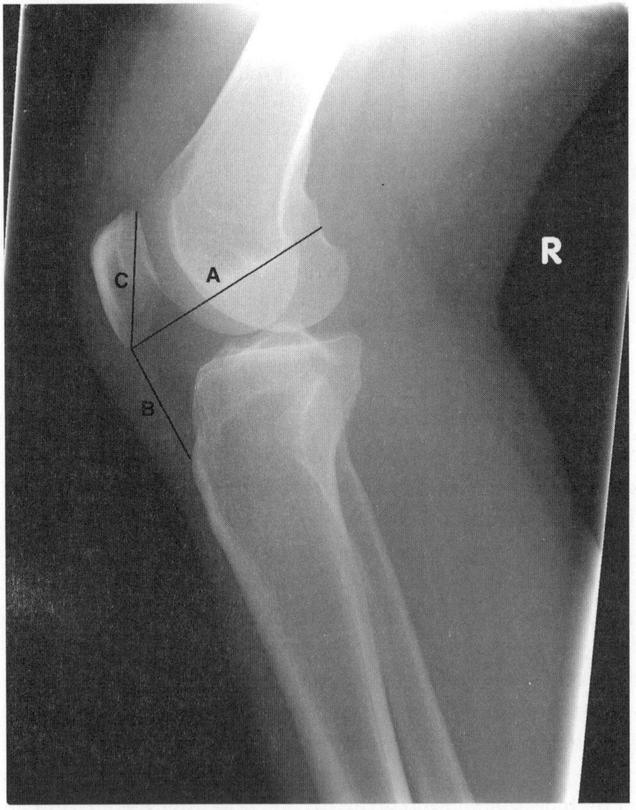

Figure 7–1. A lateral radiograph of a normal knee. The distal pole of the patella intersects Blumensaat line (A), and the Insall-Salvati ratio is approximately 1.0 (B/C).

contralateral knee for comparison. In equivocal cases in which diagnosis is unclear, ultrasound or magnetic resonance imaging (MRI) can be used. MRI can distinguish complete from partial ruptures, assist in determining the size of the tear, and also identify any concomitant injuries.

TREATMENT

Nonoperative treatment is limited to incomplete ruptures in which normal or near-normal knee extension is present. In such cases, management consists of immobilization with the knee in full extension for 4 to 6 weeks. Acute, complete tears require surgical repair unless there is a medical contraindication. **It is ideally performed within 2 weeks of the initial injury to prevent further tendon retraction, scar formation, and muscle atrophy.** Midsubstance tears are repaired end to end with a heavy nonabsorbable suture. However, ruptures most commonly occur at the osseotendinous juncture, a location that is not amenable to end-to-end repair. In this setting, the patellar tendon is reattached to its insertion using bone tunnels and heavy suture. The repair can be augmented with a cerclage suture, as is often done for midsubstance tears, in patients with systemic illnesses that have predisposed them to rupture (ie, diabetes), or in those who will likely undergo aggressive early postoperative range-of-motion exercises. Postoperative rehabilitation protocols vary from surgeon to surgeon. A common practice is to immobilize the leg in extension for 10 to 14 days, followed by progressive, protected range of motion. Isometric quadriceps strengthening may begin immediately postoperatively. The return to full activity could take up to 6 to 12 months. Furthermore, the patient will be allowed to return to sports only after a complete return of strength and range of motion has occurred.

Chronic ruptures are more difficult to repair and typically result in less favorable outcomes, as tendon degeneration and contraction make end-to-end apposition difficult to achieve. Surgery involves extensive mobilization of the tendon, lysis of scar tissue, and at times the use of an interposition flap or graft to bridge the gap and achieve a complete repair. This is a technically more demanding procedure and is less than ideal.

Complications

Complications include wound infection, patellofemoral arthritis, rerupture, and loss of knee motion. Difficulty in attaining full extension is most commonly due to quadriceps atrophy, highlighting the importance of early postoperative quadriceps strengthening.

COMPREHENSION QUESTIONS

7.1 A 22-year-old basketball player feels a painful "pop" in his knee when landing from a rebound. Immediate swelling, pain, and inability to extend his knee ensue. Radiographs depict patella alta. Treatment should include:

A. Long leg casting in extension

B. Application of a knee immobilizer followed by a slow return to play

C. Primary patella tendon repair

D. Intraarticular corticosteroid injection

7.2 Which of the following structures is not part of the knee's extensor mechanism?
   A. Quadriceps tendon
   B. Patella tendon
   C. Biceps femoris
   D. Tibial tubercle

7.3 A 55-year-old male slips on a patch of ice and falls on a hyperflexed knee. He reports hearing a "pop" during the fall and was unable to bear weight on the knee immediately after the injury. He has a large knee effusion on examination and is unable to perform a straight leg raise. You appreciate his patella baja on radiographic examination and an Insall-Salvati ratio of 0.7. What is the likely diagnosis?
   A. Patellar dislocation
   B. Quadriceps tendon rupture
   C. Patellar tendon rupture
   D. Anterior cruciate ligament (ACL) tear

ANSWERS

7.1 **C.** Sports such as basketball, football, soccer, and volleyball place high eccentric loads on the extensor mechanism and are associated with patellar tendon rupture. Primary surgical repair is always indicated for complete, acute tears.

7.2 **C.** The biceps femoris is not part of the extensor mechanism, but instead performs knee flexion. **The other muscles are part of the knee extensor mechanism.**

7.3 **B.** The differential diagnosis for any patient with a history of recent trauma to the knee and an inability to straight leg raise must include both quadriceps and patellar tendon ruptures. In patients older than 40 years, such as this patient, quadriceps tendon ruptures are more common; patella tendon ruptures are more frequently seen in patients younger than 40 years. The diagnosis of a ruptured quadriceps tendon is also supported in this patient by the radiographic finding of patellar baja and an Insall-Salvati ratio of less then 0.8. Both ACL and acute dislocations of the patella occur after noncontact pivoting injuries, making such diagnoses unlikely in this patient. Although physical exam may reveal large knee effusions in such patients, they should not lose their ability to actively straight leg raise.

CLINICAL PEARLS

- The patella's role in the extensor mechanism is to establish a mechanical advantage in knee extension by increasing the moment arm of the quadriceps muscle.
- Patellar tendon ruptures result from eccentric and violent quadriceps contraction occurring with the knee partially flexed.
- It is uncommon for the patellar tendon to rupture in healthy tendon.
- Nonoperative treatment is limited to incomplete ruptures in which normal or near-normal knee extension is present.
- Midsubstance tears are repaired end to end with a heavy nonabsorbable suture.
- Rupture at the osseotendinous juncture requires repair with bone tunnels and heavy suture.
- Acute patellar tendon tears should be repaired within 2 weeks from the injury.

REFERENCES

Frontera WR, Silver JK, Rizzo TD. *Essentials of Physical Medicine and Rehabilitation: Musculoskeletal Disorders, Pain, and Rehabilitation*. Philadelphia, PA: Saunders Elsevier; 2008:xix, 935 p.

Judd SJ. *Sports Injuries Sourcebook: Basic Consumer Health Information About Sprains and Strains, Fractures, Growth Plate Injuries, Overtraining Injuries, and Injuries to the Head, Face, Shoulders, Elbows, Hands, Spinal Column, Knees, Ankles, and Feet*. Health reference series. Detroit, MI: Omnigraphics; 2007: xix, 651 p.

Starkey C, Ryan JL. *Evaluation of Orthopedic and Athletic Injuries*. Philadelphia, PA: F.A. Davis Co; 2002: xxiv, 767 p.

CASE 8

A 43-year-old man was crossing the street when he was struck by a car moving at approximately 35 miles per hour. He was brought to the emergency department and is complaining of left knee pain. He did not lose consciousness. He has no other significant complaints. He has no significant past medical or surgical history. Findings on physical examination are notable for pain on palpation of his proximal left tibia with knee pain throughout passive range of motion. His skin is intact. His neurovascular examination is normal. His leg is circumferentially firm, but compressible. An anteroposterior (AP) radiograph is obtained and is shown in Figure 8–1.

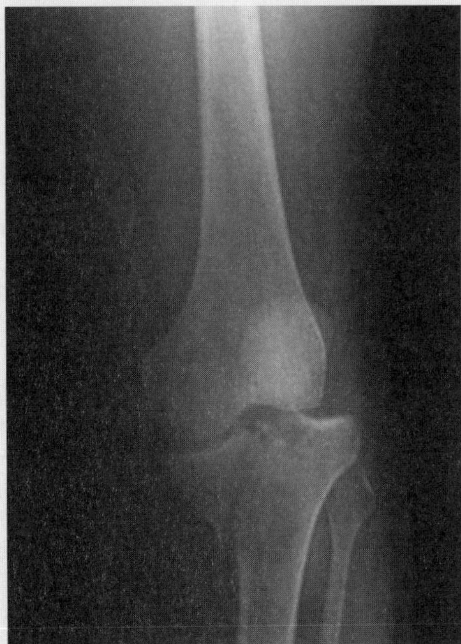

Figure 8–1. AP radiograph of the left knee.

- ▶ What is the most likely diagnosis?
- ▶ What additional injuries are you most concerned about?

ANSWERS TO CASE 8: Tibial Plateau Fracture

Summary: A 43-year-old man sustained a direct, high-energy injury to his left knee. Plain films of the left knee show a split depression of the medial condyle without lateral condylar involvement.

- **Most likely diagnosis:** Left tibia medial plateau split fracture, or a Schatzker IV injury
- **Additional injuries:** Meniscal tears, collateral and cruciate ligamentous injuries, peroneal nerve, popliteal artery injury (typically associated with medial plateau fractures), and compartment syndrome are soft-tissue injuries associated with tibial plateau fractures.

ANALYSIS

Objectives

1. Understand the anatomical and mechanistic principles behind the Schatzker classification of tibial plateau fractures.
2. Be familiar with basic treatment options for tibial plateau fractures.
3. Recognize potential complications arising from both the initial injuries and their treatments.

Considerations

This patient sustained a high-energy, direct impact injury to the region immediately below his right knee. In addition to his medial plateau fracture, he is at significant risk for several additional injuries, including collateral ligament complex, peroneal nerve injury, and popliteal artery injury. Medial meniscal tears may occur in up to 50% of plateau fractures, most commonly occurring with medial plateau injuries; likewise, lateral meniscal injuries are associated with lateral plateau fractures. Ligamentous integrity should be evaluated. A careful neurovascular evaluation is also essential. Although this patient has palpable pulses distal to his injury, a pulseless limb must be evaluated with Doppler probe and/or ankle-brachial index measurements (normal >0.9). Should audible Doppler waveforms be absent or diminished compared with the uninvolved side, vascular surgery should be consulted and the patient will likely require arteriography to evaluate the integrity of the popliteal artery.

Although this patient sustained no other obvious injuries, his mechanism warrants a complete and thorough physical exam, typically performed by a trauma team, with careful examination of all extremities and the axial skeleton performed by an orthopaedist. Although some tibial plateau fractures may be immobilized and sent away from the emergency department for outpatient follow-up, the high-energy nature of this injury necessitates admission to the hospital. As an inpatient, frequent leg compartment checks may easily be performed to ensure this patient does not develop a compartment syndrome. Intimal damage to the popliteal artery may take up to 48 hours to become symptomatic.

APPROACH TO:
Tibial Plateau Fracture

DEFINITIONS

TIBIAL PLATEAU: Term describing the weightbearing area of the proximal tibia. It is composed of the concave medial plateau and smaller convex lateral plateau. These regions are separated by the intercondylar eminence.

SCHATZKER CLASSIFICATION: A widely used classification system for tibial plateau fractures that helps orthopaedic surgeons with assessing the initial injury, formulating a management plan, and predicting prognosis. The classification divides tibial plateau fractures into 6 types.

CLINICAL APPROACH

Anatomy and Mechanisms of Injury

The tibial plateau is the predominantly cancellous region of bone that articulates with the distal femur. It includes the relatively larger, stronger, and more concave medial plateau and the relatively weaker, smaller, and more convex lateral plateau. **Medial plateau injuries, therefore, typically result from higher energy mechanisms,** which are defined as falls from greater than 12 feet or sudden-impact mechanisms such as motor vehicle collisions or bumper versus pedestrian events. Lateral plateau injuries, conversely, may occur from low-energy falls from standing in elderly osteoporotic patients. The direction and magnitude of fracture force, in addition to the underlying quality of bone, determine the fracture pattern.

Classification

The Schatzker classification is commonly used to describe tibial plateau fractures. They are classified in the following way:

Type I	Lateral split
Type II	Lateral split depression
Type III	Lateral pure depression
Type IV	Medial plateau split and/or depression
Type V	Bicondylar
Type VI	Metaphyseal-diaphyseal disassociation

Schatzker I through III fractures are generally considered low-energy injuries, whereas IV through VI injuries are high-energy injuries (Figure 8–2). Young adults with strong bone typically exhibit split fractures and have increased propensity to suffer ligamentous damage; older patients with osteoporotic bone are more inclined to suffer depression and split-depression patterns in the absence of ligamentous damage. Medial injuries (type IV) are considered by some authors to represent transient knee dislocations that have spontaneously reduced; the incidence of neurovascular injury is thus higher with these events.

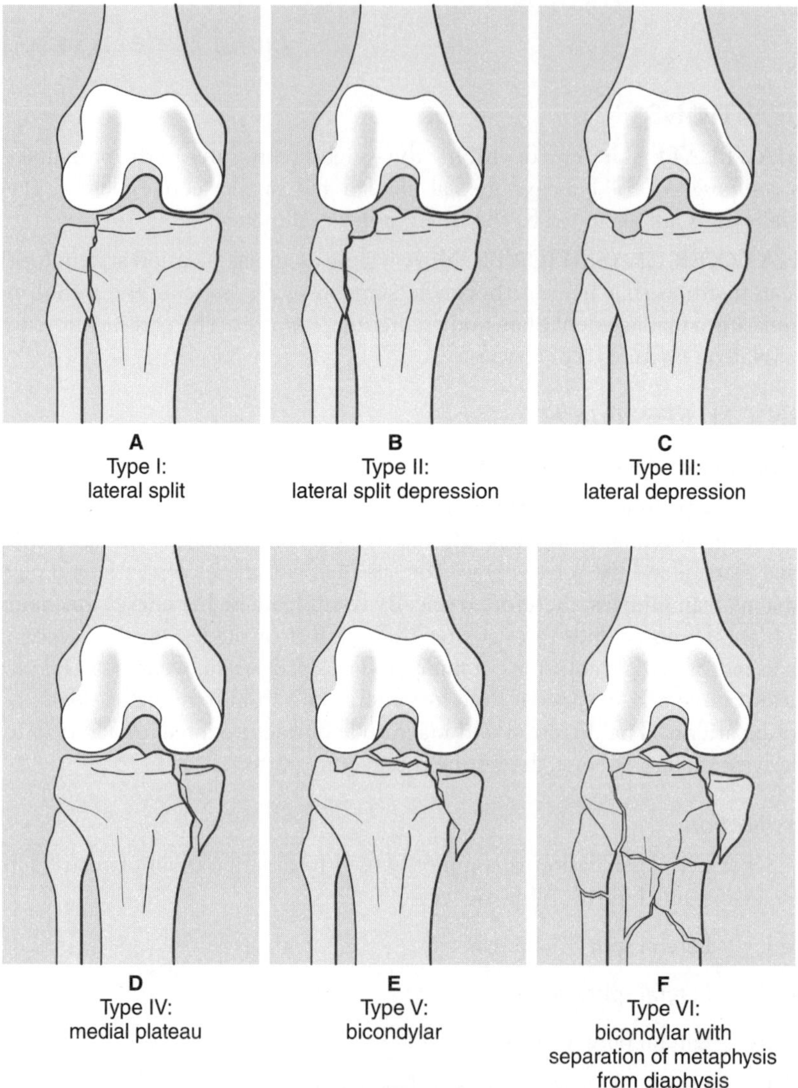

Figure 8–2. Schatzker classification of tibial plateau fractures. (**A**) Type I: lateral split, (**B**) type II: lateral split depression, (**C**) type III: lateral depression, (**D**) type IV: medial plateau, (**E**) type V: bicondylar, and (**F**) type VI: bicondylar with separation of metaphysis from diaphysis.

Radiographic Evaluation

In addition to the AP and lateral films mentioned previously, oblique views of the proximal tibia (40 degrees of internal and external rotation) should be obtained to better visualize the fracture. Computed tomography may be helpful in evaluating depressions and comminution for preoperative planning. Magnetic resonance imaging may be used to evaluate menisci and ligamentous damage.

TREATMENT

Low-energy, nondisplaced, or minimally displaced fractures may be treated nonoperatively. Patients typically receive a hinged knee brace for 8 to 12 weeks and may gradually progress to partial then full weightbearing. Nonambulating patients, patients with severely osteoporotic bone, or those not medically fit for surgery may receive similar management. **Indications for surgical fixation generally include Schatzker IV through VI fractures as well as I through III fractures exhibiting articular step-off greater than 3 mm, condylar widening greater than 5 mm, or instability with varus or valgus stress.** Typical procedures include open-reduction internal fixation, or, for cases in which a satisfactory closed reduction is achieved, percutaneous screw fixation. Depressions of the articular surface often require bone grafting to fill the voids. Depressions may be filled with autogenous bone graft, allogenic bone graft, or bone substitutes, **the strongest of which is calcium phosphate cement.**

Often, patients with tibial plateau injuries have sustained additional severe and life-threatening injuries that make them unfit for lengthy surgical procedures. These patients may benefit from temporary but fast external fixation that preserves the length and anatomical alignment of the tibia and allows for definitive fixation at a later date. Temporary external fixation is indicated similarly in patients whose severe soft-tissue swelling prohibits immediate surgical fixation.

Outcomes and Complications

Degenerative joint disease or posttraumatic arthritis of the knee is a common complication, often occurring 5 or more years after the initial injury. The incidence of arthritis is increased with significant cartilaginous or ligamentous injury and malalignment of the knee's mechanical axis or articular incongruity after repair. Additionally, Schatzker VI fractures, with their characteristic separation of metaphysis from diaphysis, may exhibit nonunion or malunion at this junction.

COMPREHENSION QUESTIONS

8.1 A 24-year-old construction worker falls 8 feet and presents to the emergency department with complaints of left wrist and knee pain. He reports landing on his left leg first, with his knee buckling inward. Given this patient's age and mechanism, which of the following best describes his risk for injury?

A. Increased chance of lateral plateau injury, increased chance of pure depression fracture, and increased chance of ligamentous and/or meniscal damage

B. Increased chance of medial plateau injury, increased chance of pure depression fracture, and increased chance of ligamentous damage

C. Increased chance of lateral plateau injury, increased chance of split fracture, and increased chance of ligamentous damage

D. Increased chance of medial plateau injury, increased chance of split fracture, and increased chance of ligamentous damage

E. Increased chance of lateral plateau injury, increased chance of split fracture, and decreased chance of ligamentous damage

8.2 A 55-year-old taxation lawyer with no significant past medical history is involved in a head-on motor vehicle collision at approximately 45 miles an hour and suffers the injury shown in Figure 8–3. He has palpable pulses distally and is neurovascularly intact. Aside from abrasions and a concussion, he has no other significant injuries. He exhibits only mild swelling at the knee. Which of the following is the best treatment for his injury?

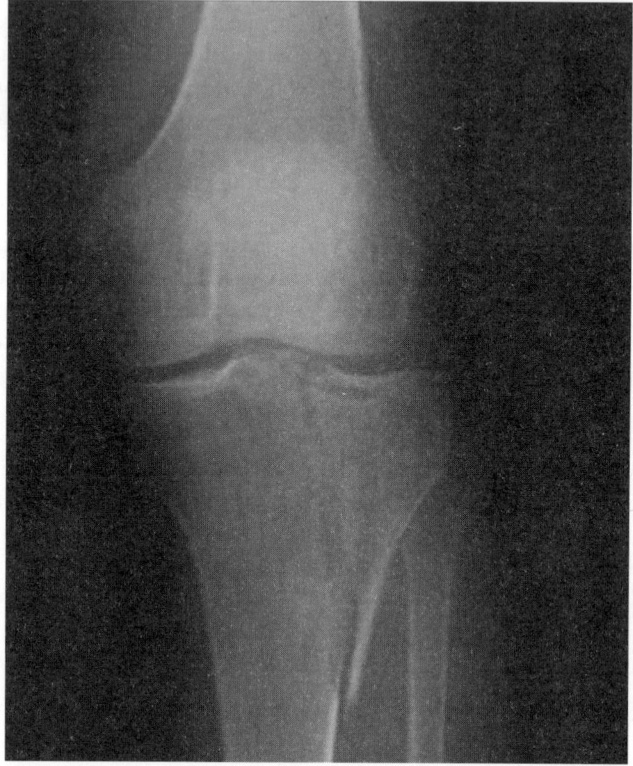

Figure 8–3. AP radiograph of the left knee.

A. Brace immobilization with early weightbearing
B. External fixation for 8 to 12 weeks, early weightbearing with fixator, active range-of-motion knee exercises
C. Closed reduction and casting, nonweightbearing for 8 to 12 weeks
D. Open reduction, internal fixation with screws and/or plates, nonweightbearing for 8 to 12 weeks
E. Functional bracing with gradual weightbearing and active range-of-motion knee exercises

8.3 A 44-year-old woman is involved in a high-speed motor accident and suffers a right-sided tibial plateau fracture. She is neurovascularly intact, and her compartments are soft. She has no other significant injuries, except for a minor concussion and several broken ribs. Which of the following, if present, is an indication for operative fixation?

A. Articular step-off 5 mm

B. Lateral meniscal tear on follow-up MRI

C. ACL tear on follow-up MRI

D. Condylar widening < 3 mm

E. Ipsilateral ankle fracture

ANSWERS

8.1 **C.** Given this young patient's relatively strong bone, he is most likely to sustain a split fracture with ligamentous injury, as compared with elderly people with softer bone, who typically sustain depression-type injuries without ligamentous damage. Furthermore, given the axial/valgus (knee inward) force as described in his fall, he is most likely to exhibit a lateral split type injury.

8.2 **D.** This is a bicondylar split fracture, or a Schatzker V. Schatzker IV, V, and VI fractures are typically treated with open-reduction internal fixation in the absence of significant swelling or other contraindications.

8.3 **A.** Indications for operative fixation for tibial plateau fractures include high-energy plateau injuries (Schatzker IV through VI) or any plateau fracture with articular step-off greater than 3 mm, condylar widening greater than 5 mm, or instability with varus or valgus stresses. Concomitant ACL, meniscal, or even ankle fractures are not necessarily indications for fixation if the reduction is adequate and the fracture is immobilized.

CLINCAL PEARLS

- High-energy tibial plateau injuries (Schatzker IV, V, VI) are frequently associated with significant comorbidities, including compartment syndrome and neurovascular injury in the affected extremity. Advanced trauma life support protocol in such situations must be followed.
- Upwards of 50% of plateau fractures are associated with meniscal tears; ACL injuries are found in approximately 30% of injuries.

REFERENCES

Buchholz RW, Court-Brown CM, Heckman JD, Tornetta P, eds. Tibial plateau fractures. In: *Rockwood and Green's Fractures in Adults*. 7th ed. 2 vol. Philadelphia, PA: Lippincott Williams & Wilkins; 2010:1790-1831.

Egol KE, Koval KJ, Zukerman JD, eds. Tibial plateau fractures. In: *Handbook of Fractures*. 4th ed. Philadelphia, PA: Lippincott Williams & Wilkins; 2010.

CASE 9

A 34-year-old man presents to the emergency department (ED) with a grossly deformed left leg after crashing his motorcycle into a fast-moving pickup truck on the freeway. He is writhing in pain. There are no other apparent injuries; he was helmeted and denies losing consciousness. There is a 15-cm soft tissue defect with protruding bone involving his anteromedial leg. Debris from the road is noted in the wound. On exam, he can flex and extend his great toe and appreciate sensation to light touch throughout his foot and has palpable dorsalis pedis and posterior tibial pulses. The patient has no past medical or surgical history, has no known drug allergies, and last ate approximately 10 hours ago. Vital signs are heart rate 125 beats/min, blood pressure 110/65 mmHg, respiratory rate 20 breaths/min, and temperature 98.1°F. Radiographs are shown (Figure 9–1).

- ▶ What is your most likely diagnosis?
- ▶ What are your next steps in management?
- ▶ What is the general operative approach to open fractures?

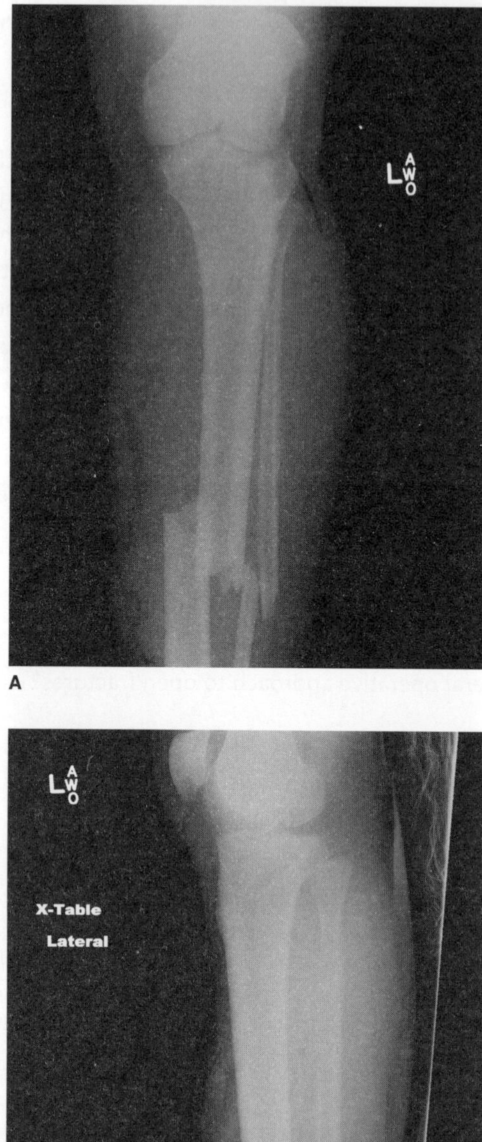

Figure 9–1. (A) AP and (B) lateral radiographs of the tibia and fibula.

ANSWERS TO CASE 9: Open Tibia Fracture

Summary: A 34-year-old man presents to the ED with a grossly deformed left leg status post a motorcycle accident in which he crashed into a pickup truck. There is an open and grossly contaminated tibia fracture, as road debris was initially found in the wound. His left lower extremity is neurovascularly intact. Although tachycardic, his other vital signs are within normal limits and he appears hemodynamically stable. No other injuries are noted.

- **Most likely diagnosis:** Open tibia and fibula fracture
- **Next steps in management:** Emergency room management including tetanus prophylaxis, administration of intravenous antibiotics, provisional irrigation, wound dressing, fracture splinting, and operative planning
- **General operative approach:** Wound debridement and fracture stabilization with an understanding of the potential need for secondary operations for skin, soft tissue, and bone reconstruction

ANALYSIS

Objectives

1. Understand the stages of care for open tibia fractures.
2. Know how to classify open fractures (Table 9–1).
3. Understand the role of emergency room management, antibiotics (Table 9–2), and operative intervention.
4. Be familiar with the potential risks and complications of open fractures.

Table 9–1 • GUSTILO AND ANDERSON OPEN FRACTURE CLASSIFICATION

Grade	Defect
I	Open fracture, clean wound <1 cm in length, simple fracture pattern
II	Open fracture, wound >1 cm in length without extensive soft tissue damage, minimal fracture comminution and contamination
III	Open fracture, extensive soft tissue damage, severe fracture comminution or segmental pattern. This type also includes farm injuries and fractures open for >8 hours before treatment
IIIa	Type III fracture with extensive soft tissue damage but adequate periosteal coverage of the bone
IIIb	Type III fracture with extensive soft tissue damage and periosteal stripping; requires soft tissue coverage procedure
IIIc	Type III fracture with an arterial injury requiring repair

Table 9–2 • OPEN FRACTURE ANTIBIOTIC SELECTION

Gustilo Grade	Antibiotic
I and II	1st generation cephalosporin (gram-positive organism coverage)
IIIa,b,c	1st generation cephalosporin *and* aminoglycoside (gram-negative coverage); add penicillin if concern for anaerobic contamination (ie, farm injury)

Considerations

This 34-year-old man presented with an open left tibia and fibula fracture after a motorcycle accident. The first priority should be for evaluation and treatment of life-threatening injuries by the ED and trauma physicians, as dictated by advanced trauma life support (ATLS) protocol. After identification and treatment of such injuries, orthopaedic assessment of the limb should ensue and includes evaluation of the soft tissue damage and neurovascular status. History, dimensions, and location of the open wounds must be documented. Obtaining a photograph may also be helpful during the initial exam.

In the ED, tetanus prophylaxis and intravenous antibiotics should be administered immediately (Table 9–2). Provisional lavage of the wound with an adequate quantity of sterile saline should be performed. Any contaminants such as dirt and grass should be removed from the wound before it is covered with a sterile dressing. Fracture reduction should occur with placement in a well-padded splint. The limb's neurovascular status should be documented before and after alignment. Pending stable labs and clearance by the trauma team, this patient should ideally be taken to the operating room within 6 to 8 hours from the time of injury for wound debridement and fracture stabilization.

APPROACH TO:
Open Tibia Fracture

DEFINITIONS

OPEN FRACTURES: Fractures that communicate with the outside environment. These complex injuries involve both the bone and surrounding soft tissues and mandate management strategies focused on prevention of infection, fracture union, and restoration of function.

GUSTILO AND ANDERSON OPEN FRACTURE CLASSIFICATION: Classification system incorporating the amount of energy, severity of soft tissue injury, and degree of contamination for determination of fracture severity.

ZONE OF INJURY: A concept describing the true dimensions of the wound, as opposed to simply the skin wound, which may only be a small opening through which the true wound communicates with the exterior. This is often seen in fractures that have significant muscle coverage, such as femoral and humeral shaft fractures.

VACUUM-ASSISTED WOUND CLOSURE (VAC): The gold standard for temporary management of open fracture wounds. It exposes the wound bed to a mechanically induced negative pressure in a closed system that facilitates granulation tissue formation while removing fluid from the extravascular space, reducing edema and improving microcirculation.

CLINICAL APPROACH

Initial Assessment

Open tibia fractures are high-energy injuries. As such, identification of other life-threatening injuries is vital. Once these injuries have been identified and adequately treated, attention must be directed toward the traumatized extremity. History and physical exam should focus on mechanism of injury, neurovascular status of the extremity, compartment syndrome, size of the soft tissue defect, periosteal stripping, fracture pattern, bone loss, and contamination. This knowledge will help to classify the fracture, determine treatment, and establish prognosis. Of note, **the degree of soft-tissue damage and contamination is important in classifying open fractures (Table 9–1).**

It is important to recognize that the diagnosis of open fractures can be missed, as seen when a small puncture wound is the only defect or when a wound is located posteriorly and the examining physician fails to inspect the limb circumferentially. Plain radiographs can also be used to aid in this diagnosis and may depict fracture comminution, displacement, bone loss, and/or subcutaneous air.

Emergency room management of an open tibia fracture requires a team-oriented approach between orthopaedic, ED, and trauma staff. Gross contaminants such as leaves and grass must be removed from the wound, and irrigation with sterile saline solution should be performed. **There is no consensus regarding optimal volume, delivery method, and irrigation solution.** After provisional lavage, a dry sterile dressing should be applied and not be removed until the operating room. The tibia should be reduced and placed in a splint. Tetanus prophylaxis, if necessary, must be administered and intravenous antibiotics given (Table 9–2).

Systemic antibiotics must be started as soon as possible, as a delay of >3 hours increases the risk of infection. Although duration of antibiotic therapy is controversial, most physicians who treat open fractures believe that it should be limited to 3 days. At wound closure, or after any major surgical procedure, an additional 3-day course of antibiotics should be given. Local therapy, in the form of antibiotic-impregnated polymethylmethacrylate beads, can be inserted into the fracture wound or inside the bone defect. This is often reserved for select grade II and III injuries.

Operative Intervention

Primary surgery ideally occurs within 6 to 8 hours from the time of injury. However, there are little data to support this timeline. In the operating room, a more thorough examination of the wound occurs, with a determination of the true zone of injury. Irrigation and debridement is performed, as the presence of nonviable tissue and foreign objects promotes bacterial growth. The ultimate goal is a clean wound with viable tissue and no infection. **In significantly contaminated wounds, additional debridement may be necessary after 24 to 48 hours.**

After wound care, the fracture reduction and fixation occurs. The decision to temporarily versus definitively stabilize the fracture depends on the general condition of the patient, extent of injury and fracture pattern. In the setting of an open tibia fracture, fixation options include temporary external fixation and intramedullary nailing. Regardless of whether temporary or definitive fixation is chosen, **the goals are to restore the tibia to its normal length and alignment, as this reduces dead space and hematoma volume.** The stabilization provided will also prevent additional damage from mobile bone fragments and promote healing. **With the exception of cases with heavy bacterial contamination, significant soft tissue damage, or vascular injury (grades IIIb and IIIc), intramedullary nailing is preferable.**

The current standard of care for open fracture wounds is for them to be initially left open, with delayed wound closure within 2 to 7 days. This is done to facilitate additional drainage and debridement and to prevent anaerobic conditions. Initial coverage of the wound includes sterile dressings and vacuum-assisted wound closure (VAC).

Secondary Surgery

Definitive fracture management may occur at a later date if only temporary fixation was performed with an external fixator. This is done when swelling has subsided and the condition of the soft tissues has improved. Soft tissue and skin coverage should occur within 7 days. Infection risk increases in wounds left open for longer periods of time.

Risks and Complications

The major risk associated with open fractures is infection, which can lead to amputation, loss of function, delayed union, malunion, or nonunion. Delayed union and nonunion are more common in open than closed fractures. The frequency of all of the preceding risk factors increases with the severity of the initial injury. Prolonged immobilization may also occur, not only because of the open fracture, but also because of other associated injuries that may have been incurred. The patient must understand these risks and that multiple surgeries may be necessary. Appropriate rehabilitation is crucial in regard to optimizing outcomes of open fractures.

COMPREHENSION QUESTIONS

9.1 A 42-year-old man is brought to the trauma center after a 6-foot fall off a ladder. Physical exam shows a slightly deformed left lower extremity with a 0.5-cm soft tissue defect over the anterolateral aspect of his leg. The wound appears relatively clean with no gross contaminants present. Radiographs depict a short oblique proximal one-third diaphyseal tibia fracture. What is his Gustilo open fracture classification grade?

A. I

B. II

C. IIIa

D. IIIb

E. V

9.2 What antibiotic should the patient in question 9.1 receive?

A. Vancomycin

B. Penicillin

C. Levaquin

D. Cefazolin

E. Cephalexin

9.3 A 70-year-old woman is brought to the trauma center with a significantly deformed right lower extremity with a 4-cm wound over the posteromedial portion of her leg. She is found to have a Gustilo and Anderson type 3A fracture. Which of the following interventions has been shown to decrease the risk of infection at the fracture site?

A. Irrigating with high-pressure pulsatile lavage

B. Immediate prophylactic antibiotic administration

C. Application of a wound VAC of the soft tissue defect in the ED

D. Operative debridement within 6 to 8 hours of injury

ANSWERS

9.1 **A.** This is a Gustilo and Anderson type I fracture. There is a simple fracture pattern in the setting of clean, <1-cm wound.

9.2 **D.** Type I fractures should receive an intravenous first-generation cephalosporin such as cefazolin (Table 9–2). Vancomycin, penicillin, and Levaquin are not cephalosporins. Cephalexin, although a cephalosporin, is an oral antibiotic and thus is not indicated for an open fracture.

9.3 **B.** The duration to beginning of antibiotic administration and adequate surgical debridement of the wound are the only factors definitively shown to reduce infection and improve outcome in open fractures. Although traditional recommendations include surgical irrigation and debridement within 6 to 8 hours of injury, there is no literature to support this time window. There is also no evidence to support pulsatile lavage over gravity flow. Finally, in this setting there is also no role for wound VAC application in the ED.

CLINICAL PEARLS

- Open tibia fractures are high-energy injuries, and as such, evaluation and treatment of life-threatening injuries per ATLS protocol is the first priority.
- Systemic antibiotics must be started as soon as possible; a delay of >3 hours increases the risk of infection.
- It is recommended that operative irrigation and debridement be performed within 6 to 8 hours from the time of injury, although there is little evidence to support this.
- Initial stabilization of open tibia fractures includes external fixation and intramedullary nailing.
- The predominant risk associated with open fractures is infection, which can lead to amputation, loss of function, delayed union, malunion, or nonunion.

REFERENCES

Melvin JS, Dombroski DG, Torbert JT, Kovach SJ, Esterhai JL, Mehta S. Open tibial shaft fractures: I. Evaluation and initial wound management. *J Am Acad Orthopaed Surg*. 2010;18:10-19.

O'Brien PJ, Mosheiff R. Open fractures: stages of care. AO *Principles of Fracture Management*. AO Foundation. Available at: https://www2.aofoundation.org. Accessed November 12, 2011.

Zalavras CG, Patzakis MJ. Open fractures: evaluation and management. *J Am Acad Orthopaed Surg*. 2003;11:212-219.

CASE 10

A 68-year-old right-hand dominant woman presented to the emergency room with a chief complaint of right shoulder pain and loss of motion. Earlier that morning, she sustained a mechanical fall onto her right side after slipping on a patch of ice. She denied any head strike or loss of consciousness and denied pain besides that in her right shoulder. Her past medical history is remarkable for osteoporosis and hyperlipidemia. She did sustain a left wrist fracture 5 years earlier, which was treated with a cast. She currently takes alendronate and simvastatin. She has no past surgical history. On examination, she appears in pain. Her vital signs are within normal limits. She has significant ecchymosis of her right upper arm. Her sensation is intact in her right arm within the radial, ulnar, median, and axillary nerve distributions. She has 5/5 strength in her biceps, triceps, wrist flexors, wrist extensors, and all finger flexors and extensors, as well as the interossei muscles. She is unable to forward flex or abduct her right shoulder. She has significant pain with any passive range of motion of the shoulder. The remainder of her exam is within normal limits. A single portable radiograph is obtained of the right shoulder and is shown in Figure 10–1.

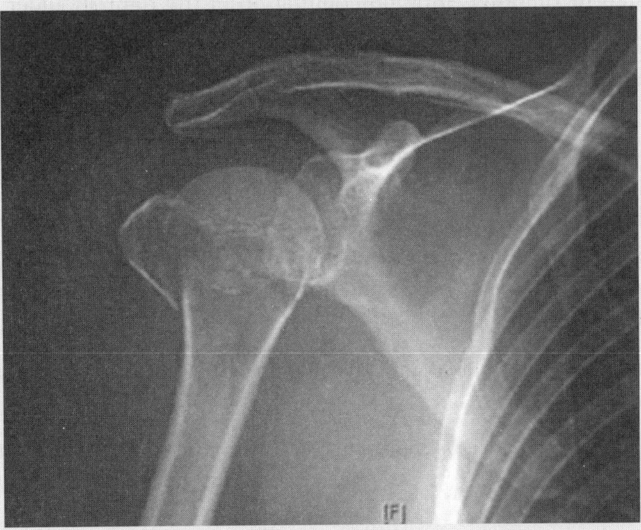

Figure 10–1. Single portable radiograph of the right shoulder.

- ▶ What is your most likely diagnosis?
- ▶ What is your next diagnostic step?
- ▶ What is the next step in therapy?

ANSWERS TO CASE 10: Proximal Humerus Fracture

Summary: A 68-year-old woman with a history of osteoporosis and previous fragility fracture presents with acute-onset right shoulder pain after a mechanical fall. Her exam is remarkable for an ecchymotic right arm and the inability to move her right shoulder due to pain. She is neurovascularly intact distally.

- **Most likely diagnosis:** The most likely diagnosis is a fracture of the proximal humerus. Other diagnostic considerations for acute shoulder pain following trauma includes fractures of the shoulder girdle (clavicle, scapula), glenohumeral dislocation (aka shoulder dislocation), acromioclavicular dislocation (aka shoulder separation), and acute rotator cuff tear.
- **Next diagnostic step:** The next step in diagnosis requires appropriate plain radiographic imaging of the right shoulder to confirm the exact fracture pattern and exclude other injuries including glenohumeral dislocation. This should include at a minimum an anteroposterior view, a scapular Y view and an axillary view. It is critical to obtain an acceptable axillary view in order to rule out dislocation of the glenohumeral joint. Based on the AP radiograph presented, this is a valgus impacted, three part proximal humerus fracture with displacement of the greater tuberosity and humeral head.
- **Next step in therapy:** Sling immobilization of the right shoulder is the next step with consideration of operative treatment depending on the amount of displacement.

ANALYSIS

Objectives

1. Understand the typical patient demographics and mechanism of injury associated with proximal humerus fractures and understand what constitutes an appropriate workup for this injury.
2. Understand the Neer classification and deforming forces for proximal humerus fractures.
3. Be familiar with the various treatment options for proximal humerus fractures.

Considerations

This 68-year-old female presented with right shoulder pain and loss of motion following a mechanical fall. The differential diagnosis must include fracture, shoulder dislocation, rotator cuff tear, and/or a combination of these injuries. A thorough physical exam and appropriate imaging studies will help distinguish these conditions. The exam is crucial, as both proximal humerus fractures and shoulder dislocations are associated with nerve injury.

Once exam and imaging confirm the diagnosis of a proximal humerus fracture, the orthopaedic surgeon must decide the appropriate treatment, which includes both nonoperative and operative modalities. The patient's general condition, functional status, comorbidities, and the specific type of proximal humerus fracture will factor into the clinical decision-making. In the ED, a sling is typically satisfactory for initial stabilization. However, in the setting of a concurrent glenohumeral dislocation, attempts to reduce the humeral head may also be required.

APPROACH TO: Proximal Humerus Fracture

DEFINITIONS

OSTEOPOROSIS: The most common metabolic bone disease, characterized by a loss in skeletal mass resulting in microarchitectural changes and increasing bone fragility.

PROXIMAL HUMERUS FRACTURE "PART": Based on the Neer classification of proximal humerus fractures. A proximal humerus is composed of 4 potential parts: the head or articular surface, the greater tuberosity, the lesser tuberosity, and the shaft. To be considered a "part," each fragment must be displaced at least 1 cm or 45 degrees. Deforming forces are applied to each part as a result of its respective muscular attachments. The greater tuberosity part is displaced by the supraspinatus and infraspinatus pulling it posteromedially, the lesser tuberosity part is displaced by the subscapularis tendon pulling it medially, and the shaft part is typically deformed in an apex anterior and abducted position by the insertions of the deltoid and pectoralis major.

NONUNION: Failure of the ends of a fractured bone to heal. Prevalence of nonunion with proximal humerus fractures is approximately 1% but is increased with certain fracture patterns, particularly surgical neck fractures with significant translation.

AVASCULAR NECROSIS: Death of osteocytes secondary to compromised blood supply. Avascular necrosis can occur after proximal humerus fractures if the blood supply to the humeral head has been sufficiently damaged. The head is predominantly supplied by the anterolateral ascending branch of the anterior humeral circumflex artery, but also receives some blood supply from the posterior humeral circumflex. This occurs most commonly after 4-part fractures. Avascular necrosis ultimately results in articular surface collapse and shoulder arthritis, which may require surgical interventions, including shoulder arthroplasty.

CLINICAL APPROACH

Etiologies

Proximal humerus fractures account for 4% to 5% of all fractures. They typically appear in a **bimodal distribution;** younger patients are typically male, and their fractures are a result of high-energy trauma (including motor vehicle accidents, falls from significant height, or gunshot injuries). Older patients who sustain this injury are much more likely to be postmenopausal women who have experienced a low-energy mechanism, such as a trip and fall from standing height, like the patient in this case.

Not surprisingly, there is a significant association with osteoporosis and proximal humerus fractures. The loss of trabecular microarchitecture and bone mass causes a significant increase in bone fragility of the humeral head, placing it at risk of fracture even with low-energy trauma. The association of osteoporosis and proximal humerus fractures is supported by the fact that the vast majority of proximal humerus fractures occur in females and individuals older than 50 years. In fact, some studies have shown that proximal humerus fractures more reliably correlate with bone fragility than do spine, hip, or wrist fractures, which are all widely regarded as classical sites of fragility fracture.

An uncommon etiology leading to proximal humerus fracture that must be excluded is malignancy. This may include benign and malignant primary bone tumors, as well as metastatic disease. Compared with nonpathologic fractures, these are extremely rare, but must be recognized if present, as this can drastically change patient management.

Clinical Presentation

Patients with a proximal humerus fracture will present with pain, swelling, and ecchymosis of the involved shoulder. They may or may not be able to move their shoulder depending on the amount of pain they have, which may be a function of how displaced their fracture is (eg, a nondisplaced fracture may be less painful than a 4-part fracture). Typically, patients will cradle the affected arm at their side.

As stated earlier, most patients presenting with a proximal humerus fracture will be older (>50 years old) and are more likely to be female. The most common mechanism is a mechanical fall. Younger patients will likely require a more violent mechanism of injury to sustain a fracture, unless an underlying metabolic bone disease is present. The history should focus on discerning the mechanism of injury and also identifying any risk factors for fracture (history of prior fracture, osteoporosis, corticosteroid use, immunocompromised status, history of malignancy or prior radiation).

Diagnosis

A thorough physical examination is the first step in diagnosis. Discerning a proximal humerus fracture from other bony and soft tissue injuries to the shoulder based on exam alone can be difficult, but some signs might point toward an alternative diagnosis. This includes deformity and crepitus of the clavicle, which would suggest a clavicle fracture, as well as deformity at the acromioclavicular joint, suggesting an acromioclavicular dislocation, or external rotation of the arm, suggesting anterior glenohumeral dislocation. Examining the entire shoulder girdle for wounds indicating an open fracture is mandatory. A good exam also assesses for the presence of a neurovascular injury. Injury to the axillary artery occurs in fewer than 5% of all cases, but is more likely with severe injuries (4-part fractures). An appropriate workup should include assessment of capillary refill and palpation of the radial pulse; Doppler ultrasound and angiography should be used on an as-needed basis when clinical suspicion is sufficiently high. Nerve injuries are also uncommon but possible, as the infraclavicular brachial plexus and peripheral nerve branches lie anteromedial to the humeral head. **Nerve injuries are more common with fracture dislocations and fractures involving the surgical neck.** An isolated axillary nerve injury is most commonly seen with a greater tuberosity fracture-dislocation as a result of its anatomic proximity. Sensory and motor testing of the axillary nerve (motor = deltoid, sensory = lateral aspect of upper arm), as well as the median (motor = FDP [flexor digitorum profundus] to index, sensory = palmar aspect thumb to half of ring finger), ulnar (motor = interossei, sensory = palmar aspect of small and half of ring finger), and radial (motor = wrist and digit extensors, sensory = dorsal aspect of first webspace) nerves should be routinely undertaken to rule out a neurologic injury.

Plain radiographs are essential to the diagnosis of a proximal humerus fracture. **An adequate plain radiographic examination should include an AP, scapular Y, and an axillary view at a minimum (Figure 10–2).** Poor or incomplete radiographs should not be tolerated. Advanced imaging may be necessary in certain cases. Computed tomography scans can be helpful in certain circumstances; they may be helpful to better understand the global fracture pattern, determine the amount of tuberosity displacement or tuberosity comminution, or determine the presence of an intraarticular "head splitting" component. Although rotator cuff tears are uncommon in combination with proximal humerus fractures, magnetic resonance imaging can be performed to evaluate the condition of the rotator cuff or any other soft tissues.

The most common classification system in use for proximal humerus fractures is the **Neer classification.** This system divides the proximal humerus into 4 potential parts. This includes the head (created by a fracture through either the anatomic or surgical neck), the greater tuberosity, the lesser tuberosity, and the shaft. **A fragment is considered a "part" if it is displaced greater than 1 cm (0.5 cm if it is the greater tuberosity) or by 45 degrees by its muscular attachments (greater tuberosity = supra and infraspinatus; lesser tuberosity = subscapularis; shaft = pectoralis major and deltoid).** Thus a fracture with minimal displacement (regardless of how many fracture lines are present) is considered a 1-part fracture. A 2-part fracture is most commonly an isolated displaced fracture at either the surgical neck or greater tuberosity; much less common 2-part fractures (although possible) include a displaced fracture through the anatomic neck or lesser tuberosity. The most common 3-part fracture involves displaced fractures through both the greater tuberosity and surgical neck. A 4-part fracture involves displacement of both tuberosities, the head and the shaft. Although this classification system is not perfect, it does serve as a means of describing the fracture and providing rough guidelines for treatment.

TREATMENT

After examining the patient, the very first step in treatment is immobilization. This consists of a simple sling or shoulder immobilizer. This enhances patient comfort and may serve as definitive treatment in some cases. If a concomitant glenohumeral

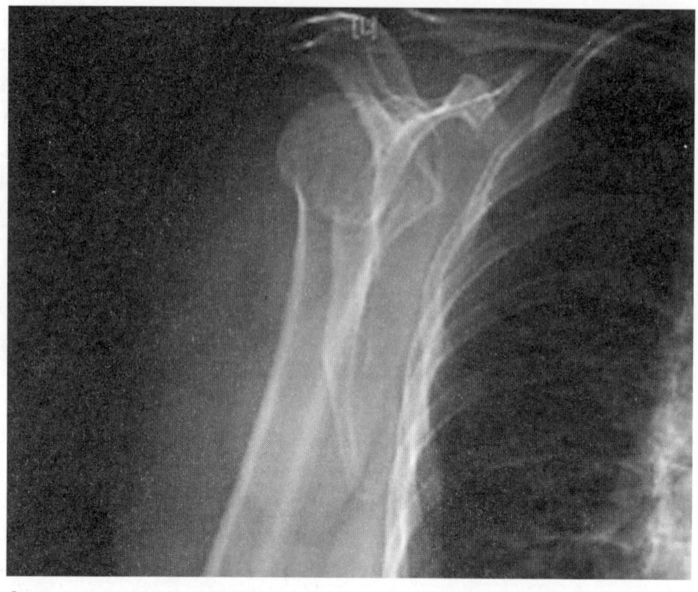

A

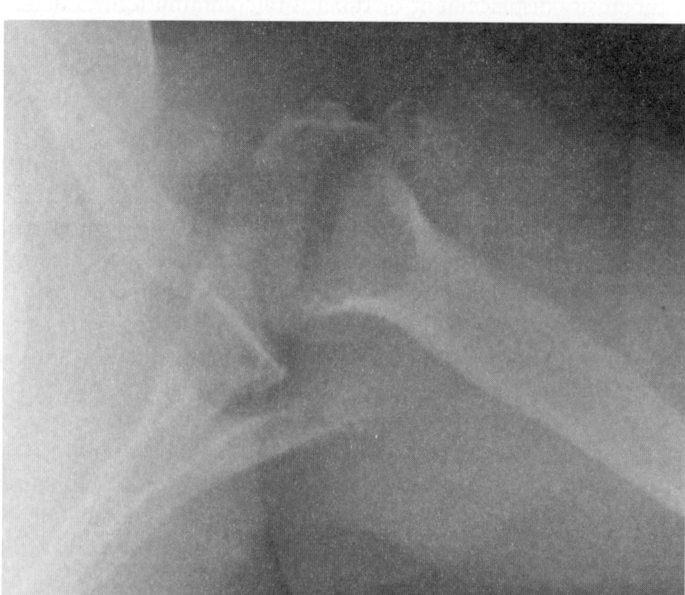

B

Figure 10–2. (**A**) Scapular Y and (**B**) axillary views of the same shoulder shown in Figure 10–1. This confirms the presence of a 3-part proximal humerus fracture.

dislocation is also present, then prompt closed reduction should be performed as soon as feasible with the assistance of local anesthesia and/or sedation.

Determining the definitive treatment for a proximal humerus fracture requires careful consideration on a case-by-case basis. Not only must the fracture characteristics be considered, but also the global assessment of the patient. A demented 90-year-old nursing home patient will perhaps require a different treatment plan compared with a healthy 30-year-old, even if their fracture patterns are similar. However, in general, the following treatment algorithm can be used to guide treatment for closed fractures.

One-part fractures → sling for 2 weeks followed by progressive range of motion with close follow-up. This is an appropriate treatment for approximately 80% of all proximal humerus fractures.

Two, 3, and valgus impacted 4-part fractures → open reduction internal fixation (particularly in younger patients). This allows for restoration of the native anatomy and early range of motion. Isolated avulsion fractures of the greater tuberosity with greater than 5-mm displacement should be treated surgically as well because of the risk of malunion leading to subacromial impingement of the displaced greater tuberosity. Of note, percutaneous pinning and intramedullary nailing are other operative interventions less commonly employed.

Fractures with significant risk of AVN (4-part fractures, head-split fractures, displaced anatomic neck fractures in the elderly) → prosthetic replacement with humeral head hemiarthroplasty. This avoids the risk of avascular necrosis and allows for early range of motion.

Open fractures and fractures with associated vascular injury should always be treated operatively with irrigation and debridement, repair of any vascular injury, and then fracture treatment as appropriate given the fracture pattern.

In general, clinical outcomes with open-reduction internal fixation are superior to hemiarthroplasty. Every effort should be made to treat displaced fractures with open reduction internal fixation unless there are a prohibitive amount of risk factors for a poor outcome with this modality (poor bone stock, high risk of AVN, poor nutritional status/healing potential, very low demand patient).

Complications

Stiffness: Loss of motion of the glenohumeral joint is a common occurrence after a proximal humerus fracture. This can occur subsequent to both operative and nonoperative treatment. Shoulder stiffness can be limited by instituting range-of-motion exercises as soon as the fracture pattern permits.

Nonunion: Most common with displaced surgical neck fractures treated nonoperatively. This can be treated with open-reduction internal fixation if no arthritis is present, with or without bone graft.

Malunion: Usually the result of inadequate closed or open treatment of displaced surgical neck or greater tuberosity fragments. When healed in a position of malalignment, bony impingement, poor motion, and weakness can result. This can be treated with an osteotomy, and internal fixation if no arthritis is present.

Avascular Necrosis: The humeral head receives its blood supply from the anterior and posterior humeral circumflex arteries. Direct injury to these vessels or fracture displacement that disrupts the intraosseous blood supply can result in avascular necrosis. This is most commonly seen after 4-part fractures. Clinical manifestations include insidious onset of shoulder pain months to years after the initial trauma. Radiographic examination typically reveals subarticular collapse of the head. This can be treated with prosthetic joint replacement (hemiarthroplasty or total shoulder replacement).

COMPREHENSION QUESTIONS

10.1 A proximal humerus fracture has the following morphology. There is 1.5-cm displacement at the surgical neck and fracture lines involving both the greater and lesser tuberosities, but without displacement. According to the Neer classification, what would this fracture be classified as?

A. One part
B. Two part
C. Three part
D. Four part
E. None of the above

10.2 Which combination of radiographs is sufficient to evaluate a proximal humerus fracture?

A. AP, internal rotation view, scapular Y
B. AP, internal rotation view, external rotation view
C. AP, scapular Y, axillary view
D. Internal rotation view, scapular Y, Stryker notch view
E. Axillary view, Velpeau view, scapular Y

10.3 An 80-year-old woman sustains a mechanical fall onto her right side. She is diagnosed with a minimally displaced right proximal humerus fracture (1 part). Which of the following is the most appropriate treatment?

A. Sling immobilization followed by early range of motion
B. Open-reduction internal fixation
C. Closed reduction and percutaneous pinning
D. Intramedullary nailing
E. Hemiarthroplasty

ANSWERS

10.1 **B.** Two-part fracture. Only the humeral head fragment is displaced (>1 cm), at the surgical neck. The tuberosity fragments are nondisplaced and thus not considered "parts." This means that the fracture has a shaft part and a head part, making it a 2-part fracture.

10.2 **C.** AP, scapular Y, and axillary view. Anything less than these views is insufficient, and the patient should be sent back for appropriate radiographs.

10.3 **A.** Sling immobilization followed by early range of motion. This is a 1-part fracture in an elderly patient. This does not require operative intervention.

CLINICAL PEARLS

- Most proximal humerus fractures occur in older individuals as a result of low-energy trauma.
- Radiographic evaluation of the shoulder must include an AP, scapular Y, and axillary view, at a minimum.
- The most commonly used classification for proximal humerus fractures is the Neer classification. This is based on the number parts that are displaced (>1 cm or 45 degrees angulated).
- The majority of proximal humerus fractures are minimally displaced and can be treated nonoperatively with sling immobilization followed by early range-of-motion exercises.
- Displaced 2- and 3-part as well as valgus impacted 4-part proximal humerus fractures are best treated operatively with internal fixation (particularly in younger patients).
- Unreconstructable fractures or fractures at risk of developing avascular necrosis (four part fractures, head splitting fractures) should be treated with hemiarthroplasty.

REFERENCES

Browner BD. *Skeletal Trauma: Basic Science, Management, and Reconstruction*. 4th ed. Philadelphia, PA: Saunders Elsevier; 2009.

Canale ST. *Campbell's Operative Orthopaedics*. 11th ed. Philadelphia, PA: Mosby/Elsevier; 2008.

Court-Brown CM, McQueen MM. Nonunions of the proximal humerus: their prevalence and functional outcome. *J Trauma*. 2008;64(6):1517-1521.

Gerber C, Schneeberger A, Vinh TS. The arterial vascularization of the humeral head: An anatomical study. *J Bone Joint Surg Am*. 1990;72:1486-1494.

Hettrich CM, Boraiah S, Dyke JP, Neviaser A, Helfet DL, Lorich DG. Quantitative assessment of the vascularity of the proximal part of the humerus. *J Bone Joint Surg Am*. 2010;92(4):943-948.

Neer CS 2nd. Displaced proximal humeral fractures. I. Classification and evaluation. *J Bone Joint Surg Am*. 1970;52(6):1077-1089.

Stableforth PG. Four-part fractures of the neck of the humerus. *J Bone Joint Surg Br*. 1984;66:104-108.

CASE 11

A 31-year-old competitive cyclist reports right shoulder pain after falling during a race. He presents to your office with his right arm guarded and held close to his body. He did not lose consciousness and denies other injuries. Findings on physical examination include a visible "bump" over his right clavicle without skin breakdown. He has intact sensation to light touch in his axillary, radial, ulna, and median nerve distributions. His motor examination of the extremity is normal below the shoulder, but passive and active motion at the shoulder itself is limited, secondary to pain. He has a palpable radial pulse. An anteroposterior (AP) radiograph of the injury site is obtained (Figure 11–1).

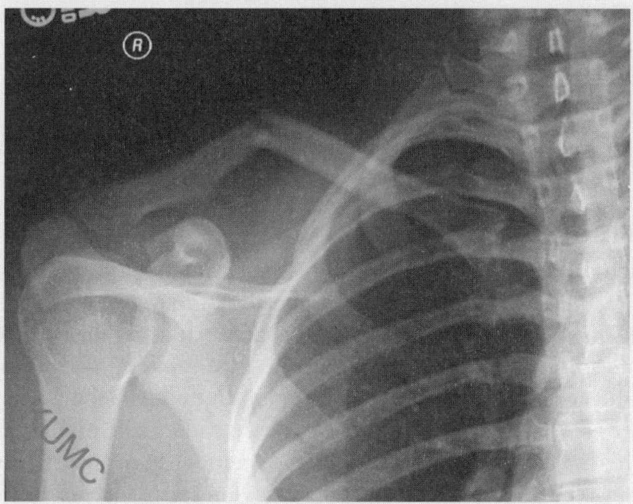

Figure 11–1. An AP chest radiograph, cropped to show the right clavicle. (Reproduced, with permission, from Simon RR, Sherman SC, Koenigsknecht SJ. *Emergency Orthopedics the Extremities*. New York, NY: McGraw-Hill; 2007:297;Fig. 11-54.)

- What is the most likely diagnosis?
- What additional concerns do you have regarding this injury?

ANSWERS TO CASE 11: Clavicle Fracture

Summary: A 31-year-old cyclist fell from his bicycle directly onto his right shoulder. An AP shoulder radiograph reveals a midshaft clavicle fracture that is angulated superiorly.

- **Most likely diagnosis:** This is a right midshaft clavicle fracture, specifically, an Allman group I injury.
- **Concerns for additional injuries:** Given the proximity of the brachial plexus and subclavian vessels to the clavicle, a careful neurovascular exam must be performed to rule out injury to these vulnerable structures.

ANALYSIS

Objectives

1. Understand the anatomy of the clavicle with regard to its ligamentous, muscular, and neurovascular relationships with the thorax and upper extremity.
2. Understand the indications and options for the treatment of clavicle fractures.
3. Understand the differences in outcomes for operative versus nonoperative management of clavicle fractures.

Considerations

Clavicle fractures are common, comprising approximately 5% to 10% of all fractures. They may be in isolation, as experienced by the cyclist in this case, but are also found in high-energy, poly-traumatic events such as motor vehicle accidents. Such patients are more likely to have thoracic cage injuries, scapula fractures, and pneumo- or hemothoraces. Low-energy mechanism injuries such as simple falls are unlikely to be associated with other fractures or intrathoracic injury.

Although the patient in the vignette sustained an isolated injury, careful attention must be focused to the neurovascular status of the extremity. The subclavian vein runs directly between the subclavius muscle and the first rib. Posterior to the subclavian vein lie the subclavian artery and brachial plexus. **The plexus is closest to the clavicle in its midportion and is at greatest risk for injury at this location.**

APPROACH TO: Clavicle Fracture

DEFINITIONS

SERENDIPITY VIEW: A radiographic image of the sternoclavicular joint obtained like an AP chest film with 40 degrees of cephalic tilt. Typically used to assess the sternoclavicular joint.

ZANCA VIEW: An AP radiographic image of the shoulder performed by centering the x-ray beam over the acromioclavicular joint with 15 degrees of cephalic tilt. Good for assessing the distal clavicle and the acromioclavicular joint.

SUPERIOR SHOULDER SUSPENSORY COMPLEX: A conceptual bone and soft-tissue complex comprising the glenoid, coracoid process, coracoclavicular ligaments, distal portion of the clavicle, acromioclavicular joint, and acromion process. Together, these structures form a supportive, stable ring from which the arm is suspended.

FLOATING SHOULDER: This may occur when two or more components of the shoulder suspensory complex (most commonly a concomitant clavicle and ipsilateral scapula neck fractures) are injured. Represents a theoretical increase in instability and displacement of the glenoid that, at least historically, was considered an indication for operative fixation.

CLINICAL APPROACH

Anatomy and Mechanism of Injury

The clavicle is an "S"-shaped bone with its medial portion apex anterior and its lateral portion apex posterior. It is wider in the axial dimension laterally where it forms the acromioclavicular joint. The clavicle acts as a **strut** connecting the upper extremity to the axial skeleton. It functions as part of the **suspensory complex** of the upper extremity and has multiple muscular and ligamentous attachments. The major muscular attachments include the **sternocleidomastoid,** which originates at the superomedial aspect of the clavicle; the **pectoralis major,** which originates anteriorly and inferomedially; the **trapezius,** inserting posteriorly and superolaterally; and the **deltoid,** originating anteriorly and inferolaterally. The medial articulation of the clavicle, the **sternoclavicular joint,** is supported by sternoclavicular (SC) ligaments. Its lateral articulation, the **acromioclavicular joint,** is supported by acromioclavicular (AC) ligaments. Additional attachments include the **coracoclavicular ligaments,** composed of both the **conoid and trapezoid ligaments** and considered the **suspensory ligaments** of the upper extremity, providing vertical support to the AC joint.

Clavicle fractures are deformed by the following forces:

- The sternocleidomastoid displaces the proximal fragment superiorly and posteriorly.
- The pectoralis major and latissimus dorsi displace medially, pulling the shoulder toward the midline and resulting in clavicle shortening.
- The weight of the arm displaces the distal fragment inferiorly.
- Such forces result in the typical presentation: the distal fragment being inferiorly displaced and medially shortened. A superficial bony "bump" may be appreciated on physical exam as a direct result of this mechanism.

Radiographic Evaluation

Standard AP radiographs are generally sufficient to evaluate and treat clavicle fractures. Additional **Serendipity** and **Zanca** views may help further evaluate proximal and lateral clavicle fractures, respectively. A computed tomography (CT) scan may be beneficial in assessing clavicle fractures when the fracture pattern is unclear or if the fracture is intraarticular. CT may also be performed later in follow-up to assess bony healing.

Classification

Clavicle fractures are commonly classified using the Allman classification as later modified by Neer. Allman originally divided the clavicle into 3 anatomical groups, based primarily on frequency of injury: middle, distal, and proximal. Neer subsequently sub-characterized group II fractures based on integrity of the coracoclavicular ligaments.

- Group I: Middle third of clavicle (approximately 80% of fractures)
  - May be nondisplaced or displaced (>100% displacement; ie, no cortical contact between ends)
- Group II: Distal third of clavicle (approximately 15% of fractures)
  - Type I: Distal clavicle fracture with the coracoclavicular ligaments intact
  - Type II: Coracoclavicular ligaments detached from the medial fragment with the trapezoid ligament attached to the distal fragment
  - Type IIA: Both conoid and trapezoid attached to the distal fragment
  - Type IIB: Conoid detached from the medial fragment
- Group III: Proximal third of clavicle (approximately 5% of fractures)

TREATMENT

Most clavicle fractures are successfully treated with simple immobilization in a sling or a figure-of-eight bandage for 4 to 6 weeks. During immobilization, active range of motion of the elbow, hand, and wrist is allowed to preserve joint motion. Passive range of motion and active assisted range of motion of the shoulder are typically initiated at approximately 2 to 3 weeks. **There are no significant differences in outcomes after sling immobilization versus figure-of-eight bandages.**

Surgical management of clavicle fractures is controversial. Absolute indications for operative intervention include open fractures, skin tenting with the potential to progress to open fracture, and associated neurovascular injuries. Relative indications for surgical fixation include displacement or shortening greater than 2 cm, significant fracture comminution, the presence of a **floating shoulder,** or bilateral clavicle fractures. Common fixation methods include plate and screw fixation and intramedullary pinning.

Postoperatively, the patients are allowed to perform **pendulum exercises** or gentle active ranging of the suspended arm with a limited motion arc for 2 weeks. At 6 to 8 weeks, muscular strengthening exercises may begin if follow-up radiographs show signs of healing. A full return to sports is generally not recommended until 12 weeks postoperatively.

When deciding between operative versus nonoperative management, there is an increasing amount of evidence supporting operative intervention for displaced midshaft clavicle fractures, especially in young, active patients. Potential benefits to operative management include decreased time to bone union, decreased rates of non- or malunion, and a faster return to work. To some patients, cosmetic factors may influence decision making. Patients, for instance, may prefer a permanent visible "bump" between partially displaced but united fractures versus prominent scars and palpable hardware from surgical intervention.

Complications

Adverse outcomes associated with management of clavicle fractures include nonunion, malunion, posttraumatic arthritis at the AC joint, infection with surgical intervention, and refracture. **A common complication of surgical management is chronic irritation from prominent hardware: Plate and screw constructs placed on the superior aspect of the clavicle are notorious for needing removal in up to 30% of patients.**

COMPREHENSION QUESTIONS

11.1 A 30-year-old professional football player gets tackled on his right shoulder and sustains a distal clavicle fracture. The patient has no neurologic or vascular abnormalities on physical exam and has no other injuries on physical exam. Initial radiographic evaluation should include:

A. CT scan
B. Bone scan
C. Chest x-ray
D. AP clavicle including Zanca views
E. Shoulder x-rays

11.2 A 17-year-old high school tennis player trips while returning a serve and sustains a right midshaft clavicle fracture. Which of the following increases the risk of nonunion in the nonoperative treatment of clavicle fractures?

A. Sling treatment
B. Figure-of-eight bandage treatment
C. Displacement and comminution
D. Male sex
E. Age < 20 years

11.3 A 53-year-old intoxicated man crashes his motorcycle into a pole. In the emergency department, he is hemodynamically stable and complains of right shoulder pain. Radiographs of the affected site are seen in Figure 11–2. Which classification best describes his injury?

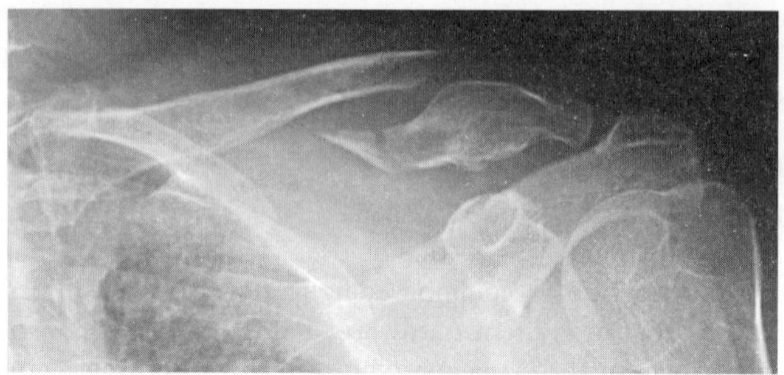

Figure 11–2. An AP radiograph of the left clavicle. (Reproduced, with permission, from Simon RR, Sherman SC, Koenigsknecht SJ. *Emergency Orthopedics the Extremities.* New York, NY: McGraw-Hill; 2007:286;Fig. 11-35.)

A. Allman group I, type IIA
B. Allman group II, type I
C. Allman group III, type IIB
D. Allman group I, type II B

ANSWERS

11.1 **D.** The best initial imaging choice to evaluate clavicle fractures is an AP view of the clavicle with Zanca views to further evaluate distal clavicle fracture pattern.

11.2 **C.** Displacement and comminution have been shown to increase risk of nonunion in nonoperative management. There are no significant differences between outcomes when using sling immobilization versus a figure-of-eight bandage.

11.3 **B.** This is a right distal clavicle fracture (group II) with coracoclavicular ligaments intact (type I): an Allman group II, (Neer) type I. Allman group I and III fractures describe the middle and proximal clavicle, respectively, and do not apply to this distal clavicle injury. Because the injury is medial to both coracoclavicular ligaments, they are intact, and thus it is a type I and not type II group II injury.

CLINICAL PEARLS

- The clavicle is distinct in being the first bone in the body to ossify (fifth week in utero) and the last to fuse its ossification center (22-25 years).
- Clavicle fractures occur in both low- and high-energy settings.
- The vast majority of clavicle fractures may be managed nonoperatively in a sling or figure-of-eight bandage.

REFERENCES

Andersen K, Jensen PO, Lauritzen J. The treatment of clavicular fractures: figure-of-eight bandage versus a simple sling. *Acta Orthop Scand*. 1987;58:71-74.

Buchholz RW, Court-Brown CM, Heckman JD, Tornetta P, eds. Clavicle fractures. In: *Rockwood and Green's Fractures in Adults*. 7th ed. 2 vol. Philadelphia, PA: Lippincott Williams & Wilkins; 2010:1106-1130.

Canadian Orthopaedic Trauma Society. Nonoperative treatment compared with plate fixation of displaced midshaft clavicular fractures: a multicenter, randomized clinical trial. *J Bone Joint Surg*. 2007;89:1-10.

Khan LA, Bradnock TJ, Scott C, Robinson CM. Fractures of the clavicle. *J Bone Joint Surg*. 2009;91: 447-460.

CASE 12

A 26-year-old man presents to the emergency department complaining of right ankle pain, swelling, and an inability to walk after twisting his ankle in a soccer tournament. He remembers making a quick cut before experiencing sharp pain and hearing a "crack" while falling to the ground. Physical exam reveals a swollen and ecchymotic right ankle with tenderness directly over the medial and lateral malleoli and over distal fibular at the level of the ankle joint. His skin is swollen, but intact. He is neurovascularly intact and has a strong dorsalis pedis pulse. Examination of the proximal leg is unremarkable. He has no past medical history. Figure 12–1 shows (A) anteroposterior (AP), (B) lateral, and (C) mortise radiographs of the right ankle.

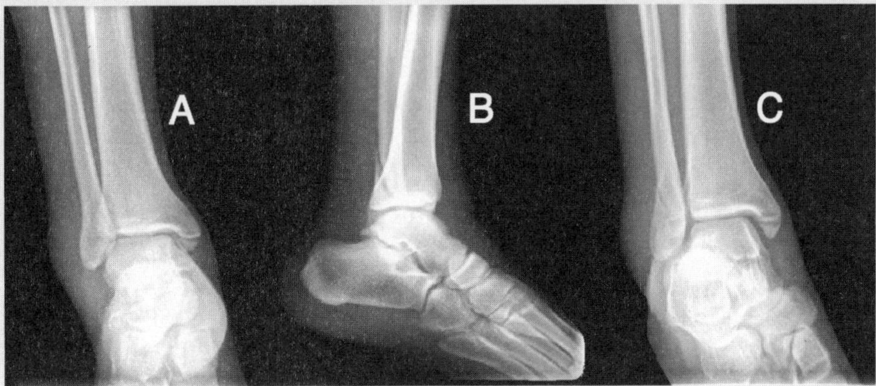

Figure 12–1. (**A**) AP, (**B**) lateral, and (**C**) mortise radiographs of the right ankle. (Courtesy of Timothy T. Roberts, MD)

- What is the most likely diagnosis?
- What is your next step in the management of this injury?

ANSWERS TO CASE 12: Ankle Fracture

Summary: A 26-year-old man suffered an acute twisting injury to his right ankle, resulting in pain, swelling, and an inability to bear weight.

- **Most likely diagnosis:** Fractures of both the lateral and medial malleoli, together known as a **bimalleolar ankle fracture.**
- **Next step in management of injury:** Administration of analgesia, systemic and/or intraarticular, and attempted closed reduction. Depending on the degree of swelling, the patient may be cast or splinted.

ANALYSIS

Objectives

1. Know the clinical presentation, physical examination findings, and appropriate initial management of ankle fractures.
2. Know which radiographic studies to order'and how to evaluate them.
3. Be familiar with the classification systems used to describe ankle fractures and recognize how different mechanisms of injury produce predictable fracture patterns.
4. Have a basic understanding of stable versus unstable ankle fractures.

Considerations

This patient presented with a twisting injury that resulted in ankle pain, swelling, and an inability to bear weight. Ankle fractures tend to occur in predictable patterns, depending on the magnitude and direction of force and the position of the foot during injury. Common ankle fracture classification schemes are derived from mechanisms of injury, and thus obtaining a careful history is helpful to understanding and treating the injury. Physical examination should include a visual inspection of the skin to rule out an open injury, to evaluate swelling or blistering, and to evaluate for signs of displacement or dislocation. A full neurovascular evaluation of the foot and ankle is mandatory.

In addition to ankle pain and swelling, this patient has tenderness over both medial and lateral malleoli and cannot bear weight—3 signs that are suggestive of fracture rather than ligamentous sprain. X-rays should therefore be ordered. The most common initial radiographic study is a 3-view ankle series. Given this patient's closed, minimally displaced bimalleolar fracture, casting or splinting (splinting is used in the setting of significant swelling or blistering) is the most appropriate next step.

APPROACH TO: Ankle Fracture

DEFINITIONS

LATERAL MALLEOLUS: The distal portion of the fibula that articulates with the talus and provides lateral stability to the ankle joint.

MEDIAL MALLEOLUS: The distal medial projection of the tibia that articulates with the talus and provides medial stability to the ankle joint.

TIBIAL PLAFOND: The distal weightbearing articulating surface of the tibia that, together with both malleoli, comprise the mortise.

MORTISE: The bony arch formed by the articulation between malleoli and the plafond, which serves to constrain the wedge-shaped talus and allows the hinge-like motion of the ankle.

SYNDESMOSIS: This describes the ligamentous complex connecting the distal fibula and tibia. It helps stabilize the ankle mortise.

CLINICAL APPROACH

Anatomy

The ankle is a complex hinge joint consisting of articulations between the distal tibia, the distal fibula, and the talus that are held in place by a complex ligamentous system. The lateral malleolus forms the lateral portion of the ankle joint and is surrounded by the strong tibiofibular ligament complex and the syndesmotic ligament complex. These ligament structures prevent the distal tibia from separating from the fibula and provide the majority of ankle stability in external rotation. Distally on the lateral side of the ankle, the talofibular and calcaneofibular ligaments provide resistance to inversion and anterior translation of the talus. **The anterior talofibular ligament is the most commonly injured ligament in ankle sprains.** On the medial side, the medial malleolus is the origin of the deltoid ligament, which provides medial ligamentous support to the ankle and is the primary medial stabilizer against lateral displacement of the talus.

Examination

Clinical evaluation of a suspected ankle fracture is necessary to ensure accurate diagnosis. First, this should include a description of the mechanism of injury. This provides insight into the position of the ankle and the forces acting on it at the time of injury. Obtaining a thorough medical history is essential, as comorbidities such as additional injuries, obesity, hypercoagulable states, diabetes, and peripheral vascular disease may affect treatment options. Evaluate the extremity closely for skin punctures or lacerations that may communicate with the ankle joint or with fracture fragments. Both open joints and open fractures are considered surgical emergencies and should be treated accordingly. An obvious deformity may represent a dislocation; reduction should be performed as soon as safely possible. As always, a complete circulatory and neurologic evaluation should be performed and clearly documented.

Radiographic Evaluation

After examining a patient, one must decide whether radiographs are needed for further evaluation. The **Ottawa Ankle Criteria** can aide in this process. The criteria state that x-rays should be ordered if there is malleolar tenderness *and:*

- Bone tenderness along the distal 6 cm of the posterior edge of the tibia or tip of the medial malleolus, *or*
- Bone tenderness along the distal 6 cm of the posterior edge of the fibula or tip of the lateral malleolus, *or*
- An inability to bear weight both immediately and in the emergency department for more than 4 steps

This algorithm demonstrates a sensitivity of nearly 100% for detecting ankle fractures and may reduce unnecessary x-ray exposure by up to 40%.

When appropriate, radiographic evaluation of the ankle should consist of a 3-view ankle series. This includes an AP view, a mortise view (oblique), and a lateral view. **The mortise view is important for evaluation of the joint space. It is obtained by internally rotating the affected extremity 15 degrees on an AP view so that the x-ray beam becomes perpendicular to the transmalleolar axis.** In a normal ankle, the mortise should show a smooth, evenly spaced gap between the plafond and malleoli and the talus (Figure 12–2A). This view is useful to determine the stability of the ankle based on several measurements. The first is the **medial clear space** (Figure 12–2C). This represents the joint space between the medial malleolus and the talus. In normal individuals, this distance should be 4 mm or less and should be equal to the space between the tibial plafond and the talus. Greater than 4 mm implies a lateral shift of the talus and possible ankle instability. Next is the **talocrural angle,** which is determined by drawing a line through the distal articular surface of the tibia and a line through the distal-most aspect of the medial and lateral malleoli (Figure 12–2B). This angle should be 83 degrees ± 4 degrees and is used to judge fibular length. The **tibiofibular clear space** may also be measured and should be less than 6 mm (Figure 12–2D). It represents the distance between the medial wall of the fibula and the incisural (posterolateral) surface of the tibia; a space greater than 6 mm suggests syndesmotic injury. If syndesmotic injury or malleolar injury is suspected, but not radiographically obvious, the examiner may obtain **stress radiographs** of the ankle after appropriate analgesia is administered. Most commonly, in the setting of a lateral malleolar fracture with concern for medial injury, the examiner stresses the ankle by dorsiflexing and externally rotating the foot, and a mortise image is obtained.

Classification

Various classification systems exist for ankle fractures. The two most commonly employed are the Weber and the Lauge-Hansen classification systems.

The Weber classification separates ankle fractures based on the location of the fibular fracture. The degree of instability is determined based on the location of the fracture. Weber A fractures describe a fracture that is distal to the syndesmosis. These are typically avulsion injuries and are usually stable. Weber B fractures occur at the level of the syndesmosis and often extend proximally, laterally, and posteriorly.

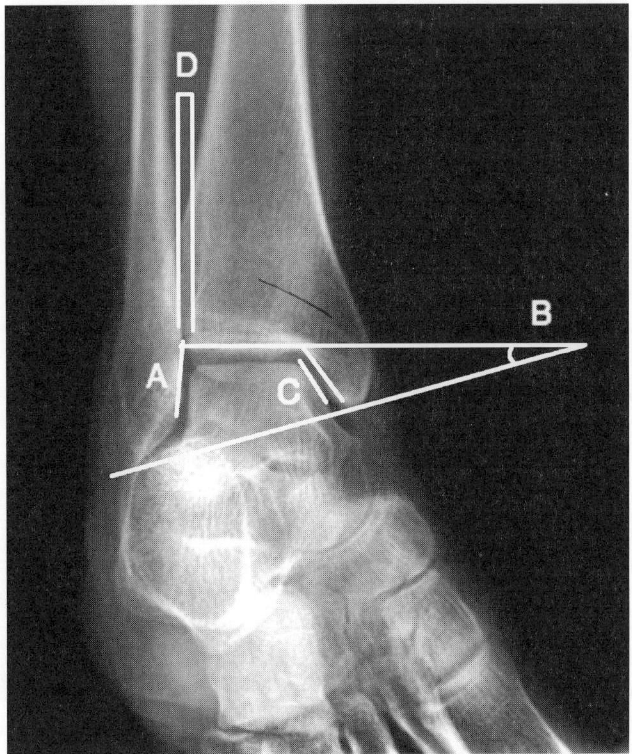

Figure 12–2. Mortise view of normal ankle showing the **(A)** mortise, **(B)** talocrural angle, **(C)** medial clear space, and **(D)** tibiofibular clear space. (Courtesy of Timothy T. Roberts, MD)

These typically result from external rotation. Fifty percent of Weber B fractures are associated with tearing of the anterior tibiofibular ligament and are unstable in such instances. Weber C fractures occur above the level of the syndesmosis and often occur with the foot in pronation at the time of injury; they are almost always associated with a medial ankle injury, whether ligamentous or bony.

The Lauge-Hansen classification describes the mechanism of injury and can be roughly correlated with the Weber system. As mentioned, this system uses 2 variables to classify the fracture pattern: the position of the foot at the time of injury (pronation versus supination) and the direction of the deforming force (external rotation versus abduction or adduction). Four patterns are described: supination-adduction (SAd), supination-external rotation (SER), pronation-external rotation (PER), and pronation-abduction (PAb). Each pattern has a relatively consistent sequence of injury, as depicted in Figure 12–3. Although seemingly complex, the fracture patterns follow simple rules: In supination injuries, the supinated foot has a relaxed deltoid ligament but taut lateral ligaments, thus regardless of external rotation or adduction forces, the initial injury begins laterally and progresses medially, depending on the degree of force, quality of the bone, and so forth. Conversely, the pronated foot has a tense deltoid ligament, and initial injury begins medially with either a medial malleolus fracture or a rupture of the deltoid ligament. Injuries

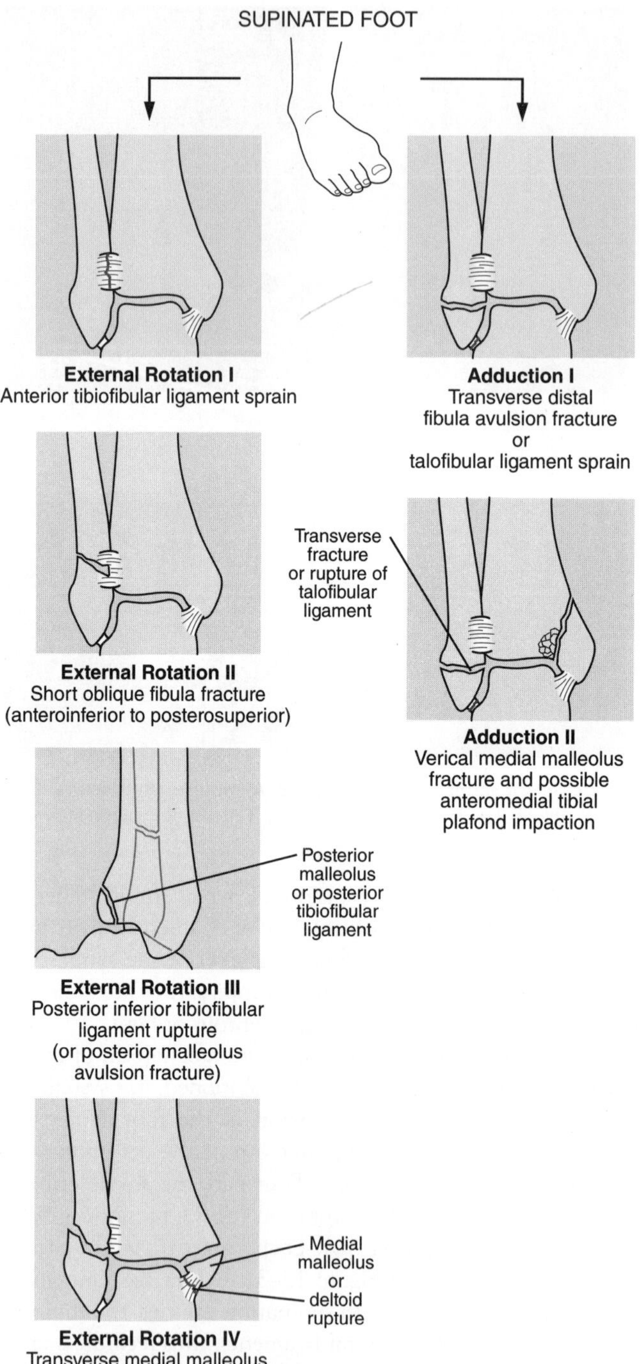

Figure 12–3. Lauge-Hansen classification of ankle fractures: 4 common sequences of injury occur based on the position of the foot at the time of injury (supination versus pronation) and the direction of the force applied (adduction with supination, abduction with pronation).

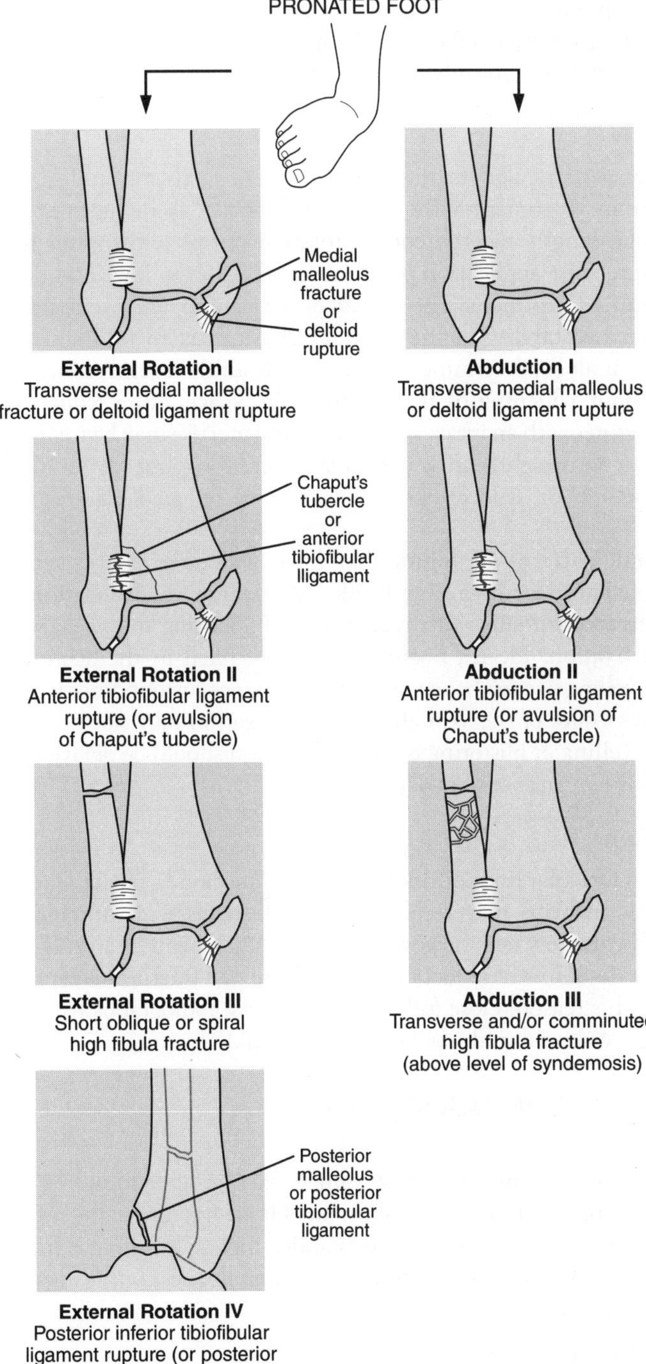

Figure 12–3. (*Continued*)

then progress proximally and laterally to the fibula, where they become analogous to Weber C injuries. Remember that the most common pattern of injury is the SER type, which correlates typically with a Weber B pattern.

TREATMENT

As with any periarticular fracture, the treatment goals for ankle fractures are to restore anatomic alignment of the joint. Additional goals include restoring or maintaining fibular length and the correct rotation of the joint. After reduction of a closed fracture, cast application or splint stabilization followed by delayed casting may be definitive treatment. The success of these nonoperative treatments depends primarily on the **stability** of the fracture. Physical exam findings, together with radiographic analysis, determine stability. **Stable ankle fractures include those presenting without widening of the mortise joint space.** After reduction, minimally displaced fractures with an intact syndesmosis and mortise may be treated with immobilization and nonweightbearing in a short leg cast or splint for 4 to 6 weeks.

Open fractures or dislocations that cannot be reduced require urgent surgical treatment.

In general, patterns of injury that have widening of the syndesmosis, an increased medial clear space, or frank subluxation or dislocation of the talus should be treated initially with reduction and splinting followed, when possible, by surgical fixation. Ideally, fractures should be fixed in the acute setting before significant swelling occurs; however, if the soft tissues surrounding the ankle become too swollen, closure of the skin after internal fixation may not be possible. When significant swelling or blistering is present, fixation should be delayed until swelling subsides. This may take several days to weeks.

Complications

As with most articular injuries, a loss of range of motion is expected to some degree. Posttraumatic arthritis may result if the ankle heals with articular incongruity. Arthritis is fortunately rare, however, when the ankle heals in an anatomic position. Finally, the rate of loss of reduction in closed-treated fractures is reportedly as high as 25%. For this reason, close follow-up with serial radiographs to assess reduction and healing is essential in the subacute care of ankle fractures.

COMPREHENSION QUESTIONS

12.1 A 35-year-old man suffers a left ankle fracture after losing his balance on a fast-moving treadmill. X-rays show an oblique fracture of the medial malleolus with widening of the syndesmosis and a high spiral fibular fracture. Which category of Weber ankle fractures is most analogous to this fracture pattern?

A. Weber A

B. Weber B

C. Weber C

D. None of the above

12.2 A 50-year-old male presents to the emergency department with right ankle pain, an inability to bear weight, and swelling over the lateral malleolus. The patient states that he twisted his ankle tripping down a flight of stairs and is complaining of "throbbing" lateral ankle pain. X-rays show a minimally displaced lateral malleolus fracture (Weber B) with a medial clear space of 3.5 mm. During your initial physical exam, palpitation of the medial malleolus also elicits tenderness. About which additional injury should you be concerned?

A. Fracture of the talar neck

B. Tear of the deltoid ligament

C. Fracture of the calcaneus

D. Tear of the anterior talofibular ligament

12.3 A 26-year-old athlete twists her right ankle while diving for a soccer ball during her tenure as goalie for a local travel league. She suffers a bimalleolar, minimally displaced closed ankle fracture. Her skin is soft and minimally swollen, and she is neurovascularly intact. Which of the following fracture characteristics is most predictive of a need for surgical fixation?

A. Degree of initial fibular fracture displacement

B. Presence of an avulsion fracture of the medial malleolus

C. Level of the fibula fracture

D. Position of the talus in the ankle mortise

12.4 A 20-year-old male patient presents to the emergency department (ED) after falling off of his mountain bike. He last ate 2 hours ago, about 15 minutes before he fell. He complains of left ankle pain and has a markedly deformed ankle with exposed bone protruding through the skin. What is the single most important and immediate step in the treatment of this injury?

A. Thorough irrigation and debridement of gross contamination from the wound

B. Reduce and splint the fracture in ED

C. Administer intravenous antibiotics and a tetanus shot/booster when applicable

D. Place nasogastric tube and proceed to the operating room for surgical stabilization

ANSWERS

12.1 **C.** *Maisonneuve* fractures, a type of pronation external rotation fracture, have a characteristic high fibular spiral fracture with a disrupted syndesmosis and tibia–fibula interosseous membrane. The medial malleolus (or deltoid ligament) is also disrupted. High fibular fractures (above the level of the syndesmosis) define Weber C fractures. Weber B fractures occur at the level of the syndesmosis, and Weber A fractures occur below it.

12.2 **B.** A tear or rupture of the deltoid ligament would be of concern in this patient. The question tells you that the mortise is intact (clear space of 3.5 mm) on x-ray; however, because the patient has tenderness over the medial malleolus, there must be concern for injury to the deltoid, which could result in an unstable ankle.

12.3 **D.** Although all of the factors here may influence the decision to surgically reduce and fix an ankle fracture, the position of the talus in the mortise is the single most important factor. Remember that widening of the ankle mortise indicates instability and is itself a surgical indication. Initial displacement is not as important as postreduction positioning.

12.4 **C.** Although urgent irrigation and debridement and provisional stabilization are important, administration of intravenous antibiotics within 6 hours of injury has been demonstrated to be most beneficial in reducing complications associated with open fractures.

CLINICAL PEARLS

- When examining a patient with an ankle injury, always perform a complete physical exam, including palpation of the lateral and medial malleolus, and a complete neurologic and vascular exam.
- When ordering ankle radiographs, obtain AP, mortise, and lateral views at minimum.
- On the mortise view, look for signs of instability. Remember that the medial clear space should be no wider than 4 mm and should be equal to the rest of the mortise clear space.
- Surgery is indicated in unstable ankle fractures and any open injuries.

REFERENCES

Buchholz RW, Court-Brown CM, Heckman JD, Tornetta P, eds. Ankle fractures. In: *Rockwood and Green's Fractures in Adults*. 7th ed. 2 vol. Philadelphia, PA: Lippincott Williams & Wilkins; 2010: P2147-P2179.

Egol KE, Koval KJ, Zukerman JD, eds. Injuries about the ankle. In: *Handbook of Fractures*. 4th ed. Philadelphia, PA: Lippincott Williams & Wilkins; 2010:76-506.

Pena F. Ankle injuries. In: Swiontkowski M, ed. *Manual of Orthopaedics*. 6th ed. Philadelphia, PA: Lippincott Williams & Wilkins; 2006:375-379.

Sanders D. Fractures of the ankle and tibial plafond. In: Lieberman JR, ed. *AAOS Comprehensive Orthopaedic Review*. Rosemont, IL: American Academy of Orthopaedic Surgeons; 2009:659-667.

CASE 13

A 55-year-old man with a history of atrial fibrillation develops a sudden sharp pain in his right leg. He presents to the emergency department, where he is found to have a cold right foot and calf, as well as nonpalpable pulses below the knee. The patient is taken to the operating room approximately 8 hours after the onset of the pain. He undergoes an embolectomy of a popliteal artery clot without complication. In the recovery room, however, he begins complaining of intense right foot and calf pain that continues to escalate, despite copious analgesia. When you evaluate the patient, he complains of 10/10 pain in his foot and calf that is constant, sharp, and without relief. On physical exam, his right lower leg is pale in comparison with the left and firm to touch. Palpable posterior tibial and dorsalis pedis pulses are present bilaterally. He experiences excruciating pain with passive dorsiflexion flexion of the right foot.

- What is the most likely diagnosis?
- How do you confirm the diagnosis?
- What is the appropriate treatment?
- What are the major complications associated with this condition?

ANSWERS TO CASE 13:

Acute Compartment Syndrome

Summary: A 55-year-old man who initially presents with 8 hours of acute lower extremity ischemia develops sharp, constant pain after undergoing successful embolectomy. The patient has a pale, firm, painful leg and foot with palpable pulses.

- **Most likely diagnosis:** Acute compartment syndrome.
- **How to confirm the diagnosis:** Measure compartment pressures in the leg.
- **Appropriate treatment:** Emergency surgical fasciotomies to relieve elevated leg compartment pressures.
- **Major complications:** Rhabdomyolysis and myoglobinemia can cause renal failure. Additionally, if ischemia is prolonged, it can lead to significant tissue damage causing diminished limb function, muscle contractures, and possible limb loss.

ANALYSIS

Objectives

1. Understand the pathophysiology underlying compartment syndrome as well as the clinical signs and symptoms of the condition.
2. Describe the diagnostic and therapeutic approach to compartment syndrome.
3. Understand the complications caused by the direct effects of elevated compartment pressures, as well as complications from myoglobinemia.

Considerations

The patient's history of prolonged lower extremity ischemia should raise the concern for the development of a compartment syndrome. Although most frequently associated with trauma, a number of nontraumatic injuries can also lead to the development of a compartment syndrome, such as reperfusion or rhabdomyolysis. This patient had an acute thrombosis of his popliteal artery with subsequent ischemia to his lower leg and foot for 8 hours. Many advocate performing prophylactic fasciotomies in any patient whose ischemia time, from an injury such as this one, exceeds 4 to 6 hours. Although the patient does not present with all of the **classic "5 Ps" (see "Definitions" in the next section)** it is rare to see a patient who in fact has all 5 signs and symptoms. The presence of all "5 Ps" typically represents a severe and *advanced* stage of compartment syndrome. The presence of palpable pulses should not impede your diagnosis of a compartment syndrome if other clinical findings suggest the diagnosis. Loss of pulses is typically the last sign and requires a significant intra-compartment pressure. Waiting for the patient to lose pulses will result in a more extensive injury to the compartmental muscle and nerves as well as increasing the risk for and severity of renal damage.

APPROACH TO: Compartment Syndrome

DEFINITIONS

COMPARTMENT SYNDROME: A clinically diagnosed condition of increased intra-compartmental pressure within a closed space, causing reduced tissue perfusion and subsequent tissue necrosis.

5 Ps: Five signs and symptoms classically found in patients with compartment syndrome, including: pain out of proportion to exam, paralysis, paresthesias, pallor, pulselessness. Sometimes poikilocytosis (coolness) is considered a sixth "P".

RHABDOMYOLYSIS: Breakdown of muscle that leads to intravascular leakage of electrolytes and proteins, including myoglobin.

CLINICAL APPROACH

Compartment syndrome results from an **increase in tissue pressure within a confined fascial space** that limits any expansion of the compartment's volume to compensate for the increase in pressure. As the pressure rises, the compartment's pressure eventually **exceeds the capillary perfusion pressure,** causing impaired oxygen delivery to tissue and subsequent tissue damage. Irreversible cellular damage, which results in breakdown of the intracellular organelles and cellular membranes, leads to leakage of intracellular electrolytes, including phosphorous, potassium, and myoglobin, as well as the activation of inflammatory cascades. This results in further swelling and tissue edema that, in turn, results in even further compartment pressure elevation. Rhabdomyolysis, the rapid breakdown of damaged muscle, may lead renal failure and dangerous electrolyte imbalances such as hyperkalemia and hypocalcemia. Hyperkalemia relates directly to intracellular potassium leakage; hypocalcemia indirectly results from the release of phosphate ions that bind and sequester available calcium.

Although compartment syndrome exists in both acute and chronic forms, it is typically thought of as an acute process. For the purpose of this discussion, acute and chronic forms of this syndrome are discussed separately.

Acute Compartment Syndrome

Although compartment syndrome is frequently associated with closed fractures, particularly comminuted fractures of the upper or lower extremities, it can be caused by any process that leads to impaired tissue perfusion. Additional causes of compartment syndrome include external compression such as constrictive casting, hematomas, arterial or venous thrombosis, intravenous (IV) infiltration, and leakage of fluid into the interstitial space (Table 13–1). Although not common, improper positioning for surgical procedures (especially prolonged positioning in lithotomy or Trendelenburg positions) can lead to impaired venous return and subsequent compartment syndrome.

The **most common fractures** associated with the development of compartment syndrome are **closed tibial fractures,** followed by **forearm fractures.** Some series

Table 13–1 • CAUSES OF COMPARTMENT SYNDROME
Arterial and/or venous obstruction
Bleeding (especially in patients on anticoagulants)
Circumferential burns
Crush and other soft tissue injury
Electrical burns
Leakage of vascular catheters
Intense exercise
Intravenous drug injections
Fractures
Penetrating trauma
Prolonged intraoperative positioning
Prolonged immobility of a limb
Reperfusion injuries
Seizures
Snake bites
Constrictive dressings (casts, tight splints, military antishock trousers [MASTs])

report the incidence of compartment syndrome after closed tibia fractures to be approximately 20%. Physicians must be highly suspicious of compartment syndrome in the patient who develops **increasing pain** following closed reduction and immobilization. Significant pain with passive stretching of the toes (or fingers, in a forearm injury) should warrant removal of the cast or splint and careful reassessment for compartment syndrome.

Compartment syndrome is a clinical diagnosis based on signs and symptoms in the appropriate clinical setting. Although the syndrome is classically described by the "5 Ps", it is rare to find a patient who has all 5 (or 6 if you include coolness) of these signs and symptoms. None of the "5 Ps" are pathognomonic for this condition, and therefore diagnosis of compartment syndrome is primarily a clinical diagnosis. For example, pain, which typically represents the first clinical complaint, is extremely nonspecific. Pulselessness, which is a late finding and does not occur until the compartment pressures are significantly elevated, may be a baseline finding in patients with peripheral vascular disease. An additional physical exam finding that is frequently seen with compartment syndrome is pain on passive movement of the muscles within the effected compartment.

Confirmation of the diagnosis is made by directly measuring the compartment pressures using either a side-port needle or a slit catheter (Figure 13–1). Compartment pressures within 30 mmHg of the patient's diastolic blood pressure warrant emergency operative intervention. Although compartment pressure measurements are extremely useful in confirming the diagnosis of compartment syndrome, it is primarily a clinical diagnosis, and therefore measurement of compartment pressures should not delay surgical intervention if the clinical picture is clear. Additionally, many advocate for prophylactic intervention with fasciotomies to prevent the development of a compartment syndrome if there has been greater than 4 to 6 hours of limb ischemia.

Surgical intervention is performed via an operative fasciotomies. Depending on the extent of injury and tissue edema, the overlying skin can either be closed at the

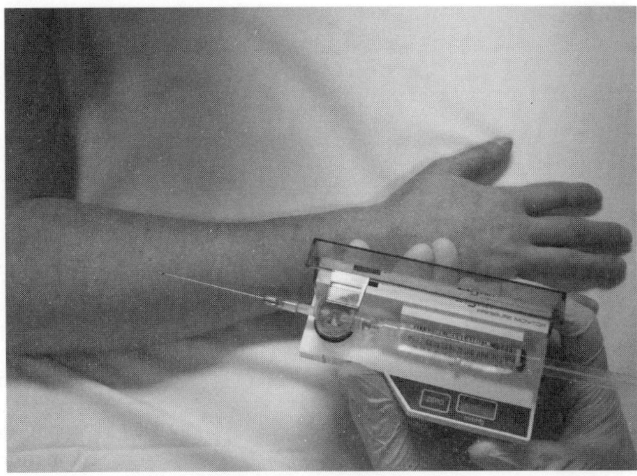

Figure 13–1. A slit catheter device used to measure compartment syndrome. (Reproduced, with permission, from Tintinalli J, et al. *Tintinalli's Emergency Medicine: A Comprehensive Study Guide*. 7th ed. New York, NY: McGraw-Hill; 2010:Fig. 275-6.)

time of surgery or can be closed once the edema has decreased. This will sometimes require the use of skin grafts at a later date. In most cases, the fasciotomies are performed through 2 skin incisions that are positioned so that all fascial compartments can be decompressed. In the leg, fasciotomies involve releasing the anterior, lateral, superficial, posterior, and deep posterior compartments (Figure 13–2). Fasciotomies of the thigh involve release of the medial, anterior, and posterior compartments. In the arm, proximal fasciotomies involve releasing the anterior and posterior compartments, whereas forearm fasciotomies require opening the dorsal and volar compartments with extension into the carpal tunnel and mobile wad compartment located on the radial aspect of the forearm (Figure 13–3). Fasciotomies are generally not performed after 48 hours unless there is remaining function documented within the muscles of that compartment. Amputation may be necessary in these settings.

When performing fasciotomies, it is important to ensure that the fascial openings are long enough to fully decompress the muscle within. If the underlying injury is severe and the openings are inadequate, compartment syndrome can recur. Failure to appreciate this fact can easily lead to further tissue damage and subsequent complications.

The cellular damage that occurs from prolonged compartment syndrome leads to release of potassium, phosphorous, and myoglobin. Evaluation of the degree of muscle damage and breakdown can be followed with serial measurements of creatine phosphokinase (CPK), which serves as an indirect gauge of the degree of myoglobinemia. Myoglobin, the oxygen storing molecule of muscles, can crystallize within the renal tubules and lead to significant renal injury. Management of this severe myoglobulinemia primarily involves aggressive hydration with IV fluids with a goal of maintaining urine output of approximately 100 mL/hr or >1 mL/kg/hr. Some advocate for IV fluid supplementation with sodium bicarbonate with the goal of increasing the pH of urine and increasing the solubility of myoglobin to reduce crystallization and subsequent renal damage.

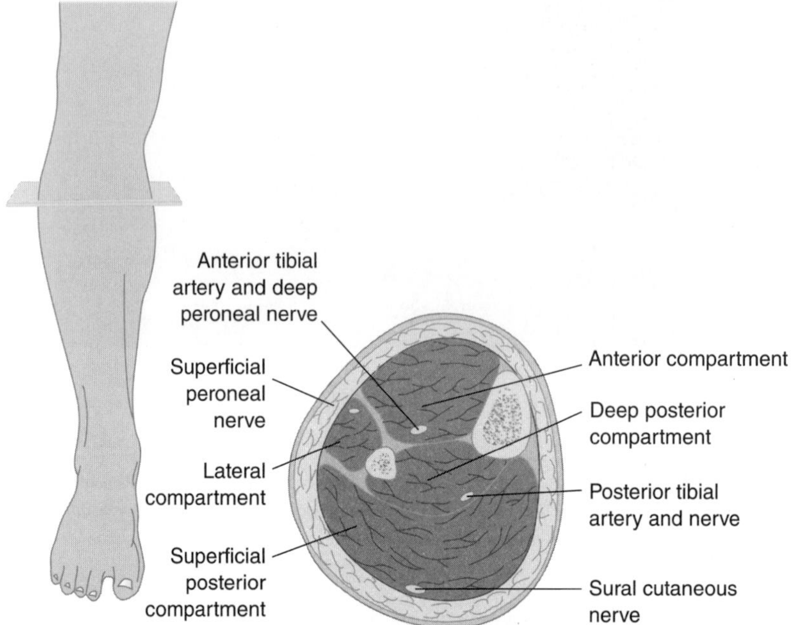

Figure 13–2. The 4 compartments of the leg. (Reproduced, with permission, from Tintinalli J, et al. *Tintinalli's Emergency Medicine: A Comprehensive Study Guide*. 7th ed. New York, NY: McGraw-Hill; 2010:Fig. 275-1.)

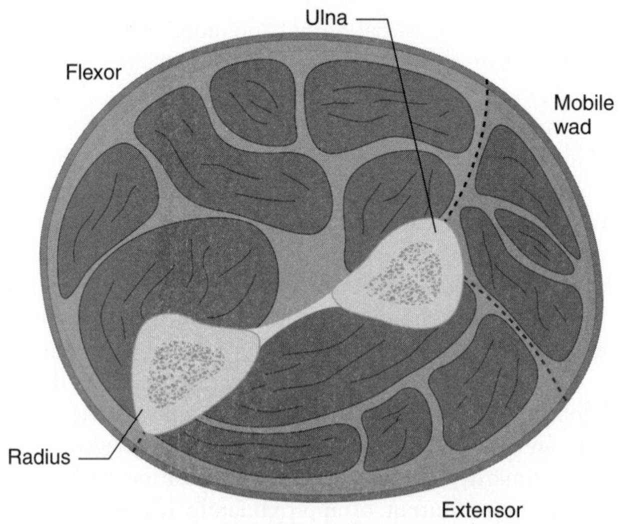

Figure 13–3. The forearm compartments. (Reproduced, with permission, from Tintinalli J, et al. *Tintinalli's Emergency Medicine: A Comprehensive Study Guide*. 7th ed. New York, NY: McGraw-Hill; 2010:Fig. 275-2.)

Patients with rhabdomyolysis also require continuous cardiac monitoring, as the hypocalcemia and hyperkalemia associated with muscle breakdown can lead to cardiac arrhythmias. Depending on the degree of hyperkalemia, patients may require further medical interventions, including calcium chloride or calcium gluconate for myocardial protection as well as insulin/glucose, sodium bicarbonate, and polystyrene sulfonate, a potassium binder.

Outcomes after the development of acute compartment syndrome are largely determined by the severity of the inciting injury, the timing of diagnosis, and the extent and severity of tissue damage. Although the majority of patients who sustain renal injury from rhabdomyolysis will eventually have a full recovery of renal function, rhabdomyolysis complicated by acute kidney injury is associated with a mortality rate as high as 20%. Furthermore, requirement for intensive care unit admission in the setting of rhabdomyolysis and acute kidney injury is associated with a mortality rate reaching nearly 60%.

Chronic Compartment Syndrome

Although compartment syndrome is most commonly seen and discussed as an acute process, it can also exist in a chronic form. The chronic form of compartment syndrome is an exercise-induced phenomenon that results in recurrent pain with activity and relief with rest. The chronic form of this syndrome is not typically associated with significant muscle necrosis nor renal damage. A diagnosis of chronic compartment syndrome is confirmed by measuring intra-compartment pressures before and after exercise. Treatment options include surgical fasciotomies for pain relief and increased exercise tolerance, prolonged periods of rest in conjunction with modifying the offending activity or exercise routine, and continuing with current exercise routines despite the pain and discomfort that they cause. Those who elect to defer surgical intervention or lifestyle modification should be made aware that chronic compartment syndrome can on occasion develop into an acute compartment syndrome.

COMPREHENSION QUESTIONS

13.1 A 24-year-old man is noted to have a urinalysis that is positive for blood. The microscopic examination of the urine is negative for casts or red blood cells. Which of the following is the most likely diagnosis?

A. Nephritic syndrome

B. Hematuria

C. Renal cell carcinoma

D. Myoglobinuria

13.2 A 55-year-old woman is noted to have a traumatic injury to her right thigh. Which of the following is most sensitive for the diagnosis of compartment syndrome?

A. Pulselessness

B. Pallor

C. Pain

D. Paresthesias

13.3 A 22-year-old roofer is brought into the ED due to hyperthermia. The urinalysis is positive for blood, and the serum CPK is markedly elevated. The patient is noted to likely have compartment syndrome and rhabdomyolysis. What is the appropriate infusion rate for IV hydration for this patient?

A. 4 mL/kg/% body surface area affected

B. 4 mL/kg/hr for the first 10 kg + 2 mL/kg/hr for the next 10 kg + 1 mL/kg/hr for each subsequent kilogram

C. Titrated to urine output of 0.5 mL/kg/hr

D. Titrated to urine output of 1 mL/kg/hr

ANSWERS

13.1 **D.** A urinalysis that is positive for blood does not distinguish between myoglobin and hemoglobin. A microscopic urine exam is necessary for a definitive diagnosis. In a patient with myoglobinuria, a microscopic evaluation will fail to show the presence of red blood cell (RBC) casts or intact RBCs. Gross myoglobinuria can lead to an abnormal coloration of the urine and is typically described as "cola colored." Hematuria and renal cell carcinoma would be expected to produce urinalysis and microscopic exam that are positive for RBCs, whereas nephritic syndrome would be expected to have RBC casts.

13.2 **C.** Pain, typically severe and even out of proportion to the injury, represents the first and most sensitive symptom of compartment syndrome. Pain, however, is extremely nonspecific. Pulselessness represents a very late finding, and therefore the finding of a palpable pulse should not exclude compartment syndrome in your differential diagnosis.

13.3 **D.** IV fluids should be titrated to maintain urine output greater than 1 mL/kg/hr to minimize the risk of myoglobin precipitation within the renal tubules and minimize the extent of kidney injury. Choice A represents a modification of the Parkland formula used in burn management (4 mL/kg/body surface area of second- and third-degree burns). Choice B represents the calculation of maintenance IV fluid. Choice C represents the typical urine output goal for most patients.

CLINICAL PEARLS

- Compartment syndrome is a clinical diagnosis. Although measurement of compartment pressures can be used to confirm the diagnosis, treatment should not be delayed for compartment pressure measurements if the diagnosis is clear.
- Pulselessness is typically a late sign, and treatment should not be delayed until it is present.
- Incomplete and/or inadequate fasciotomies can result in a subsequent redevelopment of a compartment syndrome.
- Ischemia lasting greater than 4 to 6 hours typically requires prophylactic fasciotomies to prevent development of a compartment syndrome.
- Compartment pressures within 30 mmHg of the patient's diastolic pressure are indicative of compartment syndrome and require emergency operative intervention.

REFERENCES

Bosch X, Poch E, Grau JM. Rhabdomyolysis and acute kidney injury. *N Engl J Med*. 2009;361:62-72.

Frink M, Hildebrand F, Krettek C, Brand J, Hankemeier S. Compartment syndrome of the lower leg and foot. *Clin Orthop Relat Res*. 2010;468:940-950.

Huerta-Alardén AL, Varon J, Marik PE. Bench-to-bedside review: rhabdomyolysis—an overview for clinicians. *Crit Care*. 2005;9:158-169.

Konstantakos EK, Dalstrom DJ, Nelles ME, Laughlin RT, Prayson MJ. Diagnosis and management of extremity compartment syndromes: an orthopaedic perspective. *Am Surg*. 2007;73:1199-1209.

Shadgan B, Menon M, Sanders D, Berry G, Martin C Jr, Duffy P, Stephen D, O'Brien PJ. Current thinking about acute compartment syndrome of the lower extremity. *Can J Surg*. 2010;53:329-334.

CASE 14

An 8-year-old right-hand-dominant girl presents to the emergency department (ED) with severe left forearm pain. Her mother states that the girl had been playing on their trampoline with some friends when she fell, landing on her outstretched left hand 1 hour ago. On examination, the girl is in obvious discomfort, and although her forearm is moderately swollen, the skin is grossly intact. The forearm is deformed, and she is exquisitely tender to palpation toward the distal aspect. When asked, she will gingerly flex and extend her wrist. However, she will not supinate or pronate. The radial pulse is palpable, and brisk capillary refill is noted. She has grossly intact neurologic sensation and motor function. Radiographs are obtained (Figure 14–1).

- ▶ What is the most likely diagnosis?
- ▶ What is the best treatment of this injury?

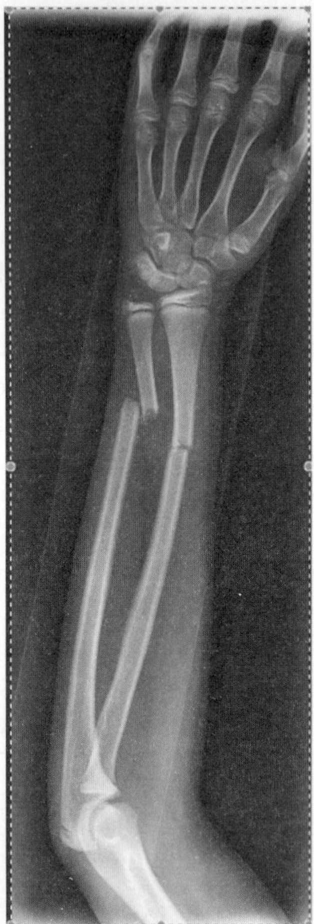

A

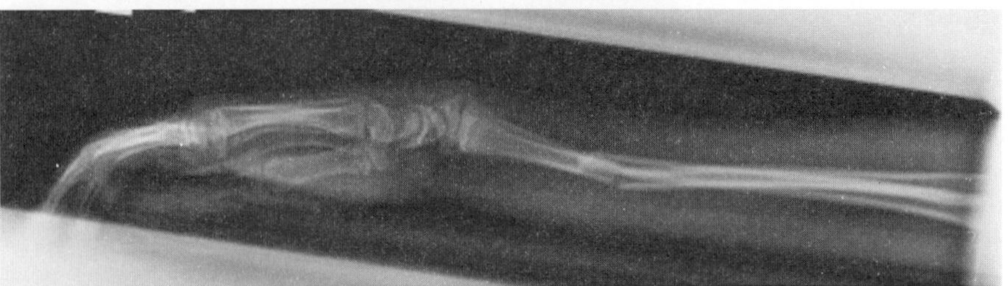

B

Figure 14–1. (**A**) AP and (**B**) lateral radiographs of a left forearm in a skeletally immature individual. (Courtesy of Andrew J. Rosenbaum, MD)

ANSWERS TO CASE 14: Pediatric Both Bone Forearm Fracture

Summary: A right-hand-dominant 8-year-old girl presents with left forearm pain and deformity after landing on her outstretched left hand following a fall from a trampoline. Motor, sensory, and vascular exams are all normal. Radiographs reveal distal one-third diaphyseal fractures of her radius and ulna.

- **Most likely diagnosis:** Both bone forearm fracture (BBFF).
- **Preferred treatment:** Closed reduction and application of a long-arm cast.

ANALYSIS

Objectives

1. Understand the mechanism of injury associated with fractures of both the radius and ulna in children.
2. Know the proper radiographic imaging to obtain in the setting of a BBFF.
3. Know the indications for both nonoperative and operative treatment of pediatric BBFF.

Considerations

This 8-year-old girl presents with pain and deformity of her left forearm after falling onto her outstretched hand while playing on a trampoline. Her severe pain and obvious deformity must make the clinician very suspicious for a fracture, specifically a BBFF. An additional physical examination finding that also supports this diagnosis is her refusal to supinate and pronate her forearm. Fortunately, this is not an open injury and she is neurovascularly intact. Plain radiographs of the forearm confirm a BBFF. The images obtained include views of both the wrist and elbow on the anteroposterior (AP) view, which do not appear to be fractured. Ideally these joints would also be included on the lateral radiograph as well. Because the girl has no specific complaints or exam findings concerning for either a wrist or elbow injury, no further imaging of these joints is needed. **Most pediatric forearm fractures, including the BBFF sustained by this girl, can be managed nonoperatively as a result of the significant remodeling potential of children's bones.** In this case, closed reduction and long-arm casting is the treatment of choice.

APPROACH TO: Pediatric Both Bone Forearm Fracture

DEFINITIONS

BOTH BONE FOREARM FRACTURE: A fracture involving both the radial and ulnar shafts. They are classified in a descriptive fashion, based on the level (distal, middle, proximal third) and the pattern (greenstick, plastic deformation, complete, comminuted).

GREENSTICK FRACTURE: A fracture in which partial bony continuity is preserved. In other words, a break that does not violate all cortices. Greenstick fractures are unique to children and can be thought of as an intermediate between a bending deformation of soft pediatric bone and a complete fracture.

CLINICAL APPROACH

Mechanism of Injury

Forearm fractures are the most common pediatric fractures associated with trampolines and the second most common fractures seen with falls from monkey bars (supracondylar fractures are first). It is usually a fall onto an outstretched hand that leads to a BBFF, with rotation influencing the location of the radius and ulna fractures. For example, when a fall is accompanied by minimal torsion or rotation, the fractures of the radius and ulna are likely to be at the same level. If the forearm is rotated during the injury, the radius and ulna usually fracture at different levels.

Classification

Classification is usually descriptive and based on the level of the fractures (distal, middle, proximal third) and the pattern (greenstick, plastic deformation, complete, comminuted). Many believe that the more proximal the forearm fracture, the more difficult it is to treat. Fracture pattern can also influence treatment options. While greenstick and complete fractures are usually amenable to closed reduction and casting, comminuted fractures in both the radius and ulna may require surgical plate fixation. A buckle fracture, which will look like a "speed bump," never occurs in isolation in the shaft but may accompany plastic deformation or greenstick fractures. A radial or ulnar shaft buckle fracture, which may appear like a "speed bump" on radiographs, almost never occur in isolation. They are typically accompanied by plastic deformation or greenstick fractures in the other forearm bone.

Workup

Physical examination and plain radiographs (anteroposterior and lateral views) of the involved forearm comprise the initial workup. **Dedicated x-rays of the wrist and elbow should be obtained only if clinical suspicion for injury at those joints exists.** On examination, soft tissue integrity, areas of tenderness, and any deformity should be noted. Range of motion at both the elbow and wrist should be assessed, as should forearm supination and pronation. Motor, sensory, and vascular exams should also be performed. A useful way to evaluate motor function distal to the injury is by asking the patient to perform the hand gestures from the game "rock, paper, and scissors." **Median nerve function is observed via the "rock" gesture; radial nerve function via the "paper" gesture; and ulnar nerve function via the "scissor" gesture.**

TREATMENT

Both nonoperative and operative interventions have the identical goal: to achieve healing within established anatomical and functional guidelines. In growing children, this must be done while taking into account the remodeling that occurs. Several mechanisms affect bone remodeling in children. **The distal radial epiphysis will correct angular deformity at approximately 10 degrees per year, independent of age, as long as the physis remains open.** As the bones lengthen through growth, remodeling will lead to decreased angulation. Bone remodeling also occurs through intramembranous apposition on the concave side and resorption on the convex side of bone. This is best accomplished in children, who inherently have thick periosteum. Of note, children older than 11 years are less effective at correcting bone angulation than younger children.

Most pediatric both bone forearm fractures are amenable to nonoperative treatment with reduction, if displaced, and long-arm casting. Young children with less than 5 to 10 degrees of angulation do not require reduction. **The following criteria serve as age-dependent guidelines:**

- **For ages <6 years, up to 15 degrees of angulation and 5 degrees of rotation can be accepted.**
- **For ages 6 to 10 years old, less than 10 degrees of angulation is preferred, as is end-to-end apposition; bayonet apposition is not ideal but may be acceptable.**
- **For ages ≥12 years, no angulation or rotation can be accepted.**
- **For ages ≥6 years, rotational deformity is never acceptable.**

Long-arm casting of BBFFs includes placing a proper interosseous mold, supracondylar mold, and appropriate padding. A complete and proximal BBFF should be immobilized in supination. This position allows the distal forearm to align with the proximal fracture fragments, which have been pulled into supination by the now unopposed biceps and supinator muscles. Fractures of the middle third of the radius should be immobilized in neutral wrist rotation, since at this level, the supination forces on the proximal fragments are neutralized by the pronator teres that remains proximally attached. Fractures in the distal third should be immobilized in pronation to similarly neutralize the effect of the pronator quadratus distally. After acceptable reduction and application of a long-arm cast, the patient is followed with x-rays at 1- to 2-week intervals.

When there is an open fracture or acceptable reduction cannot be achieved, open reduction and internal fixation, rather than casting, is the preferred treatment. Many operative techniques have been described and include plate fixation, flexible intramedullary stabilization, and percutaneous pinning.

COMPLICATIONS

Complications after treatment of BBFFs include redisplacement and loss of reduction (the most common short-term complication, typically secondary to inadequate cast molding), stiffness, refracture, malunion, delayed union/nonunion, radioulnar synostosis resulting in complete loss of forearm rotation; neurapraxia (median nerve most commonly), muscle and tendon entrapment, compartment syndrome, and infection.

COMPREHENSION QUESTIONS

14.1 An 8-year-old boy fell while riding his bike, landing on his outstretched right hand. Radiographs confirm a middle-third diaphyseal both bone forearm fracture with end-to-end cortical apposition and 12 degrees of dorsal angulation. What is the preferred method of treatment for this injury?

A. Percutaneous pinning of both the radius and ulna

B. Closed reduction and long-arm cast application in supination

C. Closed reduction and long-arm cast application in neutral

D. Short-arm cast application

14.2 Which of the following is most accurate regarding bone remodeling in children?

A. The distal radial epiphysis will correct angular deformity at approximately 20 degrees per year, independent of age, as long as the physis remains open.

B. As the bones lengthen through growth, remodeling will also occur and lead to decreased angulation.

C. Intramembranous apposition on the convex side and resorption on the concave side of bone lead to remodeling.

D. Children older than 11 years are more effective at correcting bone angulation than younger children.

14.3 A 13-year-old girl sustains a both bone forearm fracture after a fall. Which of the following statements is most accurate regarding the radiographic evaluation of anatomic forearm alignment after reduction?

A. On the AP radiograph, the ulnar styloid and the coronoid process are oriented 270 degrees apart.

B. On the AP radiograph, the radial styloid and tuberosity are oriented 180 degrees apart.

C. On the lateral radiograph, the ulnar styloid and the coronoid process are oriented 90 degrees apart.

D. On the AP radiograph, the radial styloid and tuberosity are oriented 90 degrees apart.

ANSWERS

14.1 **C.** A middle-third diaphyseal BBFF with 12 degrees of angulation in an 8-year-old is amenable to closed reduction and long-arm casting. In children 6 to 10 years old, less than 10 degrees of angulation is ideal and should be accomplished with closed reduction in this patient. The extremity should be immobilized in a neutral position via a long-arm cast, as the fracture is in the middle third.

14.2 **B.** As bones lengthen through growth, remodeling also occurs and leads to decreased angulation. Thus B is the correct answer. The distal radial epiphysis will correct angular deformity at approximately 10 degrees per year, not 20, as A states. Intramembranous apposition on the *concave* side and resorption on the *convex* side of bone lead to remodeling, the opposite of that stated in C. Lastly, children *older* than 11 years are less effective at correcting bone angulation than younger children, making D incorrect.

14.3 **B.** After proper reduction, the radial styloid and tuberosity are located 180 degrees apart. On lateral radiographs, the ulna styloid and the coronoid are 180 degrees apart.

CLINICAL PEARLS

- Classification of BBFFs is usually descriptive and based on the level of the fractures (distal, middle, proximal third) and the pattern (greenstick, plastic deformation, complete, comminuted).
- Ipsilateral wrist and elbow regions should be included on the standard forearm x-rays obtained when working up a BBFF. However, if clinical suspicion is high for additional injury to either of those joints, then dedicated wrist and elbow films must be obtained.
- Most pediatric both bone forearm fractures are amenable to nonoperative treatment with reduction, if displaced, and long-arm casting.
- **The amount of angulation and rotation that can be tolerated is age dependent, with less tolerance with increasing age.**
- When there is an open fracture or acceptable reduction cannot be achieved, open reduction and internal fixation, rather than casting, is the preferred treatment.

REFERENCE

Mehlman CT, Wall EJ. Injuries to the shafts of the radius and ulna. In: Beaty JH, Kasser JR, eds. *Rockwood and Wilkins' Fractures in Children*. 6th ed. Philadelphia, PA: Lippincott Williams & Wilkins; 2006.

CASE 15

A 6-year-old female presents to the emergency department complaining of left arm pain after falling from the monkey bars. She says she lost her grip and fell directly onto an outstretched hand. She has difficulty flexing her forearm. Her past medical and surgical histories are unremarkable. On examination of her left elbow, there is a "dimpling" of the skin in the antecubital fossa, with mild swelling around the elbow. She will not allow any range of elbow motion secondary to pain. With encouragement, the patient can extend her wrist and fingers and can spread her fingers apart. She has difficulty, however, flexing her thumb interphalangeal (IP) joint and flexing her index and middle fingers at the distal interphalangeal (DIP) joint. Sensation is intact throughout her left arm. Radial pulses are 2+. Anteroposterior (AP) and lateral plain films of the elbow are obtained (Figure 15–1).

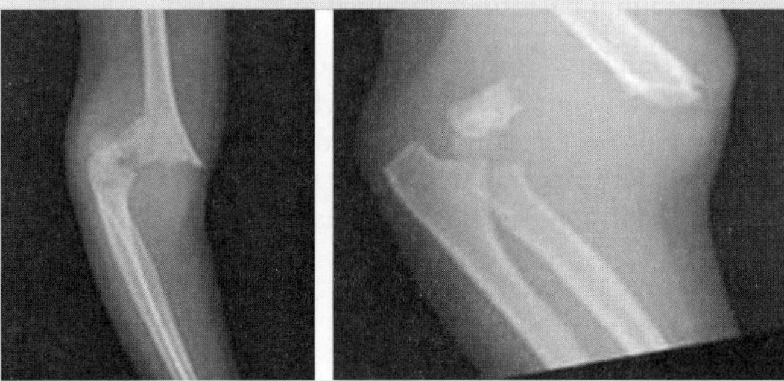

Figure 15–1. AP and lateral radiographs of a skeletally immature elbow. (Reproduced, with permission, from Tintinalli J, et al. *Tintinalli's Emergency Medicine: A Comprehensive Study Guide.* 7th ed. New York, NY: McGraw-Hill; 2010:Fig. 267-9.)

- ▶ What is the most likely diagnosis?
- ▶ Why are children most prone to this type of injury?
- ▶ What additional radiographs, if any, do you wish to order?
- ▶ What aspects of this child's exam are concerning?

ANSWERS TO CASE 15: Supracondylar Humerus Fracture

Summary: This is a 6-year-old healthy girl with left elbow pain after falling 5 feet from the monkey bars. There is dimpling in the antecubital fossa and mild swelling about the elbow. She has a motor deficit in her ipsilateral flexor pollicis longus (FPL) and flexor digitorum profundus (FDP) of the index and middle fingers.

- **Most likely diagnosis:** Extension-type supracondylar fracture.
- **Why children are most prone to this injury:** Between 5 to 8 years of age, pediatric humeri undergo remodeling in which the AP diameter of the distal humerus becomes relatively thin. With forced extension, a taut, thick anterior elbow joint capsule resists stretching as the olecranon engages the olecranon fossa. This places great stress on the supracondylar region, potentially resulting in extension-type fracture.
- **Appropriate imaging:** AP and lateral views of the elbow are essential. Additional imaging of the entire extremity is indicated for pediatric patients with symptoms that cannot be entirely localized to the elbow.
- **Physical exam findings:** This patient has obvious palsies for the FPL and the FDP of the index and middle fingers, which, in addition to the pronator quadratus, are the muscles typically innervated by the anterior interosseous nerve (AIN), a branch of the median nerve. The AIN is the most commonly affected nerve with extension-type supracondylar fractures.

ANALYSIS

Objectives

1. Recognize the clinical presentation of supracondylar fractures.
2. Understand the potential complications of supracondylar injuries.
3. Understand the treatment options for supracondylar fractures, their indications, and their potential complications.

Considerations

This patient has suffered an isolated, 100% displaced, closed extension-type supracondylar fracture. Priorities include adequate initial pain control, careful neurologic exam, and prompt immobilization. Neurologic exams should always be carefully performed and documented both before and after any form of manipulation. With 100% displaced fractures such as with this patient, it is highly likely that closed reduction with percutaneous pinning or open reduction with fixation will be required to stabilize the fracture. For this reason, steps to prepare the patient for the operating room should begin as soon as the diagnosis is made. Obtain an efficient but thorough medical history; be sure to inquire about the patient's last meal or fluid intake and to alert the OR of the potential case.

Additionally, the presence of an AIN palsy complicates treatment. Neurologic deficit may be seen in up to 10% to 20% of closed supracondylar fractures, yet the great majority of these injuries resolve spontaneously without operative nerve exploration. Although controversial, attempts may be made to close reduce this fracture in the operating room with possible percutaneous pin fixation. If closed reduction cannot be achieved, open reduction must be performed; at this point, exploration of the nerve may be indicated.

APPROACH TO:
Supracondylar Humerus Fracture

DEFINITIONS

ANTERIOR HUMERAL LINE: A radiographic line drawn along the anterior humerus on lateral radiographs of the elbow. In normal elbows, this should intersect the middle third of the capitellar ossification center.

POSTERIOR FAT PAD SIGN: A radiographic lucency located immediately posterior to the elbow on lateral elbow radiographs when a joint effusion is present. Normally, this small pad of posterior fat is radiographically invisible because it is hidden within the olecranon fossa; however, with elbow effusions, the distended joint brings the fat pad into view. In the setting of trauma, a posterior fat pad sign is up to 70% sensitive for an intracapsular fracture.

CLINICAL APPROACH

Epidemiology

Supracondylar fractures are the most common pediatric elbow fractures, accounting for approximately 55% to 75% of all pediatric elbow fractures. These injuries occur most frequently in the nondominant hand of children between 5 and 10 years of age. There is a slight male predominance. Supracondylar fractures may be either extension type or flexion type, depending on the mechanism of injury. **Extension-type injuries are by far the most common, representing up to 98% of all cases.**

Mechanism of Injury and Relevant Anatomy

The supracondylar region is located directly above the articular condyles of the distal humerus and consists of an area of cancellous bone encased within a thin cortex. **This region is especially susceptible to injury, as significant remodeling occurs roughly between the ages of 5 to 8 years of age.** A thick anterior joint capsule resists stretch when the elbow is hyperextended. As the olecranon engages the olecranon fossa, significant stress is placed on the relatively thin supracondylar region, resulting in potential extension-type fracture. Extension-type supracondylar fractures result most frequently from a fall on an extended forearm, which may result posterior displaced or posterior angulation (ie, apex anterior) of the distal fragment. A direct fall on the posterior region of a *flexed* elbow is the most common mechanism for flexion-type supracondylar fractures.

History and Physical Exam

The physician should suspect a fracture in any child who exhibits pain or reluctance to move the affected elbow. Close inspection should evaluate for open fracture. In the setting of local laceration, when one is unsure if the joint is violated, the elbow may be injected with normal saline and observed for extravasation to rule out an open joint injury. A complete neurovascular exam should be obtained, evaluating pulses and capillary refill distally with comparison to the unaffected side. Next, sensory distributions of the radial nerve (first dorsal webspace), medial nerve (palmar side of index finger), ulnar nerve (palmar side of fifth digit), and musculocutaneous nerve (lateral aspect of forearm) should be evaluated, as well as motor evaluation of the median, AIN, radial, and ulna nerves. **Neurovascular exams must be repeated and carefully documented after reduction or manipulations of any kind.**

Radiographic Evaluation

Radiographs of the pediatric elbow are among the most complex and difficult-to-interpret images in all of orthopaedics. At 5 to 10 years of age, roughly the age at which children are most prone to supracondylar fractures, there are six immature ossification centers that eventually fuse to form the mature elbow. **The order of ossification for the six ossification centers may be memorized by the acronym "CRMTOL"—capitellum, radial head, medial epicondyle, trochlea, olecranon, and lateral epicondyle. Conveniently, these begin to ossify at approximately 2, 4, 6, 8, 10, and 12 years of age, respectively.**

Radiographic evaluation of the entire affected extremity is recommended when symptoms cannot be clearly localized to a single, specific point. As stated, AP and lateral views of the elbow are essential. When obtaining lateral films of the elbow, external rotation must be avoided, as this can displace the fracture.

Classically, supracondylar fracture radiographs will have a positive **posterior fat pad sign,** indicative of joint effusion from a fracture. The sensitivity of the posterior fat pad sign is >70% in the setting of trauma without visible fractures lines. Anterior and superior fat pad signs are less sensitive. Additional radiographic assessment should include confirmation that the radial head aligns with the capitellum in all views. Finally, the **anterior humeral line** should bisect the middle third of the capitellum; in displaced extension-type injuries, the capitellum can fall posterior to the anterior humeral line.

CLASSIFICATIONS AND TREATMENT

Extension-type supracondylar fractures are classified by the Gartland classification, which is based primarily on the degree of displacement.

- Type I fractures: nondisplaced
- Type II fractures: displaced with minimal angulation/rotation, posterior cortex is intact
- Type III fractures: complete displacement

The majority of supracondylar fractures that are neither open nor complicated by neurovascular injury are treated with careful reduction followed by long-arm cast or splint immobilization. Nondisplaced, or type I fractures, are treated with a long-arm cast with the elbow flexed between 60 and 90 degrees for a minimum of 2 to 3 weeks.

Reduction

Type II and Type III fractures require careful reduction, which may be performed by hyperextending at the elbow with simultaneous traction, followed by flexion at the elbow while simultaneously applying posterior force to the reduced fragment to prevent it from slipping. Long-arm cast immobilization should follow. Both type II and III fractures that are unstable on reduction may benefit from percutaneous pinning, which should be performed under anesthesia in the operating room. Type III fractures may not always be reducible by closed methods, and therefore, open reduction and pinning or internal fixation may be necessary to achieve stabilization.

Complications

Neurovascular injury can have an incidence rate as high as 7% to 10%, typically secondary to excessive traction during injury or nerve/vessel entrapment at the fracture site. Fortunately, the majority of nerve injuries are neurapraxias—self-limited, physiologic (not structural) nerve dysfunctions that typically resolve spontaneously. **With extension-type injuries, the AIN is the most commonly affected nerve. With flexion-type injuries, conversely, the ulnar nerve is the most commonly affected nerve.**

The ulnar nerve is also especially prone to iatrogenic injury due to its prominent, superficial location over the lateral epicondyle. During cross-pinning fixation for type II and type III injuries, great care must be taken to avoid trauma to the nerve when placing medial-to-lateral pins. For this reason, many surgeons simply avoid placing medial-to-lateral pins and instead achieve fixation with 2 or more lateral-to-medial percutaneous pins in parallel. **Although biomechanical studies have demonstrated that cross-pinning techniques achieve stronger fixation than parallel pins, the clinical outcomes are essentially equivalent between the techniques.**

Although rare (<1% in isolated supracondylar injuries), it is important to evaluate for developing **compartment syndromes.** Concomitant vascular injury is uncommon with supracondylar fractures, occurring in fewer than 20% of displaced fractures—or approximately 0.5% of all cases. Typically, the brachial artery is impinged or lacerated at the fracture site, or it can become compressed secondary to swelling in the antecubital fossa. If pulses are absent on examination, but the hand is warm to touch with brisk capillary refill, the arm may be closely monitored. If the patient's hand is cool to touch with markedly pale digits compared with the unaffected side, emergency compartment release and/or angiographic studies may be indicated.

Finally, cubitus varus, sometimes referred to as a **"gunstock deformity,"** may result from inadequately reduced supracondylar fractures that heal with a malunion. This is typically a cosmetic, not functional, complication, and its incidence has been dramatically reduced with the widespread use of percutaneous pinning (2% with residual deformity) versus casting alone (8% with residual deformity).

COMPREHENSION QUESTIONS

15.1 A 10-year-old girl reports right elbow pain after a fall while running from a school bully. She has no other injuries and refuses to move the elbow out of fear of pain. Radiographs are notable for a positive fat pad sign, but show no obvious fracture line. Contralateral images of the left, unaffected elbow are obtained for comparison. Which of the following elbow apophyses is the last to appear on elbow radiographs?

A. Trochlea

B. Lateral epicondyle

C. Medial epicondyle

D. Radial head

E. Olecranon

15.2 An 8-year-old boy falls from the playground slide on a flexed left elbow and suffers a flexion type, fully displaced closed flexion-type supracondylar fracture. He complains of some finger numbness in the emergency department, but will not let anybody close enough to examine his arm. Which of the following is most likely injured in this fracture?

A. Brachial artery

B. Anterior interosseous nerve

C. Radial nerve

D. Ulnar nerve

E. Radial artery

15.3 A 5-year-old boy falls from a highchair during a rowdy game of "Go Fish" and falls onto an outstretched right hand. He presents to the emergency department with complaints that he can't move his arm. X-rays reveal a Gartland type III extension-type supracondylar fracture. His fingers are warm and well perfused, but no radial pulse is palpable. On careful examination, with which of the following motions is he most likely to have difficulty?

A. Wrist extension

B. "Thumbs up"

C. "A-okay" sign

D. Thumb-small finger opposition

E. Fanning out his fingers

ANSWERS

15.1 **B.** The lateral epicondyle should be the last apophysis to ossify in normal skeletal development. Generally, the order and age for elbow apophyseal ossification is capitellum, radial head, medial epicondyle, trochlea, olecranon, and lateral epicondyle, which ossify at approximately 2, 4, 6, 8, 10, and 12 years of age, respectively.

15.2 **D.** Although the anterior interosseous nerve is most commonly injured in extension-type supracondylar fractures (by far the most common type of supracondylar fracture), the ulnar nerve is more commonly injured in *flexion*-type supracondylar fractures. The brachial artery is potentially injured, albeit rarely, with flexion-type injuries. The radial artery does not branch until the brachial artery trifurcation, which occurs distal to the elbow. Radial nerve injury is the second most common form of nerve injury in extension-type fractures.

15.3 **C.** The "A-okay" sign, made by flexing the thumb and index finger to make a ring, tests thumb IP flexion and index finger DIP flexion, 2 tasks specific to the AIN. The AIN is most commonly injured in extension-type supracondylar fractures. "Thumbs up" and wrist extension are functions of the radial nerve—the second most commonly injured nerve with extension-type injuries. Finger fanning is a function of the intrinsic finger abductors of the ulnar nerve. Thumb and small finger opposition relies mostly on the thenar eminence (pollicis opponens), which is innervated by the recurrent median nerve.

CLINICAL PEARLS

- There is a seasonal distribution of supracondylar fractures in children, with the great majority occurring during summer-time play.
- X-rays of the pediatric elbow are complex and often difficult to interpret due to the variability of ossification centers. Images of the contralateral, normal elbow are often helpful for comparison.
- The presence of a posterior fat pad sign on lateral x-ray is helpful in determining the presence of a fracture or intraarticular pathology when no fracture line is obvious.

REFERENCES

Beaty JH, Kasser JR, eds. Supracondylar fractures of the distal humerus. In: *Rockwood and Wilkins' Fractures in Children*. 7th ed. Philadelphia, PA: Lippincott Williams & Wilkins; 2010:487-532.

Egol KE, Koval KJ, Zukerman JD, eds. Pediatric elbow. *Handbook of Fractures*. 4th ed. Philadelphia, PA: Lippincott Williams & Wilkins; 2010:598-644.

CASE 16

An 8-month-old boy is brought to the emergency department by his parents with a 48-hour history of left thigh swelling and irritability. They also state that the child has been barely moving his left lower extremity over this time. The parents do not recall any injury or recent trauma. After further discussion, the mother does recall that approximately 2 days ago, the child fell from the changing table (~3 feet off the ground) onto the carpeted floor of their apartment. On examination, the child is developmentally appropriate but irritable. His left thigh is swollen and exquisitely tender. He will not move his leg. You also note several other bruises on the child's right arm. Radiographs are taken (Figure 16–1).

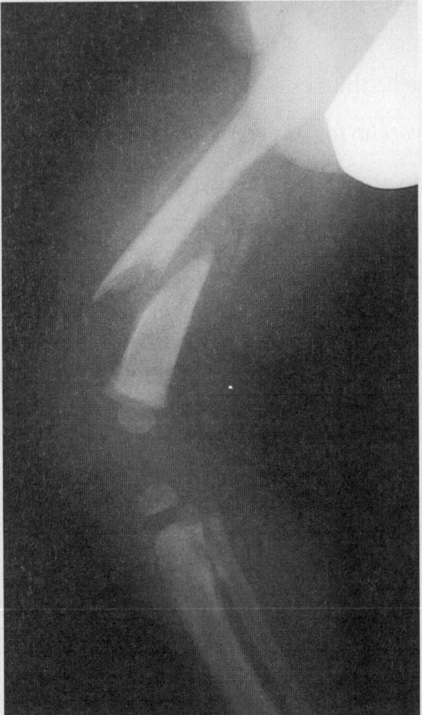

Figure 16–1. Spiral femur and proximal tibia fracture. Note displaced spiral femur fracture with faint callus formation and more solid (older) periosteal reaction of the proximal tibia. Child abuse is likely because there are 2 injuries that occurred at different times and no treatment was obtained. (Reproduced, with permission, from Knoop KJ, Stack LB, Storrow AB, et al. *Atlas of Emergency Medicine*. 3rd ed. New York, NY: McGraw-Hill; 2009:Fig. 15-26. Photo contributor: Alan E. Oestreich, MD.)

- ▶ What is the most likely diagnosis?
- ▶ What is your next diagnostic step?

ANSWERS TO CASE 16:
Child Abuse

Summary: An 8-month-old boy presents with a 48-hour history of irritability and left thigh swelling. The parents at first deny any recent trauma but then recall the child falling from his changing table 2 days prior. On examination, the thigh is swollen and the child is irritable. You also note bruising of the right upper extremity. Radiographs of the left femur reveal a spiral fracture and an older proximal tibia fracture.

- **Most likely diagnosis:** Physical abuse.
- **Next step:** Skeletal survey.

ANALYSIS

Objectives

1. Recognize orthopaedic injuries associated with child abuse.
2. Know the proper workup for suspected child maltreatment.
3. Understand the importance of reporting suspected child abuse.

Considerations

The proposed mechanism of injury, a fall from a changing table only 3 feet off the ground, is unlikely to cause a femur fracture. Furthermore, the **spiral nature** of the fracture is inconsistent with the mother's story, as these fractures typically result from twisting injuries and not simple falls. Additional concerns include the bruising observed on the child's right upper extremity, the older proximal tibia fracture, and the mother's delay in seeking medical attention for 2 days from the initial accident. **Many pediatricians who frequently encounter child abuse advocate for clinicians to assume that any long bone fracture in a child under 3 years of age is child abuse until proven otherwise.** Therefore, it is imperative that after a complete skeletal survey of this child to assess for other bony injuries, this case be reported to children's protective services for suspected abuse.

APPROACH TO:
Child Abuse

DEFINITIONS

SKELETAL SURVEY: Dedicated radiographs of every anatomic region of the body used to look for signs of previous and/or acute injuries when abuse is suspected. Anteroposterior (AP) and lateral images of the axial skeleton and frontal projections of each extremity are included.

CHILDREN'S PROTECTIVE SERVICES: Local governmental agency responsible for conducting civil investigations of children alleged to have been abused or neglected.

THE CHILD ABUSE PREVENTION AND TREATMENT ACT: Defines child abuse as "at a minimum, any act or failure to act resulting in imminent risk of serious harm, death, serious physical or emotional harm, sexual abuse, or exploitation of a child by a parent or caretaker who is responsible for the child's welfare."

CLINICAL APPROACH

Each year more than 1 million children are the victims of abuse or neglect, and more than 1200 of them die as a result of the abuse. Although health care providers are mandated to report all cases of suspected abuse as dictated by civil statutes, the diagnosis is rarely straightforward. It often requires consideration of sociobehavioral factors and clinical findings. Fractures are the second most common presentation of physical abuse after skin lesions. It is therefore pivotal that the orthopaedist understand the signs of nonaccidental trauma to increase the likelihood of recognition and proper management.

General Considerations

A thorough history and complete general and orthopaedic examination is necessary in cases of suspected child abuse. An abused child may be either **overly passive** or **overly aggressive.** Irritability, hyperactivity, and destructive behavior may all be observed on exam. Age-appropriate questions must be asked. Leading questions should be avoided. The parents' behavior may also provide clues regarding whether this is a case of abuse. **Red flags** include a vague history that lacks detail, providing an injury mechanism inconsistent with the physical findings, or parents who are hostile or too casual during questioning (Table 16–1).

Table 16–1 • CONCERNING FEATURES THAT MAY BE ASSOCIATED WITH CHILD ABUSE
Evolving or absent history about injury
Delay in seeking care for concerning condition
Unusual interactions between child and parent
Overly compliant child with painful medical procedures
Overly affectionate behavior from child to medical staff
Protective of abusing parent
Parental substance abuse or intoxication
Poor self-esteem in parent
History of abuse in parent's childhood
History of domestic violence
Loss of control of parent triggered by child's behavior

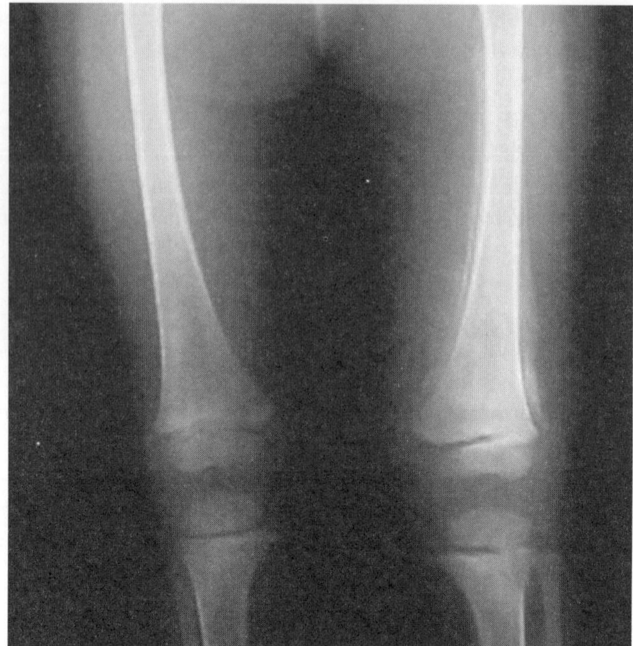

Figure 16–2. Classic metaphyseal lesions of the distal left femur and proximal left tibia in a 27-month-old child. (Reproduced, with permission, from Tintinalli J, et al. *Tintinalli's Emergency Medicine: A Comprehensive Study Guide*. 7th ed. New York, NY: McGraw-Hill; 2010:Fig. 290-4.)

Musculoskeletal Features

Approximately one third of children who are victims of nonaccidental trauma require orthopaedic care, with fractures most common in younger children due to the vulnerability of their developing skeletons and defenselessness. Although multiple fractures in various stages of healing are very common in abused children, many will present with only 1 fracture.

Long bone (femur or humerus) fractures are the most commonly fractured bones in child abuse. Certain types, such as the midshaft spiral femur fracture, were once thought of as indicative of nonaccidental trauma. **However, studies have found that no specific fracture pattern in the femur is pathognomonic of abuse and that all patterns can be observed.** Fractures of the hands, feet, and clavicle are uncommon in abuse, as are physeal fractures. The lone exception is transphyseal fractures of the distal humerus in children less than 1 year old. Metaphyseal fractures are less common than diaphyseal injuries, but are very concerning for physical abuse (Figure 16–2).

DIFFERENTIAL DIAGNOSIS AND WORKUP OF SUSPECTED ABUSE

Any condition that can lead to bruising, fracture, or periosteal changes must be considered in the differential diagnosis of child abuse. Biomechanical testing for metabolic markers for bone disease (ie, calcium, phosphate, alkaline phosphate, copper, parathyroid hormone, and 25-hydroxyvitamin D) should be performed. **Osteogenesis imperfecta** may present like nonaccidental trauma and should also be investigated with genetic testing and biochemical analysis. When bruising is present, a complete blood count, differential blood count, and coagulation studies must be performed. Occasionally, children with **leukemia, hemophilia,** or other hematologic disorders are brought in for suspected abuse due to multiple bruises. Other rare pediatric conditions that can present like abuse include **Caffey disease, rickets,** and **congenital syphilis.** It is important to note that the practitioner must also always consider accidental trauma and normal radiographic variants as potential causes of the clinical presentation of a patient for whom abuse is suspected.

A skeletal survey should be used in addition to imaging of obvious deformities to detect other acute or healed fractures in potentially abused children. **The American Academy of Pediatrics Section on Radiology recommends a mandatory survey in all cases of suspected abuse in children less than 2 years of age. In those between 2 and 5 years of age, a skeletal survey should be done based on clinical indications. In children older than 5 years, the skeletal survey has minimal value.** Radionuclide bone scanning for detection of physical abuse is controversial and should be reserved for use when skeletal surveys are negative despite high suspicion for abuse. Additionally, a repeat skeletal survey 2 weeks after initial presentation may reveal injuries not evident in the initial survey in cases with high suspicion for abuse.

MANAGEMENT

In most states, physicians are required to report suspected cases of child abuse based on reasonable suspicion of nonaccidental trauma or maltreatment. **Reporters are immune from civil and criminal liability, even if it is ultimately determined that no abuse has occurred.**

The treatment of abuse fractures is identical to those incurred accidentally and are typically amenable to closed, nonoperative treatment. However, the orthopaedic management of the abused child is only one component of treatment, and a team-oriented approach is essential. This includes pediatricians, other subspecialists, and social workers.

When the orthopaedist is the first physician to see a potentially abused child, communication with the nearby emergency department or local child abuse agency must be swiftly initiated. Hospital admission is often required to care for the acute injuries and to provide a safe environment where a full workup can be conducted.

COMPREHENSION QUESTIONS

16.1 A 3-year-old girl presents shortly after a right arm injury. The patient's father reports that he was playing with his daughter by swinging the girl in circles while holding on to her arms when she suddenly complained of pain in the left arm. The patient immediately held the injured arm close to her body with the help of her noninjured arm. Which of the following is most accurate regarding this injury?

A. Represents child abuse

B. Requires a skeletal survey

C. Is a common accidental injury

D. Is inconsistent with the described mechanism of injury

16.2 Osteogenesis imperfecta (OI) may present similarly to child maltreatment. However, there are features of OI that may help differentiate the 2, including blue sclera and osteopenia. Which of the following is another distinguishing feature?

A. Polydactyly

B. Patent foramen ovale

C. Multiple fractures in the setting of minimal trauma

D. Dental involvement

16.3 The pediatrician of a 2-year-old girl orders a skeletal survey because of suspected abuse. The imaging identifies multiple fractures, including the right humerus, left tibia, and right femur. Because it is important to distinguish between those that are acute versus those that are older and already healing, the pediatrician calls her colleagues in the Orthopaedics Department, who reviews with her the age-based features of fracture healing. At what point does new periosteal bone formation become apparent on plain radiographs?

A. 4 to 14 days

B. 1 to 2 months

C. 1 year

D. Within hours

ANSWERS

16.1 **C.** This case represents a nursemaid's elbow, which is caused by a traction force on an outstretched arm. This is a common accidental injury in which the patient presents with a slightly flexed and pronated arm. The injury is reduced by flexion and supination of the patient's forearm with concurrent pressure over the radial head. A successful reduction should return the patient to full use of the arm immediately.

16.2 **D.** Multiple medical conditions can present similarly to nonaccidental trauma, including OI. This autosomal dominant genetic disease often presents with multiple fractures in the setting of minimal trauma. However, distinguishing features include osteopenia, blue sclera, family history, and dental involvement. Polydactyly and a patent foramen ovale are not typical features of OI.

16.3 **A.** To estimate the age of a fracture, it is important to know the age-dependent radiographic features of healing fractures. Listed below is a timeline for the appearance of various radiographic features:

Days 2 to 10: Soft tissue swelling subsides

Days 4 to 14: New periosteal bone formation becomes apparent

Days 10 to 21: Loss of definition of fracture line, presence of soft callus

Days 14 to 42: Presence of hard callus

Months 3 to 12: Fracture remodeling

CLINICAL PEARLS

- Although multiple fractures in various stages of healing are very common in abused children, many will present with only 1 fracture.
- Any condition that can lead to bruising, fracture, or periosteal changes must be considered in the differential diagnosis of child abuse.
- The American Academy of Pediatrics Section on Radiology recommends a mandatory survey in all cases of suspected abuse in children less than 2 years of age.
- A team-oriented approach to the abused child is crucial and involves pediatricians, subspecialists, and social workers.

REFERENCES

Jayakumar P, Ramachandran M. Orthopaedic aspects of paediatric non-accidental injury. *J Bone Joint Surg Br*. 2010;92:189-195.

Kocher MS, Kasser JA. Orthopaedic aspects of child abuse. *J Am Acad Orthop Surg*. 2000;8:10-20.

CASE 17

A 13-year-old African American male patient presents to the emergency department with pain in his left knee after falling on his side during a soccer game. He is unable to ambulate and is in significant discomfort. His mother states that he has been experiencing several weeks of pain in his left knee before his fall, but x-rays and repeated exams of his knee at his primary care physician's office had failed to demonstrate any pathology. The patient has no known past medical history. He denies fevers, chills, and recent illness, and he recalls no history of traumatic injury to his left lower extremity. On examination, the child is obese and is comfortable after administration of appropriate analgesia. His left lower extremity is held in slight external rotation. His knee is without effusion and has a full range of painless motion. Motion at the hip, however, is painful, especially with passive internal/external rotation. He is neurovascularly intact throughout his bilateral extremities. Exam of the right lower extremity is unremarkable. Laboratory studies are significant for a thyroid-stimulating hormone (TSH) level of 7.3 mIU/mL (normal 0.6-5.5 mIU/mL). An anteroposterior (AP) pelvis and bilateral frog-leg lateral views are shown in Figures 17–1 and 17–2, respectively.

- ▶ What is the most likely diagnosis?
- ▶ What aspects of this patient's history put him at risk for this injury?
- ▶ What is the next step in the management of this patient?

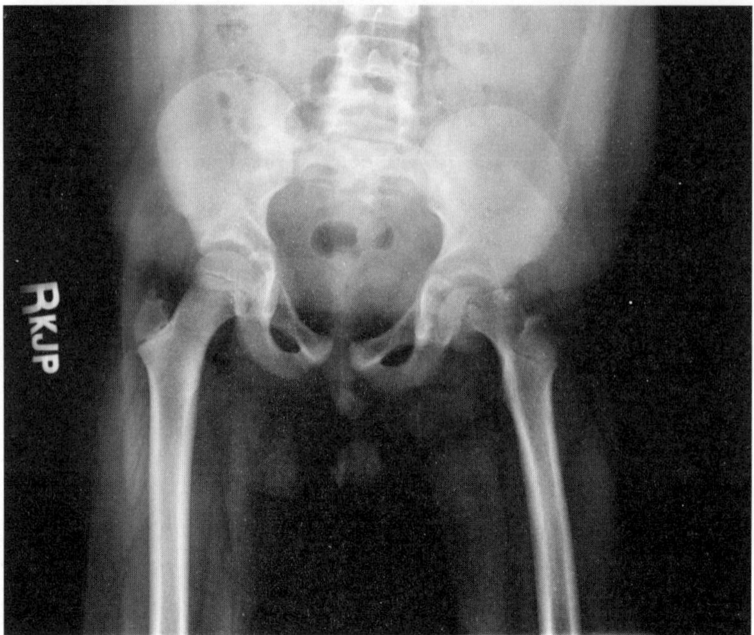

Figure 17–1. AP radiograph of the pelvis.

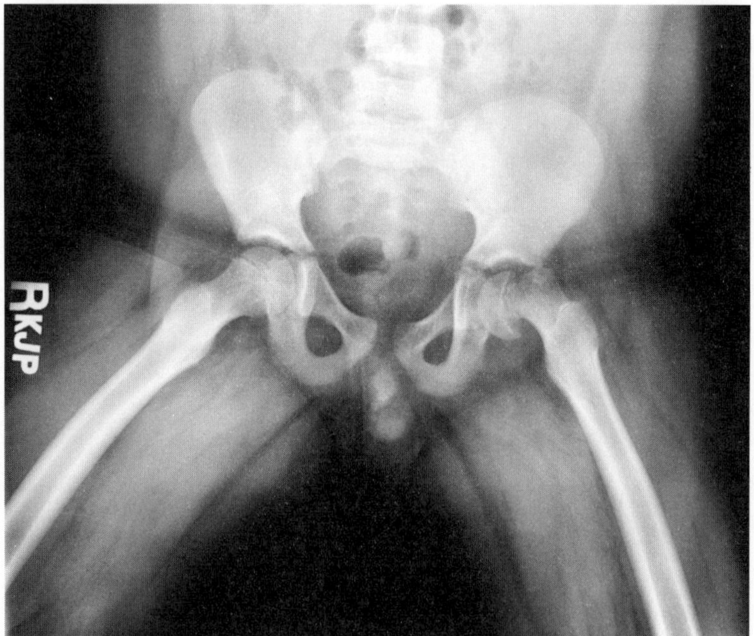

Figure 17–2. Frog-leg lateral radiograph of the pelvis.

ANSWERS TO CASE 17: Slipped Capital Femoral Epiphysis (SCFE)

Summary: A 13-year-old obese, African American male presents with several weeks of left lower extremity pain, exacerbated by a recent fall. Exam demonstrates left hip pathology that is referred to the knee. Additionally, the patient has previously undiagnosed hypothyroidism.

- **Most likely diagnosis:** Left slipped capital femoral epiphysis.
- **Historical risk factors:** Obesity, male, African American, adolescence, with concomitant endocrinopathy (hypothyroidism).
- **Next appropriate step:** Percutaneous screw fixation.

ANALYSIS

Objectives

1. Recognize the presentation of SCFE.
2. Understand the workup for SCFE and patient population.
3. Be familiar with the treatment for SCFE and its potential long-term complications.

Considerations

This is an overweight, African American male adolescent with a history of pain in his left knee. Up to 46% of patients with SCFE will present initially with complaints of distal thigh or knee pain. It is essential to recognize that hip pathology can often be referred to the distal thigh or knee. Complaints of knee pain should warrant complete and thorough physical exam, and typically radiographic evaluation, of the ipsilateral hip. Patients with SCFE typically present with an externally rotated, subtly foreshortened lower extremity, with a markedly decrease range of painful internal rotation.

Hip x-rays should include, at a minimum, an AP view of the pelvis as well as lateral views of each femoral head and neck, typically achieved through a frog-leg lateral view. Although this patient's SCFE is clearly visible on both AP and lateral films, early SCFE lesions are often subtle and are generally apparent on lateral views before they are obvious on the AP.

Patients with newly diagnosed SCFE lesions should be immediately made non-weightbearing on the effected extremity. Complete workup for SCFE secondary to underlying medical conditions should be performed, including initial laboratory testing for TSH, a complete metabolic panel, and a complete blood count. Patients undergoing potential operative fixation should always receive blood type and screening and coagulation (prothrombin time/partial thromboplastin time) studies.

APPROACH TO:
Slipped Capital Femoral Epiphysis (SCFE)

DEFINITIONS

OSTEONECROSIS: The cellular death of bone, typically resulting from a prolonged disruption of blood supply.

STABLE SCFE: Defined simply by the patient's ability to ambulate, even with crutch assistance. Less than 10% of patients with a stable SCFE develop osteonecrosis.

UNSTABLE SCFE: Defined as SCFE in patients who are unable to ambulate. These patients have a high incidence of osteonecrosis, upward of 50%.

CLINICAL APPROACH

SCFE (often pronounced "skiffy") is a disorder of **adolescence** in which a fracture—or, technically, a disruption—occurs through the growth plate of the femoral head. The epiphysis, or region of developing bone above the growth plate (physis), is therefore mobile and tends to "slip" from the neck of the femur under the repetitive loading of body weight. The "slipping" process is actually a misnomer, however, as **it is not technically the epiphysis that slips from the femur, but rather the femur that displaces from the anatomically stable epiphysis.**

Epidemiology

SCFE typically affects children between **10 and 17 years of age,** occurring at an average of 13.4 years for boys and 12.2 years for girls. Its prevalence in the United States is 10 in 100,000 people annually. SCFE has a slight male-to-female predominance of 3:2 and occurs at increased incidences of 2.2 in patients of African ancestry, 4.5 in those of Pacific Islander ancestry, and 0.1 for North African and Indian subcontinental ancestry, versus 1.0 for white controls. Racial differences are closely related to average adolescent body weights.

Pathogenesis

As stated, SCFE is a failure of the physis, with separation of the epiphysis from the proximal femoral metaphysis. Biomechanical factors such as obesity, femoral retroversion (increased posterior angulation of the femoral neck), and increased physeal obliquity (an increasingly angulated growth plate that is vulnerable to shearing forces when body weight is loaded) all contribute to physeal weakening. In younger children, the physis is protected by a perichondral ring that resists shearing forces. This protective ring weakens in adolescence, however, and increases the risk of SCFE. SCFE occurs during puberty, when rapid cellular expansion is occurring at the **physeal zone of hypertrophy.** Failure is thought to occur at this slightly weakened zone of rapid, immature expansion. Finally, hormonal and endocrine changes are associated with SCFE, but the mechanisms by which they contribute to the disease process are not fully understood. There are data to show that **hypothyroidism, growth hormone supplementation, and hypogonadism increase one's risk of SCFE.**

Radiology

The direction of a typical "slip" causes the femur to fall into **varus, extension, and external rotation.** Typically, the epiphysis tends to move **posteriorly first,** a translation that is **most apparent on frog-leg lateral views.** With the femurs externally rotated, abducted, and flexed, an unobstructed lateral view of the femoral neck shows early posterior displacement of the epiphysis. For this reason, frog-leg lateral images are considered most sensitive for the diagnosis.

Several radiographic measurements can be made to diagnose and grade SCFE. The Klein line, or a line drawn parallel to the superior femoral neck, should intersect the epiphysis in normal individuals. In patients with advanced slips, however, the Klein line contacts the edge of, or is superior to, the migrating epiphysis. The metaphyseal blanch sign of Steel is a blurring of the proximal femoral metaphysis that may be visualized on an AP pelvis film. This is caused by overlapping of the normal metaphysis with the posteriorly displaced epiphysis.

CLASSIFICATION

Although several classification schemes exist, the most practical and prognostically relevant classification divides the disease into stable and unstable SCFE. SCFE stability is defined simply by whether or not the patient is able to tolerate weightbearing on the affected extremity. Stability includes those who are able to partially weight bear with crutches. Patients with unstable SCFE are so uncomfortable with movement of the hip that they refuse to ambulate. **Up to 50% of patients with unstable SCFE have an incidence of osteonecrosis of the femoral head.**

TREATMENT

Intervention should occur as soon as the diagnosis is made. For patients with mild or moderate stable disease, **in situ fixation is the method of choice.** Attempts to forcefully reduce the deformity are not recommended; however, sometimes the slip will spontaneously reduce or improve when the patient is positioned for surgery. Regardless, the goal or treatment is to stabilize the slipped epiphysis, as remodeling often occurs and patients can tolerate a certain degree of residual external rotation. **Single-screw percutaneous fixation is the most common mode of treatment,** although double-screw fixation techniques are sometimes performed. For single-screw fixation, the goal is to place the screw through the middle of the epiphysis and perpendicular to the growth plate. Patients with stable slips are typically allowed to bear weight after fixation. Bilateral fixation may be indicated in patients with underlying endocrinopathies, even if the contralateral hip is asymptomatic and without radiographic evidence of the disease. **Although controversial, some authors also advocate for the prophylactic pinning of the contralateral hip in children less than 10 years of age with unilateral SCFE or in those with open triradiate cartilage.** The impetus behind prophylactic fixation of the unaffected hip stems from the elevated rates at which young children and patients with endocrinopathies develop bilateral disease.

In patients with unstable SCFE, there is significant controversy over whether reduction manipulations should be employed versus in situ fixation, whether capsulotomy or arthrocentesis should be performed versus no joint decompression, and whether single- versus multiple-screw fixation techniques should be used. Most surgeons advocate relatively urgent treatment in these patients, as greater than 24 hours between acute injury and fixation may be associated with increased risk of osteonecrosis. A common treatment regimen for unstable SCFE involves single-screw fixation after joint aspiration to relieve intracapsular pressure and promote vascular perfusion. These patients are generally made nonweightbearing with crutches for 6 to 8 weeks postoperatively.

Complications

Osteonecrosis is a severe, debilitating complication, for which risk is increased with unstable SCFE, delayed surgical fixation of acute unstable SCFE, attempted reduction manipulations, and improper placement of pins, specifically in the posterior-superior femoral neck, leading to disruption of vasculature. Osteonecrosis is initially managed with nonweightbearing, nonsteroidal anti-inflammatory drugs, and gentle range-of-motion exercises. When severe, however, reconstructive intervention may be necessary. Slip progression after initial fixation is another potential complication that, fortunately, occurs in only 1% to 2% of patients after single-screw fixation. Although double-screw fixation may theoretically reduce this complication, elevated potential risks of osteonecrosis with multiple-screw fixation favors single-screw techniques for most surgeons.

COMPREHENSION QUESTIONS

17.1 A 13-year-old boy is referred to your office with a right-sided SCFE after workup over several weeks by his pediatrician for insidious right knee pain. On exam, he has obligatory external rotation with hip flexion and is refusing to bear weight. His TSH is 8.5 mIU/mL. Which of the following is the most appropriate treatment for this patient?

A. Percutaneous pinning of the right hip

B. Open reduction and capsulotomy of the right hip with plate and screw fixation

C. Percutaneous pinning of the left hip

D. Percutaneous pinning of bilateral hips

E. Administration of levothyroxine with follow-up TSH levels in outpatient setting and bed rest until resolution of pain

17.2 Through which of the following physeal zones does the disruption in SCFE typically occur?

A. Reserve zone

B. Proliferative zone

C. Hypertrophic zone

D. Zone of provisional calcification

17.3 An 8-year-old obese girl of Pacific Island ancestry is referred to your office for a right-sided unstable SCFE lesion after a fall while playing kick-ball. She had no previous pain in this extremity. On examination, she has an externally rotated right lower extremity that is severely painful with passive range of motion. Frog-leg lateral x-rays show a displaced right SCFE lesion with a normal-appearing left femoral head. Which of the following factors is indication to prophylactically fix this patient's *left* hip?

A. Obesity

B. Age

C. Unstable nature of the right-sided SCFE

D. Acute, traumatic right-sided SCFE without preexisting symptoms

E. Pacific Island ancestry

ANSWERS

17.1 **D.** Bilateral percutaneous screw fixation is appropriate in this patient due to the patient's history of undiagnosed hypothyroidism. His right hip, most urgently, requires fixation, but the presence of endocrinopathy is a generally accepted indication for additional fixation of the unaffected contralateral side. Management of hypothyroidism is important in this patient, but bed rest is generally an unsuitable treatment for SCFE.

17.2 **C.** SCFE classically occurs through the zone of hypertrophy, a region of rapid cellular expansion during the adolescent growth spurt that is especially vulnerable to shearing injury.

17.3 **B.** Indications to prophylactically fix the contralateral hip in a patient with a unilateral SCFE lesion are limited to patients with obvious endocrinopathies and those younger than 10 years of age or with open triradiate cartilage. This patient's age is reason enough to strongly consider preemptively pinning the left hip. Her obesity and ethnicity are risk factors for SCFE; however, they are not indications for prophylactic fixation. The unstable and acute nature of her SCFE lesions does not necessarily correlate with a need for prophylactic intervention.

CLINICAL PEARLS

- Remember that hip pathology can often be referred to the distal thigh or knee and thus a complete exam of both joints is essential. Almost 50% of SCFE patients present with distal thigh or knee pain.
- Percutaneous single-screw in situ fixation is the treatment of choice for SCFE.
- Prophylactic fixation of the contralateral hip, regardless of whether or not it is symptomatic, is generally advocated in patients with SCFE secondary to endocrinopathies or in SCFE patients younger than 10 years at presentation. Admittedly, this is controversial.

REFERENCES

Aronsson DD, Loder RT, Breur GJ, Weinstein SL. Slipped capital femoral epiphysis: current concepts. *J Am Acad Orthop Surg*. 2006;14:666-679.

Flynn, JM, ed. Hip, pelvis, and femur disorders: pediatrics. In: *Orthopaedic Knowledge Update: Ten*. Rosemont, IL: American Academy of Orthopaedic Surgeons; 2011:739-752.

CASE 18

A young couple's 14-month-old daughter is referred to the pediatric orthopaedic clinic by their general pediatrician because of a limp they noticed when their child ambulates. The parents cannot recall an inciting event or specific day that this began and deny any recent trauma. They state that their daughter does not appear to be in pain when she walks and has had no recent illnesses or sick contacts. The child is in good health and has met all developmental milestones up to this point, including taking her first steps at 9 months and walking independently at 12 months. Of note, this is the parent's first child. Although the pregnancy was uncomplicated, the child was ultimately delivered at full term via cesarean section as a result of a breech presentation. The parents also state that ultrasonography for "some type of hip problem" was performed at 5 weeks of age and was normal. On exam, the left leg appears shorter than the right. Additionally, a greater degree of hip abduction is noted on the right versus the left.

- ▶ What is the most likely diagnosis?
- ▶ What is the next step in workup?
- ▶ What is the appropriate treatment of this condition?
- ▶ What physical exam maneuvers are used to diagnose this condition in newborns?

ANSWERS TO CASE 18:

Developmental Dysplasia of the Hip

Summary: An otherwise healthy 14-month-old girl is brought to the clinic by her parents due to a limp. On exam, the left hip has decreased abduction compared with the right, and the left leg is shorter than the right. The parents state that this is their first child and that she was born full term via cesarean section as a result of a breech presentation. She has met all developmental milestones to this point. They also recall an ultrasound for "some type of hip problem" performed at 5 weeks of age that was negative.

- **Most likely diagnosis:** Developmental dysplasia of the left hip (DDH).
- **Next step in workup:** Anteroposterior (AP) radiograph of the pelvis.
- **Treatment:** Closed reduction of the left hip under general anesthesia followed by spica cast placement.
- **Diagnostic maneuvers in the newborn:** Ortolani and Barlow maneuvers.

ANALYSIS

Objectives

1. Understand the "classic" history and presentation of DDH.
2. Know the diagnostic approach to DDH.
3. Understand treatment and how it differs based on patient's age.
4. Appreciate the complications associated with DDH.

Considerations

This 14-month-old child has a constellation of findings concerning for left hip pathology. The differential diagnosis of a limp in this age group must be considered here and includes both infectious and noninfectious causes. The former includes conditions such as a septic hip or osteomyelitis, whereas the latter includes transient synovitis, trauma, and DDH. Per the patient's family, the patient has had no recent illness or been exposed to any sick contacts, making infectious causes and transient synovitis unlikely. The parents also deny any recent trauma. When entertaining the diagnosis of DDH in this patient, the birth history is significant, as DDH risk factors include female sex, breech presentation, and first-born status; this patient has all of these. The parents also state that an ultrasound done when their daughter was 5 weeks old, presumably to evaluate for DDH, was negative. This should not deter the orthopaedist from a diagnosis of DDH, as diagnosis can be delayed for multiple reasons, including late development of the pathologic changes associated with it. The same can be said for negative physical exam findings for DDH during the initial newborn screening, which is performed on all infants and includes the Ortolani and Barlow tests. Because of the significant long-term complications of DDH, a complete workup must ensue, with treatment initiated as soon as possible.

APPROACH TO:
Developmental Dysplasia of the Hip

DEFINITIONS

DEVELOPMENTAL DYSPLASIA OF THE HIP: Term describing a spectrum of developmental abnormalities of the hip joint that lead to subluxation and dislocation, predisposing patients to the development of early degenerative changes.

TRENDELENBURG GAIT: An abnormal gait associated with hip abductor weakness (ie, gluteus medius). It is characterized by the dropping of the pelvis on the unaffected side of the body at the time of heelstrike on the affected side. This lasts until heelstrike on the unaffected side, at which time lateral protrusion of the affected hip occurs. This gait can be seen in children with DDH.

GALEAZZI TEST: Test to evaluate for DDH that is performed by flexing the infant's knees in the supine position so that the ankles touch the buttocks (Figure 18–1).

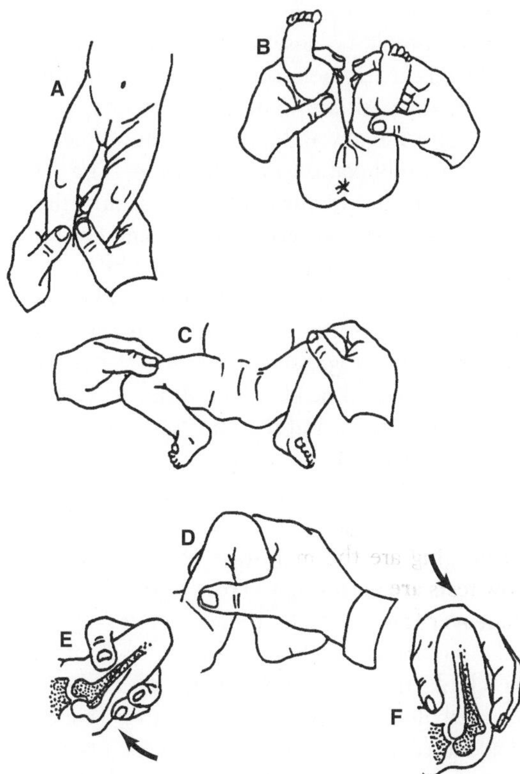

Figure 18–1. Clinical examination of developmental dislocation of the hip. In all pictures, the child's left hip is the abnormal side. (**A**) Asymmetric skin folds; (**B**) Galeazzi test; (**C**) limitation of abduction; (**D, E, F**) Ortolani and Barlow tests (see text). (Reproduced, with permission, from Skinner HB. *Current Diagnosis & Treatment in Orthopedics*. 4th ed. New York, NY: McGraw-Hill; 2006:Fig. 11-4.)

If the knees are not level, the test is considered positive and indicates a possible congenital hip malformation. The test is also known as the **Allis sign.**

ORTOLANI AND BARLOW SIGNS: Two maneuvers used to evaluate for DDH. The Ortolani exam is a reduction maneuver that restores normal hip joint anatomy, whereas the Barlow exam is a provocative maneuver that detects an unstable hip (Figure 18–1). These tests may be negative beginning at 3 months of age, despite DDH being present, due to the development of soft-tissue contractures.

CLINICAL APPROACH

Etiology

DDH is the most common orthopaedic abnormality in newborns and is the result of a disruption in the normal relationship between the acetabulum and femoral head. The incidence of DDH is reported anywhere from 1 to more than 35 per 1000 live births. DDH is most common in Native Americans and is also seen in whites. It is rare in African Americans. **It is considered a multifactorial trait and is more common in females (females comprise ~80% of cases), firstborn infants, and those born in the breech presentation.** The risk for DDH is increased 12-fold if a first-degree relative has it.

The neonatal hip is unstable because of the undeveloped muscle, ligamentous laxity, and easily deformed cartilaginous surfaces comprising the joint. This relative instability, coupled with any positioning in utero that may stretch the hip capsule (as seen with the excessive flexion and adduction in a breech presentation), will predispose the neonate to subluxation or dislocation. **The left hip is more frequently involved because the left femur is adducted against the mother's lumbosacral spine when in the left occiput anterior (most common) intrauterine position.** Instability results as less femoral epiphysis is contained by the acetabulum.

The femoral head displaces posteriorly and superiorly because of the pull of the gluteal and hip flexor muscles. When subluxated, this causes an asymmetric pressure that leads to a dysplastic, progressive flattening of the posterior and superior acetabular rim and medial femoral head. When dislocated, the normal, concentric motion seen at the hip joint is lost, and the joint surfaces become dysplastic with a deformed and shallow configuration.

Diagnosis

Physical exam and imaging are the mainstays of diagnosis. **In the newborn, the Ortolani and Barlow tests are performed as part of the standard newborn screens.** In the Ortolani maneuver (Figure 18–1), the examiner will feel the dislocated hip reduce as the flexed hip is abducted while the greater trochanter is lifted anteriorly. A positive sign is a "clunk" that is often heard and felt as the femoral head reduces anteriorly into the acetabulum. In the Barlow maneuver (Figure 18–1), the infant's thigh is flexed and adducted as the examiner applies a posteriorly directed pressure. It is positive if the hip dislocates from this. Another diagnostic maneuver is the **Galeazzi test,** which identifies a dislocated hip via a difference in knee levels when the patient's knees are flexed in the supine position so that the ankles touch the buttocks. This test can be used for diagnosis in older patients, unlike the Ortolani and Barlow maneuvers, which are rarely helpful after 3 months of age because of the development of soft-tissue contractures. Other physical exam findings consistent with DDH include asymmetric or limited abduction of the dysplastic hip (approximately < 70 degrees from the midline), asymmetric thigh folds and buttock creases, and leg length discrepancies in which the shorter leg is indicative of dysplasia. Once a child can walk, a Trendelenburg gait may be observed, as may a leg length discrepancy with asymmetric toe-walking on the affected side. A waddling, wide-based limp may suggest bilaterally dislocated hips.

Radiography and ultrasonography are used for confirming the diagnosis. **In the newborn, ultrasound is very sensitive and provides a dynamic view of the cartilaginous femoral head and acetabulum. However, it should be used only after 4 to 6 weeks of age because of the initial hip laxity associated with birth and concern for overdiagnosis.** Furthermore, imaging should only be used on infants with a risk factor or physical findings concerning for DDH. Universal screening of newborns with ultrasound is not cost effective and would also lead to overdiagnosis. **Plain radiographs cannot distinguish the cartilaginous components of the hip joint and should therefore only be performed when children are at least 4 to 6 months old, which is when the ossific nucleus of the femoral head can be seen on radiographs (it appears on ultrasonographic images at 12 weeks).** Several lines and angles can be drawn on AP pelvic radiographs to identify DDH (Figure 18–2).

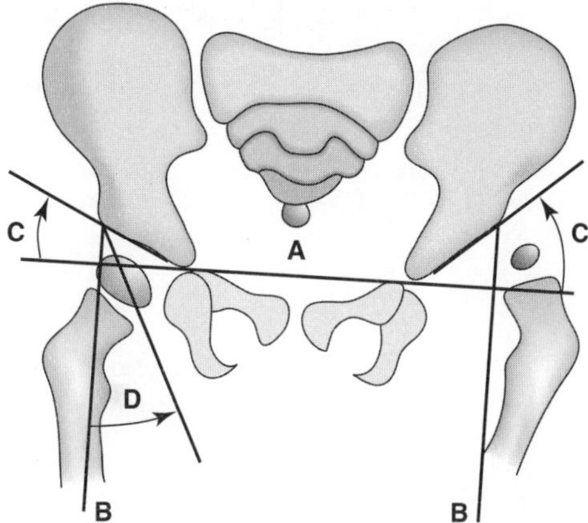

Figure 18–2. Lines drawn for measurement in developmental dysplasia of the hip. In the figure, the patient's left hip (on the right of the figure) is the subluxated one. (A) Hilgenreiner line is a horizontal line of the pelvis, drawn between the triradiate cartilages. The proximal femoral ossification center should be below this line. (B) Perkins line is a vertical line (perpendicular to Hilgenreiner line) drawn down from the lateral edge of the acetabulum. The femoral head ossification center, as well as the medial beak of the proximal metaphysis, should fall medial to this line. (C) The acetabular index is the angle between Hilgenreiner line and a line joining the acetabular center (triradiate) with the acetabular edge as it intersects Perkins line. It measures acetabular depth and should be below 30 degrees by 1 year of age and below 25 degrees by 2 years of age. (D) The center-edge angle is the angle between Perkins line and a line joining the lateral edge of the acetabulum with the center of the femoral head. It is a measure of lateral subluxation that becomes smaller as the hip subluxates laterally. Normal is 20 degrees or greater. (Reproduced, with permission, from Skinner HB. *Current Diagnosis & Treatment in Orthopedics.* 4th ed. New York, NY: McGraw-Hill; 2006:Fig. 11-5.)

TREATMENT

The goal of treatment for DDH is to reestablish a concentric relationship between the femoral head and acetabulum. It must begin as soon as the diagnosis is made to decrease the risk of aseptic necrosis and permanent dysplastic changes and depends on the patient's age. **From 0 to 6 months of age, treatment involves splinting the hips in flexion and abduction, which is achieved with a Pavlik harness** (Figure 18–3). In this position, a dislocated hip may spontaneously reduce over several weeks. The harness is used for 6 to 8 weeks or until normal hip anatomy develops. If concentric reduction is not achieved after 2 to 4 weeks, other treatment should be administered, such as closed reduction with spica casting. **Closed reduction under general anesthesia with spica cast application is a treatment option for ages 6 to 18 months,** as the infants are too large and strong to be controlled by a Pavlik harness. An arthrogram is used during this procedure to confirm a concentric reduction before cast application. The spica cast typically remains on for 12 weeks. If unable to obtain a concentric reduction at this time, open reduction techniques may be necessary. **After 18 months of age, the femoral head and acetabulum will have developed abnormally, and open reduction is required to maintain reduction.**

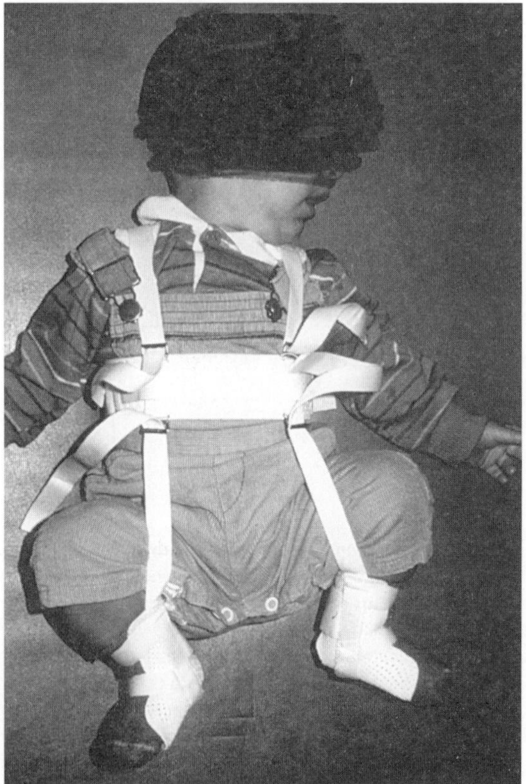

Figure 18–3. The Pavlik harness, a device used for treatment of hip dislocation, subluxation, and dysplasia. (Reproduced, with permission, from Skinner HB. *Current Diagnosis & Treatment in Orthopedics.* 4th ed. New York, NY: McGraw-Hill; 2006:Fig. 11-6.)

When DDH is untreated after 2 years of age, bony procedures involving either the acetabulum (ie, Salter, Pemberton, and Dega osteotomies), femur (ie, femoral varus derotational osteotomy), or both are required and attempt to create an environment conducive to remodeling to a more normal joint.

Complications

Ischemic necrosis is the most severe complication of DDH and can occur despite treatment. It results from compression of the vasculature supplying the capital femoral epiphysis and extreme direct pressure on the femoral head. Increased rates of ischemic necrosis are seen with forceful or excessive abduction, repeat surgery, and multiple attempts at closed reduction. Diagnosis is made based on radiographic findings, including the failure of the ossific nucleus of the femoral head to develop within 1 year after reduction, broadening of the femoral neck 1 year after reduction, and an increased density and fragmentation of an ossified femoral head.

COMPREHENSION QUESTIONS

18.1 A 15-month-old girl presents to your office for evaluation of her right hip. Which of the following is *most* associated with a diagnosis of developmental hip dysplasia?

A. Negative Barlow maneuver
B. Asymmetry of hip abduction
C. Negative Ortolani maneuver
D. Increased hip abduction

18.2 Which of the following is associated with developmental dysplasia of the hip?

A. Male sex
B. Vertex occiput posterior delivery
C. Polydactyly
D. First born

18.3 An otherwise healthy 5-month-old infant diagnosed with developmental dysplasia of the right hip is treated in a Pavlik harness with the hips flexed to 90 degrees and abduction of 50 degrees. An AP radiograph of the pelvis at 4-week follow-up shows that the hip remains dislocated. What is your next step in management?

A. Continue treatment as is; the hip should reduce within the next 2 weeks
B. Closed reduction with hip arthrogram and hip spica casting
C. Open reduction with femoral shortening osteotomy
D. Open reduction with pelvic acetabular osteotomy

ANSWERS

18.1 **B.** There are many maneuvers used to diagnose DDH, including the Ortolani and Barlow tests. However, they are rarely helpful after 3 months of age because of the development of soft-tissue contractures. Therefore, in older children one must rely on other exam findings. This includes asymmetric and limited hip abduction on the affected side.

18.2 **D.** Polydactyly is not associated with DDH. However, being the firstborn, female, and/or breech at birth are.

18.3 **B.** A 6-month-old infant who has failed treatment of DDH with a Pavlik harness after 2 to 4 weeks should be treated with closed reduction of the hip and spica casting. Continued treatment with the harness may lead to posterior acetabular erosion, a severe and devastating consequence. Both femoral and pelvic osteotomies are unnecessary in this patient and are often reserved for those 2 years of age and older with untreated DDH.

CLINICAL PEARLS

- DDH is considered a multifactorial trait and is more common in females (females comprise ~80% of cases), firstborn infants, and those born in the breech position.
- The risk for DDH is increased 12-fold if a first-degree relative has it.
- Diagnosis involves several exam maneuvers, including the Ortolani, Barlow, and Galeazzi tests.
- Plain radiographs cannot distinguish the cartilaginous components of the hip joint and should therefore only be performed when children are at least 4 to 6 months old, which is when the ossific nucleus of the femoral head can be seen on radiographs (it appears on ultrasonographic images at 12 weeks).
- The goal of treatment for DDH is to reestablish a concentric relationship between the femoral head and acetabulum.
- Treatment is age-dependent and includes use of a Pavlik harness when patients are <6 months old, closed reduction and spica casting when patients are 6 to 18 months old, and open reduction when patients are >18 months of age. After 24 months of age, reconstructive osteotomies involving the femur and/or acetabulum are often required.
- Ischemic necrosis is the most severe complication of DDH and can occur despite treatment.

REFERENCES

Guille JT, Pizzutillo PD, MacEwen GD. Development dysplasia of the hip from birth to six months. *J Am Acad Orthop Surg*. 2000;8:232-242.

Vitale MG, Skaggs DL. Developmental dysplasia of the hip from six months to four years of age. *J Am Acad Orthop Surg*. 2001;9:401-411.

CASE 19

A 56-year-old obese man presents to the emergency department for a 2-day history of progressive pain, swelling, and inability to bear weight on his right knee. The patient denies a history of recent trauma, prior knee surgery, sick contacts, or similar symptoms in the past. The patient states he has had fevers and chills over this time. His past medical history is notable for poorly controlled non–insulin-dependent diabetes and alcohol abuse. He is febrile with a temperature of 102.7°F and has an elevated heart rate of 110 beats/minute. His blood pressure is 160/95 mmHg, respiratory rate is 16 breaths/min, and oxygen saturation is 100% on room air. Examination of the knee demonstrates a swollen, erythematous, and diffusely tender right knee that is warm to palpation with painful and limited passive range of motion. Radiographs of the knee are negative for an acute fracture or dislocation but do show an effusion. The patient's laboratory values include a white blood cell (WBC) count of 19,100 cells/μL, erythrocyte sedimentation rate (ESR) of 48 mm/hr, and C-reactive protein (CRP) of 20 mg/L. Blood cultures are pending.

- ▶ What is the most likely diagnosis?
- ▶ What is your next diagnostic step?
- ▶ What is the most appropriate initial treatment for this patient?

ANSWERS TO CASE 19: Septic Knee

Summary: A 56-year-old man with medical history significant for obesity, diabetes, and alcohol abuse presents to the emergency department febrile and tachycardic with a 2-day history of right knee pain, swelling, and an inability to bear weight. He denies any trauma or previous right knee surgery. Radiographs show an effusion but no fracture or dislocation of his right knee. Additionally, his WBC, ESR, and CRP are all elevated. Blood cultures are pending.

- **Most likely diagnosis:** Septic arthritis. However, the differential diagnosis also includes crystalline arthropathies (ie, gout, pseudogout) inflammatory arthridites (ie, rheumatoid, psoriatic, and reactive arthritis), tumor, occult fracture, Lyme disease, and osteoarthritis.
- **Next diagnostic step:** Obtaining joint fluid aspirate for analysis, including a cell count with differential, Gram stain, glucose level, and crystal analysis.
- **Initial treatment:** Intravenous antibiotic therapy (after obtaining blood cultures and joint fluid aspirate) and operative irrigation and drainage.

ANALYSIS

Objectives

1. Be familiar with the multitude of diseases and conditions that can present similar to a septic joint.
2. Understand the appropriate workup for septic joint.
3. Know the treatment for a septic joint.

Considerations

This 56-year-old male developed a grossly swollen, erythematous, and painful right knee with an inability to bear weight over the prior 48 hours. He is also febrile to 102.7°F and tachycardic. His laboratory values are abnormal and are representative of an acute infectious or inflammatory process. Furthermore, the patient's history of poorly controlled diabetes makes him vulnerable to systemic infection. The suspicion for a septic right knee in this patient must be high. Given the history of alcohol abuse, gout is a possibility. However, his fevers and chills again favor an infectious cause of his knee pain and swelling. The patient has no history of inflammatory arthridities, such as rheumatoid arthritis, and this diagnosis is unlikely. A diagnosis of Lyme disease should always be considered in the differential for septic arthritis, but is more likely in the setting of a positive tick exposure history where the disease is endemic. Synovial fluid aspirate from this patient's right knee will likely be consistent with septic arthritis (Table 19–1), at which time intravenous antibiotics must be started and operative irrigation and drainage performed.

Table 19–1 • CLASSIFICATION OF SYNOVIAL FLUID IN AN ADULT KNEE JOINT

	Normal	Septic	Noninflammatory (ie, osteoarthritis)	Inflammatory (ie, rheumatoid arthritis)	Crystalline Arthropathy (ie, gout)
Volume (< 3.5 mL)	< 3.5	> 3.5	> 3.5	> 3.5	> 3.5
Viscosity	High	Mixed	High	Low	Low
Clarity	Clear	Opaque	Clear	Cloudy	Cloudy
Color	Colorless/ straw	Mixed	Straw/yellow	Yellow	Yellow
WBC/mm^3	< 200	> 50,000	< 2000	5000-75,000	5000-75,000
Polys (%)	< 25	> 70	< 25	50-70	50-70
Gram stain	Negative	Often positive	Negative	Negative	Negative, but crystal analysis will be positive

APPROACH TO: Septic Knee

DEFINITIONS

SEPTIC ARTHRITIS: An orthopaedic surgical emergency most commonly caused by bacterial seeding of a joint.

OSTEOMYELITIS: An infection of bone that can cause a septic arthritis or occur as a sequela of it.

ARTHROCENTESIS: Term describing the process by which synovial fluid is obtained; also referred to as joint aspiration.

CLINICAL APPROACH

Pathophysiology

Septic arthritis most commonly occurs in the knee, followed in frequency by the hip, elbow, ankle, and, least commonly, the sternoclavicular joint. It typically occurs after bacterial seeding of the joint, but can also be caused by fungi and viruses. The 3 predominant ways by which this occurs are through direct inoculation from trauma or surgery, contiguous spread from an adjacent osteomyelitis, or in the setting of bacteremia, which is more likely to arise in immunocompromised and hospitalized individuals who have recently undergone invasive procedures.

Septic arthritis causes rapid and irreversible articular hyaline cartilage destruction in the involved joint due to the release of proteolytic enzymes from the

Table 19–2 • COMMON ORGANISMS ASSOCIATED WITH SEPTIC ARTHRITIS

Organism	
Staphylococcus species	*Staphylococcus aureus* most common, seen in > 50% cases
Neisseria gonorrhea	Most common bacteria in otherwise healthy sexually active young adults
Salmonella	Seen in patients with sickle cell disease
Pseudomonas aeruginosa	Seen in patients with history of IV drug abuse
Eikenella corrodens	Seen in patients after human bite
Pasteurella multocida	Seen in patients after dog or cat bite
Streptococcus	More common in children than adults
Fungi, tuberculosis	Seen in immunocompromised patients

bacteria as well as host synovial cells, chondrocytes, and inflammatory cells. **Cartilage damage occurs within 8 hours of bacterial inoculation of the joint.** Certain bacteria produce proteolytic enzymes such as collagenase, elastase, hyaluronidase, lipase, and lipoproteinase, which lead to cartilage destruction. Bacterial virulence factors also contribute to cartilage destruction. An example is the coagulase produced by *Staphylococcus aureus*, the most common pathogen responsible for bacterial septic arthritis (Table 19–2). It is believed that the coagulase impairs intracapsular vascular supply due to small vessel thrombosis. The subsequent increased intracapsular pressure impedes an effective host immune response.

Clinical Presentation and Workup

Most patient's with septic arthritis present with a relatively acute onset of a hot, swollen, and tender joint with restricted and limited range of motion and weight-bearing. Systemic signs, such as fevers and chills, may also be present. In patients with concurrent bacteremia, they may appear toxic.

Radiographs are useful for ruling out other acute processes that can cause joint effusions, such as fractures and dislocation. Ultrasound is useful for confirming effusions in large joints such as the hip and for guiding aspirations. Magnetic resonance imaging will also show joint effusions and can also detect adjacent osteomyelitis.

Laboratory findings consistent with a septic joint include an elevated WBC with a left shift, ESR >30 mm/hr, and a CRP >5 mg/L. Although an elevated peripheral WBC count with increased number and percentage of polymorphonuclear leukocytes is *indicative* of infection, **the absence of an elevated WBC *does not* rule out infection.** Both ESR and CRP are acute-phase response markers that are elevated in the presence of infection and/or inflammation. CRP rises within a few hours of infection, reaching values up to 400 mg/L within 36 to 50 hours. It normalizes within 1 week after initiation of appropriate treatment. ESR rises within 2 days of the onset of infection and continues to rise for 3 to 5 days after appropriate antibiotic treatment is instituted. It normalizes after 3 to 4 weeks. Blood cultures should also be obtained, as bacteremia can cause septic arthritis.

Joint fluid aspiration is the gold standard for diagnosing a septic joint and helps guide antibiotic treatment and determine the need for operative intervention. **It should be analyzed for cell count with a differential, Gram stain, culture, glucose level, and crystal analysis (Table 19–1).**

TREATMENT AND OTHER CONSIDERATIONS

Only after obtaining blood cultures and a joint aspirate should broad-spectrum, empiric antibiotic therapy commence. With organism speciation and antibiotic sensitivities, more focused antibiotic treatment and duration can be determined. Depending on institutional availability, consultation with infectious disease specialists often proves invaluable in assisting with the management of these oftentimes complicated clinical cases. **Because of the rapid and irreversible cartilage damage, the diagnosis of septic arthritis requires emergent operative irrigation and drainage.**

A septic joint can quickly lead to bacteremia or a systemic inflammatory response syndrome (SIRS), particularly in the immunocompromised patient. Thus, beyond orthopaedic evaluation and intervention, it is essential as a practitioner to recognize the signs of systemic compromise (ie, tachycardia, tachypnea, hypotension, end organ damage) when evaluating a patient for a septic joint.

Bacterial septic arthritis has a reported mortality of approximately 10%. Patient outcome depends not only on the type of organism involved and the general health of the individual, but also on the speed and decisiveness with which the diagnosis is made.

COMPREHENSION QUESTIONS

19.1 A 70-year-old man with a history of osteoarthritis presents to the emergency department with a 2-day history of right knee pain and swelling. He has no history of similar symptoms. He denies trauma, fever, or pain in any other joints. On examination, he is afebrile. The right knee is swollen, erythematous, and painful with passive range of motion. The remainder of the examination is unremarkable. An arthrocentesis is performed, which shows purulent fluid and a leukocyte count of 90,000/μL with 90% neutrophils. No crystals are seen on polarized microscopy. Gram stain and culture are pending. What is the most likely cause of this patient's symptoms?

A. Gout

B. Pseudogout

C. Rheumatoid arthritis

D. Septic arthritis

19.2 A 40-year-old intravenous drug user presents to the emergency department with a 2-day history of right knee pain with associated swelling and erythema. The patient is febrile with a holosystolic murmur at the right lower sternal border. Complete blood count reveals a leukocytosis. Blood and synovial fluid cultures are sent, and broad-spectrum antibiotics are started. Synovial fluid analysis is pending. What is the most likely pathogen causing these symptoms?

A. *Neisseria gonorrhoeae*

B. *Staphylococcus aureus*

C. *Pseudomonas aeruginosa*

D. *Borrelia burgdorferi*

19.3 A 50-year-old woman diagnosed with rheumatoid arthritis many years ago presents to your clinic with acute on chronic left knee pain. Her knee pain has been well controlled with anti–tumor necrosis factor therapy. She denies recent trauma, fevers, or rash. She is afebrile, and examination of the knee reveals swelling and pain with passive range of motion. What is the next most appropriate step in managing this patient's symptoms?

A. Intraarticular steroidal injection

B. Add methotrexate

C. Add nonsteroidal anti-inflammatory drugs (NSAIDs)

D. Arthrocentesis

ANSWERS

19.1 **D.** Although the patient's clinical presentation is consistent with a septic joint, one must consider other causes of a joint effusion in the early stages of the workup. However, the arthrocentesis, which yielded gross pus, makes a septic knee the most likely of the answer choices.

19.2 **B.** Gram-positive bacteria remain the most common cause of septic arthritis. *Staphylococcus aureus* accounts for the majority of culture-positive septic arthritis, especially within certain patient subgroups such as hemodialysis patients and intravenous drug abusers. The predominance of *S. aureus* in septic arthritis has remained unchanged for many years.

19.3 **D.** The most appropriate next step would be arthrocentesis to rule out a joint infection. Patients with rheumatoid arthritis have consistently accounted for a high percentage of patients with septic arthritis. These patients may be predisposed to septic arthritis because of poor clearance of bacteria from abnormal joints or because of phagocytic defects acquired secondary to drugs or disease.

CLINICAL PEARLS

- There is considerable overlap in the clinical presentation of the most common etiologies of acute joint inflammation.
- A detailed history and physical exam is vital to eliciting risk factors for septic arthritis.
- Always investigate a source of infection in suspected septic arthritis, since the pathophysiology most often involves hematogenous spread to the joint.
- Do not depend on serum markers to rule out septic arthritis.
- Arthrocentesis is vital to determining the etiology of an acutely erythematous, swollen, and painful joint.
- Do not initiate empiric antibiotic treatment without first having obtained both blood and synovial fluid specimens.

REFERENCES

Ateschrang A, Albrecht D, Schroeter S, Weise K, Dolderer J. Current concepts review: septic arthritis of the knee pathophysiology, diagnostics, and therapy. *Central Eur J Med*. 2011;123:191-197.

Carpenter C, Schuur J, Everett W, Pines J. Evidence-based diagnostics: adult septic arthritis. *Acad Emerg Med*. 2011;18:781-796.

Lieberman JR, ed. *American Academy of Orthopaedic Surgeons Comprehensive Orthopaedic Review*. Rosemont, IL: American Academy of Orthopaedic Surgeons; 2009.

Salter RB. *Textbook of Disorders and Injuries of the Musculoskeletal System*. 2nd ed. Baltimore, MD: Williams & Wilkins; 1983:178-181.

CASE 20

A 62-year-old female is referred to your office for a 3-week history of right foot pain. The patient denies recent trauma to the area, but states she had her second toe amputated by her podiatrist 6 months ago, secondary to an infection she contracted "from a pebble in [her] shoe." Although her foot had healed, she has begun experiencing a recurrence of pain in this area, despite a change in footwear and diligent monitoring of her feet for ulcers. She admits to mild fevers over the past 10 days, but denies other symptoms. On further history, the patient has type 2 diabetes mellitus. She admits that she stopped seeing her primary care physician last year since he started prescribing "painful insulin shots" for her. On physical exam, erythema is noted at the plantar-medial aspect of her right forefoot. This region is warm to the touch, mildly edematous, and firm, but without any obvious fluctuance or drainage. She has chronic neuropathies in her toes and feet, bilaterally. Recent laboratory results from her primary care provider's office are remarkable for a white blood cell (WBC) count of 7.4 thousand/μL, erythrocyte sedimentation rate (ESR) of 55 mm/hr, and C-reactive protein (CRP) of 65 mg/L. An anteroposterior (AP) x-ray and a T2-weighted magnetic resonance imaging (MRI) of the right foot are shown in Figures 20–1 and 20–2.

- ▶ What are the radiologic findings?
- ▶ What is the most likely diagnosis?
- ▶ What risk factors predispose her to such a diagnosis?

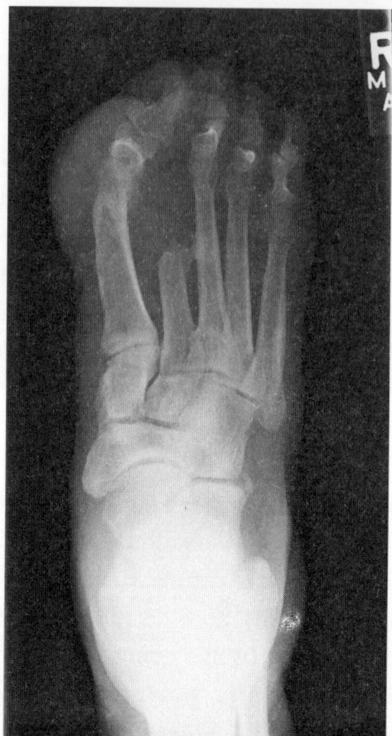

Figure 20–1. AP radiograph of the right foot, status post second ray resection.

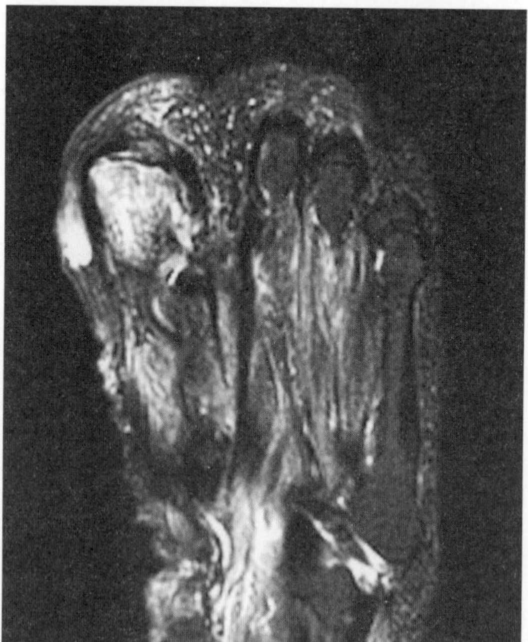

Figure 20–2. T2-weighted axial MRI slice of the right foot.

ANSWERS TO CASE 20: Osteomyelitis

Summary: A 62-year-old woman with uncontrolled diabetes and peripheral neuropathy presents with atraumatic, insidious right foot pain, 3 weeks in duration. She has mild systemic symptoms (fever) and has experienced similar symptoms in the past for which she underwent an amputation of her second toe.

- **Radiologic findings:** This AP radiograph of the right foot shows chronic bone and soft tissue loss in the second ray, consistent with the patient's history of osteomyelitis and toe amputation. There is significant soft tissue swelling over the head of the first metatarsal and base of the great toe. There is also significant bony erosion in this region, with a loss of normal cortical bone, periosteal elevation, and lytic changes consistent with osteomyelitis. On T2-weighted MRI, the head and distal shaft of the first metatarsal are hyper-resonant, consistent with edema and inflammation in the region. There is also adjacent hyperintensity of the soft tissues medial to the great toe, consistent with soft tissue inflammation and possibly an abscess collection.
- **Most likely diagnosis:** Osteomyelitis of the first ray.
- **Predisposing factors:** Poorly controlled type 2 diabetes mellitus, peripheral neuropathy, and history of previous osteomyelitis.

ANALYSIS

Objectives

1. Understand the pathogenesis of osteomyelitis and recognize its clinical and radiographic presentation.
2. Be familiar with the differential diagnoses for, and diagnostic workup of, osteomyelitis.
3. Be familiar with basic treatment options for osteomyelitis, both operative and nonoperative.

Considerations

This patient presents with a soft tissue infection that has progressed to involve the underlying metatarsal bone. She has a history of uncontrolled diabetes and neuropathy. As a risk factor for osteomyelitis, neuropathies predispose patients to microtrauma because the body's pain-protective response to skin-damaging repetitive wear is lost. Previously, this patient's neuropathy left her susceptible to skin ulceration from a pebble in her shoe, which wore through the protective dermal barrier and introduced bacteria into the soft tissues overlying the second metatarsal. Poorly controlled diabetes impedes the body's wound healing and infection-fighting capabilities, rendering diabetics susceptible to bacterial colonization, particularly in their feet. Radiographic studies should be used to further investigate and diagnose osteomyelitis: plain radiographs, computed tomography (CT) scans, MRI, WBC scans, and/or bone scans are used to make the diagnosis. In this patient's case, plain x-rays clearly show erosive bony changes in the first ray, while T2-weighted MRI shows edematous changes in the bone and surrounding soft tissues consistent with osteomyelitis. This patient has an elevated ESR and CRP, which are elevated in more than 90% of cases of osteomyelitis. An elevated WBC count, although positive in many types of infections and inflammatory states, is only positive in approximately 40% of cases.

Once the diagnosis is made, the patient should be admitted to the hospital and intravenous antibiotic therapy should commence. If deep tissue or bone biopsy can be easily obtained, and if the patient remains stable, antibiotic therapy may be delayed until biopsies or aspirations are acquired. This is especially true in patients for whom osteomyelitis represents one in several possible diagnoses or when osteomyelitis is occurring in particularly difficult to debride regions such as vertebral bodies. Biopsy before antibiotic administration optimizes the chance that an adequate sample of bacteria will be acquired for culture and that an appropriate, targeted antibiotic agent may be selected. Unstable patients with evidence of sepsis, however, should receive prompt systemic antibiotic treatment, regardless of whether biopsy can be performed. An additional caveat involves the culturing of superficial tissues, as these cultures tend to grow out benign, typical skin flora, which sometimes leads to the unnecessary and misdirected treatment.

For this patient, with extensive involvement of deep tissues, surgical drainage and debridement should be performed. Amputation may also be considered. Intravenous antibiotic therapy typically continues for 4 to 6 weeks, with infectious disease consultation useful for assistance with antibiotic selection and management.

APPROACH TO:

Osteomyelitis

DEFINITIONS

ACUTE OSTEOMYELITIS: Presence of bacteria or infectious pathogens in bone or bone marrow without the chronic histologic changes described below. Defined in some literature as a bone infection lasting less than 6 weeks. Acute osteomyelitis most commonly occurs in children.

CHRONIC OSTEOMYELITIS: May be defined by histologic changes such as the presence of a sequestrum or an involucrum, or by duration of infection greater than 6 weeks. Chronic osteomyelitis is characterized by the presence of bacterial biofilm and bacterial resistance to host defenses and antibiotic agents and often requires surgical debridement and long-term systemic antibiotic therapy.

BIOFILM: An aggregate of microorganisms embedded within an adherent polysaccharide matrix that provides bacterial immunity to host cellular defenses and antiobiotic agents.

SEQUESTRUM: A region of devitalized bone that serves as a nidus for continual infection; a hallmark of chronic osteomyelitis.

INVOLUCRUM: The formation of new, reactive bone around an area of septic necrosis; another hallmark of chronic osteomyelitis.

CLINICAL APPROACH

Pathophysiology

Osteomyelitis is an infection of **bone or bone marrow.** This highly variable disease may be classified as acute versus chronic, hematogenous versus contiguous, and with or without vascular compromise (Lee and Waldvogel classification). Osteomyelitis may also be classified by its location and extent (Cierny and Mader classification).

Osteomyelitis can result from a **continuous spread** of an infection from soft tissue or joints, trauma causing **direct bacterial inoculation** into bone or adjacent soft tissues, or **hematogenously spread** from an infection elsewhere in the body.

Patients with **vascular diseases, poorly controlled diabetes, and those in states of immunocompromise are at elevated risk** for developing acute osteomyelitis. Immunocompromised individuals are also at risk for developing chronic osteomyelitis. Other risk factors for **chronic osteomyelitis** include history of **intravenous drug abuse** and **failure of treatment of acute osteomyelitis.**

Osteomyelitis can be caused by bacteria, fungi, and viruses. By a great majority, the **most common causative agents are bacterial,** with *Staphylococcus aureus* being the most commonly identified offending organism. Other common inoculants include *Pseudomonas aeruginosa*, *Escherichia coli*, coagulase-negative staphylococci, enterococci, and propionibacteria. *Salmonella* species are commonly identified pathogens in patients with sickle-cell anemia; however, staphylococcal species are still most common in these patients.

Diagnosis

Osteomyelitis may present as an occult infection in patients of all ages. Its most common presentation is in patients with **deep bone pain** and **without significant systemic symptoms.** When systemic symptoms are present, fever and chills predominate. **Soft tissues surrounding an infection may be edematous, warm, and erythematous.** Patients may present with a history of recent trauma or infection or with a history of an invasive procedure. Osteomyelitis should be included in the differential diagnosis of other musculoskeletal pathologies such as gout, ischemia, arthritis, neuropathy, and degenerative disc disease in the spine. Delay in diagnosis and treatment of acute infection may lead to chronic osteomyelitis, a relapsing and remitting indolent infection characterized by intermittent pain attacks and systemic symptoms.

Radiographic Evaluation

Plain radiographs should be obtained before more advanced imaging is considered. On plain films, acute osteomyelitis may be identified by cortical bone destruction with a surrounding area of periosteal elevation. Acute osteomyelitis will typically have a lytic, or radiolucent, appearance, whereas chronic infections may be distinguished by the presence of a mixed lytic and blastic, or radio-opaque, appearance. Radiographs are not sensitive for osteomyelitis, however, as up to **30% to 40% of bone destruction must occur before osteomyelitic changes are visible on**

plain x-rays. Symptoms of the disease typically are present before x-ray changes are apparent.

MRI with intravenous (IV) gadolinium contrast is far more sensitive for diagnosing osteomyelitis. MRI offers a clear view of soft tissue pathology and is currently the gold standard in the diagnosis of osteomyelitis. Be wary that in the presence of metallic implants, the sensitive/specificity of MRI is decreased; in such situations, IV contrast CT scans may be helpful in elucidating bony pathology.

Finally, radioisotope tagged WBC scans are very specific for osteomyelitis and are often used to follow treatment progression. Bone scans may be used in a similar fashion, but are less specific.

TREATMENT

Acute osteomyelitis, typically presenting in children and IV drug abusers with erythematous and painful limbs, requires prompt antibiotic therapy, often 4 to 6 weeks' duration. Such patients may not require surgical debridement, but should be followed closely to ensure successful therapy.

Chronic osteomyelitis also requires long-term IV drug therapy, but typically requires additional open surgical procedures to debride necrotic tissue, drain abscesses, and remove sequestra or nonviable bone serving as nidi for bacteria.

In chronic osteomyelitis, IV antibiotic is typically administered for 4 to 6 weeks and may be administered in an outpatient setting once a patient has been stabilized. In patients with extensive disease or immunocompromised states, longer courses of IV drug therapy may be indicated. Initial antibiotic coverage should be broad, with tailored antibiotic selection once, and only if, reliable bacterial cultures and drug sensitivities are available. Initial antibiotic selection must cover *S. aureus*, the most commonly identified pathogen in osteomyelitis. In patients with a history of recent hospitalization, initial therapy must cover methicillin-resistant *S. aureus*, a prevalent nosocomial infection. Serial CRP and ESR studies, although not especially specific for osteomyelitis, are sometimes followed as markers for successful treatment.

In addition to a thorough surgical debridement, several adjunctive surgical treatments may be indicated, including the placement of antibiotic-eluting polymethyl-methacrylate (PMMA) beads. PMMA, the same bone "cement" used in the implantation of joint prostheses, may be mixed with antibiotic agents such as gentamycin, molded into round beads or fashioned into an antibiotic spacer, and placed into the debrided cavity. After resolution of infection, the beads are typically removed.

The placement of orthopaedic implants such as screws, plates, rods, and prostheses pose a special challenge to the orthopaedist, as artificial implants may serve as a nidus for chronic infection. In such cases, the surgeon must weight the benefits of removing infected hardware with the risks of losing stability or function. As a general rule, infected hardware should be removed when possible.

Outcomes and Complications

Musculoskeletal infection that has been treated with antibiotics and surgical debridement can lead to functional deficit in the given extremity. This is dependent on the amount of tissue debrided and if vital structures have been violated and destabilized. When this occurs, it is usually in an attempt to perform a limb-salvage procedure, as both patients and surgeons try to avoid amputation if at all possible. However, in the setting of severe and recurrent musculoskeletal infections, amputation may be the only means by which to permanently eradicate the infection.

COMPREHENSION QUESTIONS

20.1 A 34-year-old, HIV-positive male presents to the emergency department (ED) with complaints of several weeks of neck pain. The patient admits to using recreational drugs, but does not willingly discuss what substances he uses. He has recently begun feeling numbness in his bilateral hands and states he is now unable to properly write with a pen. On exam, he has point tenderness along the lateral aspect of his neck. An MRI is obtained, showing edema and prevertebral swelling in his C3 and C4 vertebrae. There is T2-weighted hyperresonance of the C3-4 disc space, with swelling posterior to C3 that is impinging on the cord. What is the best treatment for this patient?

A. Inform the patient that he should follow up as an outpatient for further workup.

B. Physical therapy and warm compresses, as the patient has no symptoms of myelopathy.

C. Admit to the hospital promptly for antibiotic therapy and evaluation for surgical intervention.

D. Bone scan and CT scanning of the chest abdomen and pelvis to evaluate for other lesions.

E. Biopsies to classify the lesions and determine their source.

20.2 A 44-year-old truck driver is almost 1 year in recovery from knife wound to his left distal thigh after an altercation at a local bar. He had initially been treated with debridement in the ED and wound closure and was treated with a short course of oral antibiotics. He was neurovascularly intact after the injury. He presents now to your clinic with serous drainage through a sinus tract on the medial aspect of his distal thigh. The area is erythematous and edematous and is mildly tender to palpation. He has been able to bear weight on it, but states that it is causing increasing discomfort while trying to drive his truck. Plain radiograph films are obtained and are equivocal. An MRI is also obtained and shows a region of hyperintensity in the metaphysis of the distal left femur surrounding an area of hypointense bone. What is the best treatment for this patient?

A. Long (14-day) course of oral antibiotics with close follow-up

B. Needle biopsy and targeted oral antibiotics

C. CT scan of the affected extremity

D. Needle biopsy and IV antibiotics

E. Surgical debridement and IV antibiotics

20.3 A 12-year-old African American male with a history of sickle cell disease is admitted to the hospital with severe left upper extremity pain and fevers. Blood cultures are obtained, and broad-spectrum IV antibiotics and fluid resuscitation are initiated. What is the most likely causative organism in this patient?

A. Viral infection

B. *Salmonella*

C. *Streptococcus* species

D. *Staphylococcus aureus*

E. *Escherichia coli*

ANSWERS

20.1 **C.** This patient has osteomyelitis of the cervical spine with discitis at C3-4, and evidence of epidural abscess. Given the patient's myelopathic state, the patient should be admitted immediately to the hospital and IV antibiotic therapy should begin promptly, ideally after a biopsy is obtained. If symptoms do not remit on broad-spectrum antibiotic treatment, or if myelopathy worsens, prompt surgical evacuation of the abscess should be performed.

20.2 **E.** This patient has history and radiographic findings consistent with a chronic osteomyelitis. The region of bone involved on MRI is consistent with a sequestrum that must be surgically debrided. After culture, broad-spectrum IV antibiotics should be initiated and targeted according to susceptibility testing of the cultures. Although needle biopsy may help target the appropriate organism, it is insufficient to effectively eradicate the infection. Similarly antibiotics alone, whether oral or broad-spectrum IV, are insufficient without a thorough surgical debridement.

20.3 **D.** Although *Salmonella* species are commonly associated with sickle cell patients with osteomyelitis, the most common causative agent is actually *S. aureus*. *Escherichia coli* and streptococcal species infections also occur in these populations; however, they are less common. Viral osteomyelitis is exceedingly rare.

CLINICAL PEARLS

- Osteomyelitis is sometimes referred to as the "great imitator" because it can radiographically mimic almost any neoplastic or inflammatory process.
- Osteomyelitis must destroy 30% to 40% of a given region of bone before it is evident on plain x-ray.
- Elevated WBC counts are found in only 40% of patients presenting with chronic osteomyelitis; elevated CRP and ESR are found in approximately 90%.
- Acute osteomyelitis usually requires prolonged IV antibiotic therapy. Chronic osteomyelitis generally requires surgical debridement as well as prolonged antibiotics.

REFERENCES

Forsberg JA, Potter BK, Cierny III G, Webb L. Diagnosis and management of chronic infection. *J Am Acad Orthop Surg*. 2011;19(suppl 1):S8-S19.

Frassica FJ, Frassica DA, McCarthy EF. Orthopaedic pathology. In: Miller MD, ed. *Review of Orthopaedics*. 5th ed. Philadelphia, PA: Saunders Elsevier; 2008.

Srinivasan RC, Tolhurst S, Vanderhave KL. Orthopedic surgery. In: Doherty GM, ed. *Current Diagnosis & Treatment: Surgery*. 13th ed. New York: McGraw-Hill; 2010.

Tice AD. Osteomyelitis. In: Longo DL, Fauci AS, Kasper DL, Hauser SL, Jameson JL, Loscalzo J, eds. *Harrison's Principles of Internal Medicine*. 18th ed. New York: McGraw-Hill; 2012.

CASE 21

An otherwise healthy, right-hand-dominant, 25-year-old man is seen in the emergency department after slipping on the front steps of his house 2 days ago. He states that he landed on an outstretched right upper extremity and immediately began experiencing shoulder pain. He has been unable to move his shoulder since the fall and has had his arm in a sling that a friend gave him. On physical exam, you note no ecchymosis, abrasions, or any other deformity. However, shoulder range of motion, especially internal rotation, is significantly limited. Anteroposterior, axillary, and scapular-Y radiographs of his right shoulder reveal no abnormalities. The patient is most concerned about his ability to return to his competitive tennis league by next week, as he is playing for the club championship.

- ▶ What is the most likely diagnosis?
- ▶ What are the imaging studies of choice for evaluating this patient's problem?
- ▶ What is the most appropriate treatment for this patient?

ANSWERS TO CASE 21: Rotator Cuff Injury

Summary: An otherwise healthy and active 25-year-old man slips and lands on his right shoulder. He is unable to raise his arm and has limited active range of motion. Neurovascular examination is normal. Radiographs are negative for a fracture and dislocation.

- **Most likely diagnosis:** Acute tear of the rotator cuff.
- **Imaging studies of choice: Plain radiographs must always be obtained first in the setting of acute trauma to the shoulder, as has been done here. When rotator cuff tear (RCT) is suspected,** magnetic resonance imaging (MRI) should also be performed. It is extremely accurate (93%-100%) in detecting full-thickness tears and can evaluate tear size, tendon retraction, muscle atrophy, and related intra-articular pathology. However, it cannot be used in patients with pacemakers, aneurysm clips, metal in the eye, or other metal implants within the body.
- **Treatment:** The appropriate treatment for an acute, full-thickness RCT in an otherwise healthy and physically active young patient is primary repair.

ANALYSIS

Objectives

1. Understand rotator cuff anatomy.
2. Properly diagnose a rotator cuff tear.
3. Be familiar with treatment options for rotator cuff tears.

Considerations

This 45-year-old man sustained an injury to his right shoulder after slipping on his front steps. He presents with pain and weakness of the right shoulder in the setting of normal radiographs. This constellation of findings is concerning for an acute RCT.

A complete history and physical exam of the neck and involved extremity must be done. Although active range of motion is typically decreased because of pain and/or weakness, passive range of motion is expected to be normal. Shoulder strength in elevation, abduction, external rotation, and internal rotation should be assessed, and specific provocative maneuvers can be performed to evaluate the individual muscles of the rotator cuff (Table 21–1, Figure 21–1).

An MRI, which is the gold standard for diagnosis of RCTs, should be obtained (Figure 21–2). However, if a contraindication to MRI exists, an arthrogram or ultrasound can be done. MRI in this patient will confirm an RCT. Given the patient's described mechanism of a hyperabduction/external rotation injury during a fall, he has likely torn his subscapularis tendon.

Although nonoperative management is appropriate for some people, this patient will benefit from a rotator cuff repair, as he is young and active.

Table 21–1 • PROVOCATIVE MANEUVERS USED TO EVALUATE SPECIFIC MUSCLES OF THE ROTATOR CUFF

Lift-off test (subscapularis)	The patient's arm is internally rotated with the elbow flexed to 90 degrees and hand held posteriorly at the waist with the palm facing out. The patient then attempts to move his arm away from his body against pressure from the examiner. The test is positive if the patient experiences pain or weakness during this maneuver.
Empty can test (supraspinatus)	The patient's arm should be held in 90 degrees of elevation in the plane of the scapula, with the elbow extended, upper extremity internally rotated, and the forearm pronated. This results in the patient's upper extremity in a thumbs-down position, as if he were emptying a can. In this position, the examiner stabilizes the shoulder while applying a downward directed force on the arm. The patient will try to resist this force. The test is positive if the patient experiences pain or weakness with resistance (Figure 21–1).
Infraspinatus test	The patient stands with his arm at the side with the elbow at 90 degrees and the arm internally rotated to 45 degrees. The examiner applies a medial rotation force that the patient resists. Pain or the inability to resist further internal rotation indicates a positive test for infraspinatus pathology.

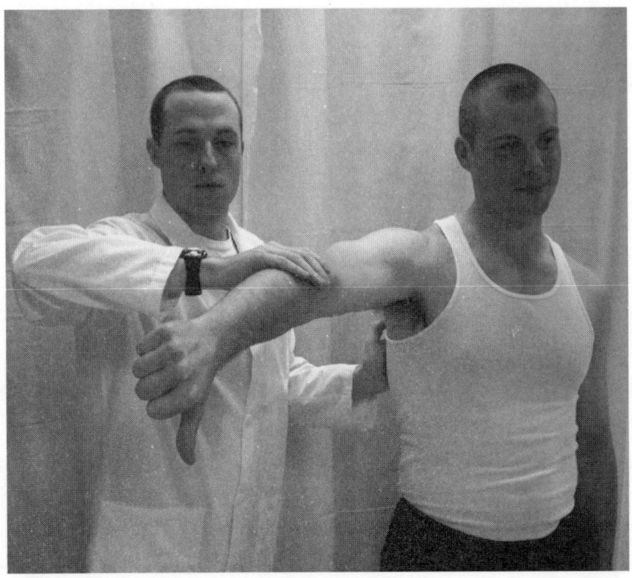

Figure 21–1. The empty can test, which evaluates supraspinatus pathology. (Reproduced, with permission, from Tintinalli J, et al. *Tintinalli's Emergency Medicine: A Comprehensive Study Guide.* 7th ed. New York, NY: McGraw-Hill; 2010:Fig. 277-5.)

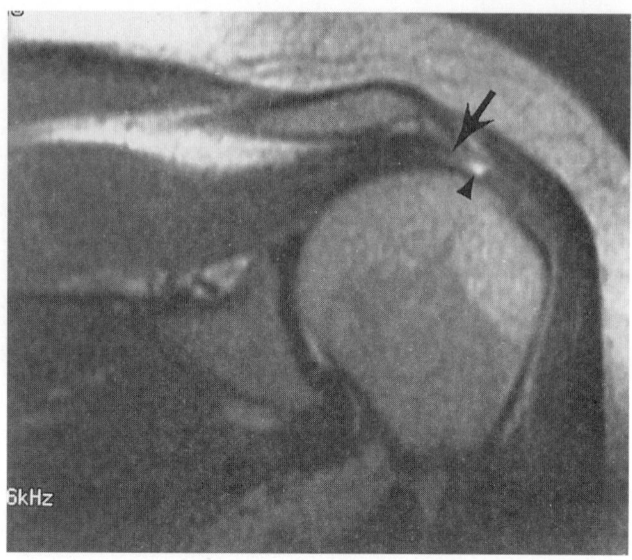

Figure 21–2. Rotator cuff tear. MRI coronal image of the shoulder reveals a tear in the supraspinatus tendon (*arrow*) with edema (*arrowhead*). (Reproduced, with permission, from Tintinalli J, et al. *Tintinalli's Emergency Medicine: A Comprehensive Study Guide*. 7th ed. New York, NY: McGraw-Hill; 2010:Fig. 277-7.)

APPROACH TO:
Rotator Cuff Tears

DEFINITIONS

ROTATOR CUFF: A confluence of 4 muscles (supraspinatus, infraspinatus, teres minor, and subscapularis) that arise from the scapula and insert on the humeral head. The main functions of the rotator cuff are to stabilize the glenohumeral joint and to rotate the humerus outward.

ROTATOR CUFF TEAR: A common cause of shoulder pain that can involve an individual tendon or a combination of tendons. The supraspinatus is the most commonly torn rotator cuff tendon.

ROTATOR CUFF ARTHROPATHY: A condition of the shoulder in which glenohumeral arthritis develops secondary to a chronic, irreparable rotator cuff tear. It is typically seen in older individuals with loss of shoulder motion and strength.

SUBACROMIAL IMPINGEMENT: Term used to describe the process and continuum by which rotator cuff tendons become irritated and inflamed as they pass through the subacromial space. This is secondary to impingement of the humeral head and rotator cuff beneath the coracoacromial (CA) arch of the shoulder. With the arm in neutral position, the greater tuberosity (where the supraspinatus inserts) lies anterior to the CA arch. With forward flexion and internal rotation, the subacromial bursa and supraspinatus tendon become entrapped between the anterior acromion/coracoid and greater tuberosity.

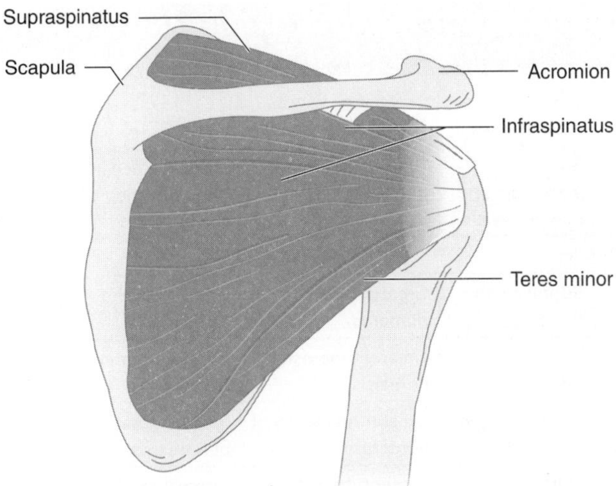

Figure 21–3. Posterior view of the shoulder illustrating rotator cuff muscles. (Reproduced, with permission, from Tintinalli J, et al. *Tintinalli's Emergency Medicine: A Comprehensive Study Guide.* 7th ed. New York, NY: McGraw-Hill; 2010:Fig. 277-1.)

CLINICAL APPROACH

Shoulder Anatomy and Biomechanics

The shoulder complex is comprised of the glenohumeral (GH), sternoclavicular (SC), acromioclavicular (AC), and scapulothoracic (ST) joints (Figures 21–3 and 21–4). **There is a 2:1 ratio of shoulder motion between the GH and ST joints (ie, 180 degrees of abduction consists of 120 degrees of GH motion and 60 degrees of ST motion).** Both static stabilizers (ie, bony structures, labrum, joint capsule, ligaments) and dynamic stabilizers (ie, rotator cuff, periscapular muscles) help in maintaining

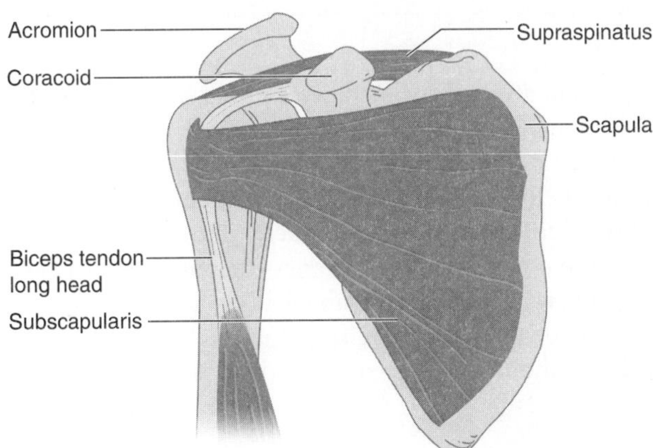

Figure 21–4. Anterior view of the shoulder illustrating the supraspinatus muscle and the long head of the biceps. (Reproduced, with permission, from Tintinalli J, et al. *Tintinalli's Emergency Medicine: A Comprehensive Study Guide. 7th ed.* New York, NY: McGraw-Hill; 2010:Fig. 277-2.)

Table 21–2 • MUSCLES OF THE ROTATOR CUFF AND GLENOHUMERAL JOINT

Muscle	Proximal Attachment	Distal Attachment	Action	Innervation
Deltoid	Spine, acromion, and lateral clavicle	Deltoid tuberosity of humerus	Flexion, extension, and abduction of the humerus	Axillary n. (C5-6)
Rotator Cuff Muscles				
Supraspinatus	Supraspinatus fossa	Greater tuberosity of humerus	Abduction of humerus	Suprascapular n. (C5-6)
Infraspinatus	Infraspinatus fossa	Greater tuberosity of humerus	External rotation of humerus	Suprascapular n. (C5-6)
Teres minor	Lateral margin of scapula	Greater tuberosity of humerus	External rotation of humerus	Axillary n. (C5-6)
Subscapularis	Subscapular fossa	Lesser tuberosity of humerus	Internal rotation of humerus	Upper and lower subscapular nn. (C5-6)
Intertubercular Groove Muscles				
Teres major	Inferior angle of scapula	Intertubercular groove humerus	Adduction, extension, and internal rotation of humerus	Lower subscapular n. (C5-6)
Pectoralis major	Clavicle, sternum, and costal cartilage	Intertubercular groove humerus	Adduction, extension, flexion and internal rotation of humerus	Medial and lateral pectoral nn. (C5-T1)
Latissimus dorsi	T7-T12, sacrum, and thoracolumbar fascia	Intertubercular groove humerus	Adduction, extension, and internal rotation of humerus	Thoracodorsal n. (C6-8)

congruity and providing GH joint stability. Static stabilizers can function in the setting of intrinsic muscle damage and neuromuscular injury, whereas the dynamic stabilizers cannot. Table 21–2 outlines the muscles vital to shoulder function.

The rotator cuff helps to maintain a stable fulcrum for shoulder motion via its role as a dynamic stabilizer of the glenohumeral joint. The cuff balances the force couples in the coronal and transverse planes. In the coronal plane, the inferior rotator cuff (infraspinatus, teres minor, subscapularis) balances the support moment created by the deltoid. In the transverse plane, the anterior cuff (subscapularis) functions to balance the moment created by the posterior cuff (infraspinatus and teres minor).

Etiology

The incidence of RCTs ranges from 5% to 40% and increases with age. Of note, 55% of asymptomatic patients ≥60 years of age will have rotator cuff pathology evident on MRI. **RCTs should be thought of as part of a continuum of disease involving the shoulder.** The continuum includes subacromial impingement, subcoracoid impingement, calcific tendonitis, rotator cuff tears, and rotator cuff arthropathy.

Tears can be acute, iatrogenic, or secondary to chronic degenerative changes. Acute avulsion injuries include subscapularis tears in younger patients after a fall and supraspinatus, infraspinatus, and/or teres minor tears in those older than 40 years after a shoulder dislocation. Overhead throwing athletes are susceptible to cuff tears secondary to the high tensile forces that the rotator cuff is subjected to during the deceleration phase of throwing. Iatrogenic injuries are commonly seen after repair failure of the subscapularis tendon after an open anterior shoulder surgery. Chronic degenerative tears are seen in older patients and typically involve the supraspinatus, infraspinatus, and/or teres minor.

Presentation and Diagnosis

Patients with RCT present either after an acute trauma and inability to move the arm and shoulder (ie, shoulder dislocation or fall) or with the insidious onset of symptoms such as **night pain** and **difficulty performing overhead activites.** Physical examination of the shoulder should begin with inspection of the skin for scars, atrophy, swelling, droop, and scapular winging. Palpation of the bony prominences and muscles of the shoulder girdle should be done next. The patient should then be placed supine, at which time active and passive range of motion of both shoulders is assessed. Planes of motion to be evaluated include forward elevation (150-180 degrees is considered normal), abduction, internal rotation to vertebral height (T4-8 is considered normal), internal rotation at 90 degrees of abduction, external rotation at side, and external rotation at 90 degrees of abduction. A neurovascular exam of the entire upper extremity should also be done, as should the specific tests that isolate the individual muscles of the rotator cuff (Table 21–1).

Imaging studies are ordered based on the findings from the history and physical exam, with plain radiographs the first ones obtained. **Findings on plain x-ray associated with rotator cuff pathology include calcific tendonitis, proximal migration of the humerus (seen with chronic RCT), or a hooked acromion. MRI, when obtained, evaluates muscle quality and the tear size, tear shape, and degree of tendon retraction. Other findings on MRI consistent with RCT include muscle atrophy, medial biceps tendon subluxation (indicative of a subscapularis tear), and cysts in the humeral head (seen in the majority of patients with a chronic RCT).**

Classification

Classification of cuff tears can be done based on anatomical location, tear size, amount of cuff atrophy, tear shape, thickness, and chronicity. **Partial-thickness** tears often appear as fraying of an intact tendon, whereas **full-thickness** tears are through-and-through. These can be small pin-point defects, large buttonhole tears (the tendon still remains attached to the humeral head and thus retains function), or tears in which the tendon is completely detached from the humeral head. When classified by chronicity, they can be described as **acute** (due to a sudden, powerful movement or trauma), **subacute,** or **chronic** (develops over a longer period of time, seen in individuals who frequently participate in overhead activities).

TREATMENT

Rotator cuff tears can be managed via both operative and nonoperative means. The patient's age, activity level, overall health, cuff status (ie, size and age of tear, amount of retraction, muscle quality), and presence of GH arthritis must be considered when determining the best treatment for a given patient. **In general, young, active patients presenting with an acute tear and a primary complaint of weakness are best treated with early surgical repair, whereas older patients complaining of pain in the setting of chronic, degenerative tears are most responsive to nonoperative treatment.**

Nonoperative treatment includes nonsteroidal anti-inflammatory drugs, (NSAIDs), activity modifications, subacromial corticosteroid injections, and physical therapy. Corticosteroid injections into the subacromial space are done with failure of other conservative modalities for greater than 4 to 6 weeks. The goal of these injections is to decrease pain. They may be repeated after several months if initially effective. **However, the patient should receive no more than 3 injections per year.** Physical therapy focuses on aggressive rotator cuff and periscapular muscle strengthening.

Operative repair of an RCT can be done through either open or arthroscopic approaches, which have been shown to have equivalent results. With both techniques, the goal is to restore the native tendon(s) insertional footprint area on the tuberosities. It is thought that a larger, more anatomic footprint improves healing and the mechanical strength of the repair. Biologic healing of the cuff is estimated to take approximately 8 to 12 weeks; this is the rate-limiting step for recovery. Anatomic footprint restoration is often achieved with double-row suture techniques. Of note, animal models have *failed* to show increased repair strength with the addition of a trough in the greater tuberosity.

Complications after rotator cuff repair include recurrence, deltoid detachment (with open procedures), acromiclavicular joint pain, axillary nerve injury, and suprascapular nerve injury. **Worker's compensation patients report worse outcomes with higher postoperative disability and lower satisfaction.**

There are several procedures that may be performed at the time of rotator cuff repair or as independent operations before repair. Subacromial decompression is done if impingement is thought to have contributed to tendon irritation and tearing. AC joint resection is performed via distal clavicle excision in patients whose AC joint is tender to palpation and painful. A long head of the biceps tenotomy (detachment of the tendon origin from the labrum or glenoid) or tenodesis (releasing of the tendon origin and suturing it to the proximal humerus) is done in patients with a symptomatic biceps tendon.

Irreparable and massive rotator cuff tears require special consideration. In patients with this but an otherwise normal GH joint, tendon transfer can be performed with the goal of restoring overhead function. For irreparable or chronic subscapularis tears, pectoralis major transfer is performed. For large tears of the supraspinatus and infraspinatus, a latissimus dorsi transfer is performed. In this procedure, the latissimus is attached to the cuff muscles, subscapularis, and greater tuberosity. The given extremity is then immobilized in a brace for 6 weeks in 45 degrees of abduction and 30 degrees of external rotation. **Of note, the best candidate for a latissimus dorsi transfer is a young laborer.**

COMPREHENSION QUESTIONS

21.1 A 45-year-old man has a fall from his motorcycle and is complaining of shoulder pain. Radiographs are negative for fracture and dislocation. On exam, you note a positive lift-off test. What is the most likely diagnosis?

A. Teres minor tear

B. Supraspinatus tear

C. Infraspinatus tear

D. Subscapularis tear

21.2 An 80-year-old man sustained an anterior shoulder dislocation 2 weeks ago. He was reduced in the emergency department acutely and has been treated in a sling by his primary care physician. Radiographs after reduction appear normal. He now presents with severe pain and weakness of his shoulder. What is the most likely diagnosis?

A. Continued anterior subluxation of the humerus

B. Rotator cuff tear

C. Cervical spine radiculopathy

D. Proximal humerus fracture

21.3 A 65-year-old woman presents to the clinic complaining of worsening pain in her left shoulder that is most severe at night. She is an avid swimmer and states that she has been unable to swim for the last 3 weeks because of the pain. She denies any recent trauma and has brought plain radiographs of her shoulder in 3 views (ordered by her internist) with her, which are negative. You suspect a torn rotator cuff and order an MRI. However, the patient tells you that she cannot have one, due to her pacemaker. Which of the following imaging modalities is the most appropriate for this patient?

A. Ultrasound

B. PET scan

C. Arthrogram

D. Additional plain radiographs

ANSWERS

21.1 **D.** A positive lift-off test is consistent with a subscapularis injury. In this maneuver, the patient's arm is internally rotated, the elbow flexed to 90 degrees, and hand held posteriorly at the waist. If the patient experiences pain or weakness as he tries to move his arm away from his body against resistance, the test is positive.

21.2 **B.** Forty percent of patients older than 60 years with a shoulder dislocation will have a concomitant RCT. However, it is also important to recognize that even in the absence of trauma, RCT is very common in older individuals. Sixty-five percent of patients older than 70 years have a full-thickness RCT.

21.3 **C.** Arthrograms are used when MRI is contraindicated. They improve sensitivity and specificity in the diagnosis of an RCT. It is a fluoroscopic examination of the shoulder joint after the introduction of contrast media into the joint. Extravasation of the dye from the joint would support the clinical diagnosis of an RCT. Although ultrasound is also an alternative imaging modality in the setting of a contraindication to an MRI, an arthrogram is a better choice. There is no role for PET scans in the diagnosis of RCT. Additional plain radiographs will likely be of no benefit unless the originals are of poor quality.

CLINICAL PEARLS

- The rotator cuff is an important dynamic stabilizer of the shoulder and provides humeral head depression, rotation, shoulder abduction, and GH joint compression.
- The supraspinatus is the most commonly torn tendon.
- MRI is extremely accurate in detecting full-thickness tears of the rotator cuff and can evaluate tear size, tendon retraction, muscle atrophy, and related intraarticular pathology.
- Young, active patients presenting with an acute tear and a primary complaint of weakness are best treated with early surgical repair of a rotator cuff tear.
- Open and arthroscopic techniques are used to repair the rotator cuff.

REFERENCES

Bassett RW, Cofield RH. Acute tears of the rotator cuff: the timing of surgical repair. *Clin Orthop*. 1983;175:18-24.

McMahon P. *Current Diagnosis and Treatment in Sports Medicine*. New York: McGraw-Hill; 2007:120-155.

Rockwood CA, Matsen FA. *The Shoulder*. Philadelphia: WB Saunders; 1998:755-795.

Sperling JW, Cofield RH. Rotator cuff repair in patients fifty years of age and younger. *J Bone Joint Surg Am*. 2004;86:2212-2215.

Vaccaro AR. *Orthopaedic Knowledge Update* 8. Washington, DC: American Academy of Orthopaedic Surgeons; 2005:257-350.

Wilk KE, Reinold MM, Andrews JR. *The Athlete's Shoulder*. New York: McGraw-Hill; 2008:25-60.

CASE 22

An 18-year-old female athlete presents after injuring her right knee during a soccer game. She states that she was running for a ball downfield when she planted her right foot to cut inside a defender, heard a "pop," and fell to the ground in pain. She was unable to leave the field on her own power. Over the next 10 to 15 minutes, her right knee swelled considerably compared with her left. She was placed into a knee immobilizer by her trainer and presents to your office the day after the injury.

On physical exam, the patient has a significant effusion and holds her knee in approximately 10 degrees of flexion; she is unable to flex past 90 degrees. She is uncomfortable and guarding throughout your examination. Her knee is aspirated, and 40 mL of blood is extracted. She is more comfortable after this and her range of motion is improved. She has no joint line tenderness. Her knee is stable to varus and valgus stress. On Lachman exam, there is significant anterior translation compared with her left, uninjured knee without a firm end point. Anterior drawer testing reveals increased tibial translation, whereas posterior drawer testing shows symmetric posterior translation.

- ▶ What is the most likely diagnosis?
- ▶ What physical exam finding confirms your diagnosis?
- ▶ What imaging study should be ordered to confirm your diagnosis?
- ▶ What is the most appropriate treatment for this patient?

ANSWERS TO CASE 22:

Anterior Cruciate Ligament Reconstruction

Summary: An 18-year-old female soccer player presents 1 day after injuring her right knee after a noncontact pivoting injury during a soccer game. She had immediate pain and quickly developed an effusion. She was unable to leave the field under her own power. Arthrocentesis produced a large hemarthrosis. She has no joint line tenderness. Lachman and anterior drawer tests are positive. Her knee is stable to varus and valgus stress.

- **Most likely diagnosis:** Anterior cruciate ligament (ACL) rupture.
- **Confirmatory physical finding:** Positive Lachman test.
- **Imaging:** Knee x-rays followed by magnetic resonance imaging (MRI).
- **Treatment:** ACL reconstruction after regaining knee motion.

ANALYSIS

Objectives

1. Know the anatomy and function of the ACL.
2. Understand the pertinent physical exam findings, differential diagnosis, and confirmatory imaging modalities for ACL injury.
3. Be familiar with the rationale for nonoperative and operative treatment of ACL injuries.

Considerations

This 18-year-old female athlete presents with concern for an ACL injury. The mechanism, a noncontact pivoting injury with the foot firmly planted on the ground, is consistent with this. The "pop" she heard, coupled with the rapid development of a joint effusion, also supports this diagnosis. In the office it is important to obtain a reliable physical exam, which can be impeded by a hemarthrosis, as seen in this case. Joint effusions are painful, limit both active and passive range of motion, and complicate the practitioner's ability to accurately perform a complete exam of the knee. After aspiration, the patient's range of motion improves, and Lachman and anterior drawer tests are found to be positive. The next step in the workup includes plain radiographs and an MRI. The ACL tear must be confirmed and associated fractures and other injuries ruled out. After this, a treatment plan can be established.

APPROACH TO:
Anterior Cruciate Ligament Reconstruction

DEFINITIONS

LACHMAN TEST: The most reliable and clinically sensitive physical exam test for detecting an ACL tear. To perform the test, place the patient supine on the exam table with the knee in approximately 30 degrees flexion. The examiner should place one hand behind the tibia with the thumb on the tibial tuberosity. The other hand is placed on the patient's thigh. As the tibia is pulled anteriorly, an intact ACL should prevent forward translation on the femur. When the ACL is intact, a firm end point is observed. Findings consistent with a positive Lachman test include anterior tibial translation with a soft end point, more than 2 mm of anterior translation compared with the contralateral knee, and greater than 10 mm of total anterior translation.

ANTERIOR DRAWER TEST: Test performed to evaluate for ACL injury. The patient is placed supine with the hip flexed to 45 degrees and the knee to 90 degrees. The examiner should sit on the patient's feet and grasp the tibia, pulling it forward (or backward in the posterior drawer test, which is used to diagnose posterior cruciate ligament [PCL] injury). Increased forward tibial translation and end point laxity suggest a ruptured ACL (increased posterior translation suggests a PCL injury).

PIVOT SHIFT TEST: Test used to assess rotational stability of the knee. It is performed by applying slight distal traction on the extended leg with a valgus and internal rotation force then applied. In this position, the tibia will be subluxated anteriorly in an ACL-deficient knee. The knee is then flexed to 30 degrees, at which time the iliotibial band transitions from a knee extensor to flexor, helping to reduce the subluxated tibia. General anesthesia is often required to perform this test in the acute setting because of pain and guarding.

CLINICAL APPROACH

Epidemiology

ACL injuries are highly publicized and researched. They comprise nearly half of all knee ligament injuries and are more common in the young, athletic population, with 70% occurring secondary to sporting activities. Skiing and soccer have the highest risk of ACL rupture, with female athletes being 2 to 8 times more likely to tear their ACL than men.

Anatomy and Biomechanics

The ACL originates from the medial wall of the lateral femoral condyle and travels obliquely, inserting on the tibia in the anterior aspect of the intercondylar eminence of the tibia (Figure 22–1). This location is adjacent to the anterior insertion of the lateral meniscus. **It is made up of 2 distinct components, the anteromedial (AM) and posterolateral (PL) bundles, which are named for their tibial insertions.** The ligament is intraarticular but extrasynovial and receives its blood supply from the

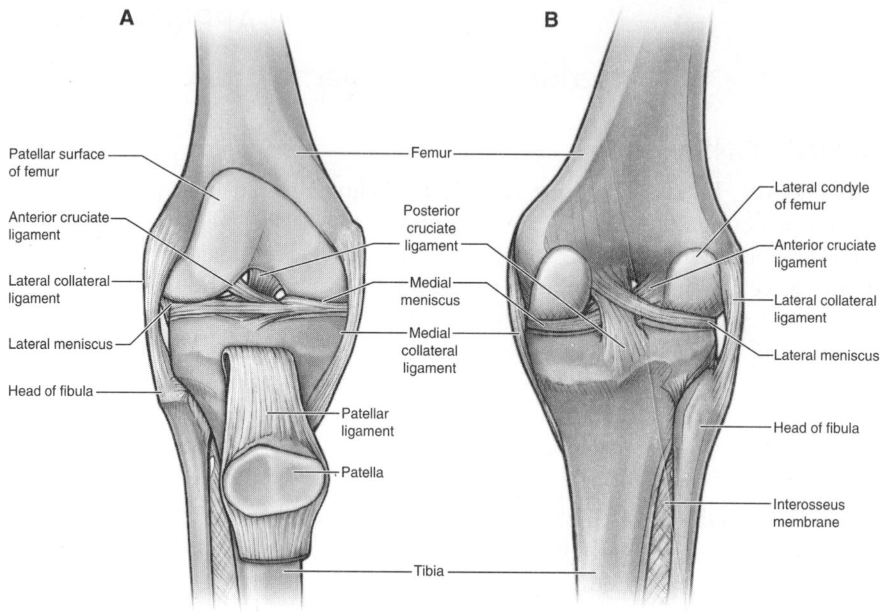

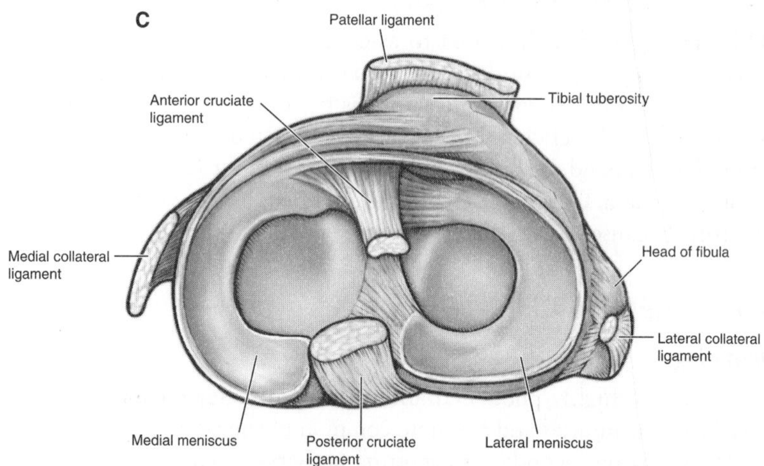

Figure 22–1. **(A)** Anterior view of the right knee joint with the joint capsule open showing the patella reflected inferiorly. **(B)** Posterior and **(C)** superior views of the right knee joint. (Reproduced, with permission, from Morton DA, Foreman KB, Albertine KH. *The Big Picture: Gross Anatomy.* New York, NY: McGraw-Hill; 2011:Fig. 36-5.)

middle geniculate artery. The ACL is approximately 33-mm long and 11 mm in diameter. It can resist a load of approximately 2200 newtons.

The primary function of the ACL is to restrict anterior translation of the tibia relative to the femur. Secondarily, it provides a restraint to tibial rotation and varus or valgus stress. **The AM bundle is the larger of the 2, is tighter in flexion,** and provides the majority of the restraint against anterior translation of the tibia on the femur, particularly at mid-ranges of knee flexion. **The PL bundle is more taut in extension and plays a greater role in countering rotational forces.**

Differential Diagnosis

The history given by the patient of an injury occurring during a cutting move, the audible "popping" or tearing sensation, and large postinjury effusion represent a classic presentation of an ACL tear. **Included in the differential diagnosis are patellar dislocation, meniscal injury, posterior cruciate ligament injury, and osteochondral fracture.** Most of these diagnoses can be confirmed with a thorough physical exam. An arthrocentesis of the affected knee can also add information, as the presence of fat within the fluid suggests a fracture, as opposed to a pure hemarthrosis, which is seen in a multitude of knee injuries.

Physical Exam

Physical exam of any joint should begin with simple inspection. Range of motion is assessed, and lack of extension can suggest a locked knee from a meniscal tear or loose body. The joint lines are palpated for presence of pain that would suggest meniscal injury. Varus and valgus stability is assessed at 0 degrees and 30 degrees to confirm the integrity of the medial and lateral collateral ligaments. The ACL is examined using the **Lachman test.** This is performed by attempting to translate the proximal tibia anteriorly with respect to the distal femur with the knee held in 30 degrees of flexion. This tests the translation of the tibia as compared with the noninjured knee as well as evaluating for a firm end point. The **anterior and posterior drawer tests** examine the ACL and PCL, respectively. The knee is flexed to 90 degrees, and translation anteriorly (anterior drawer) of the proximal tibia assesses the ACL, whereas posterior translation (posterior drawer) assesses the PCL. Care must be taken to recognize any posterior sag of the tibia before performing the anterior drawer test, as this would indicate a PCL injury and ultimately lead to a false-positive anterior drawer. The **pivot shift test** is another sensitive test for ACL rupture and assesses the secondary rotatory restraint of the ACL. In the acute setting, this is quite painful and is most often used intraoperatively during an exam under anesthesia.

Imaging

Anteroposterior (AP) and lateral views of the knee should be the first imaging studies obtained to rule out any associated fractures. This includes tibial eminence fractures, which can mimic a ligamentous injury, and the **"Segond fracture,"** which is a lateral capsular avulsion fracture that is considered pathognomonic for an underlying ACL injury. Merchant, or "sunrise," views are special views of the patella that evaluate the bony architecture of the patellofemoral articulation for fracture or dislocation.

After initial radiographic evaluation, **MRI of the injured knee is highly sensitive and specific in confirming injury to intraarticular structures** (Figures 22–2A and 22–2B). In addition to visualizing the ligaments, the MRI allows for evaluation for chondral injuries and bone bruises, which can also be indicative of ligamentous injury. The menisci may also be evaluated for injury with an MRI.

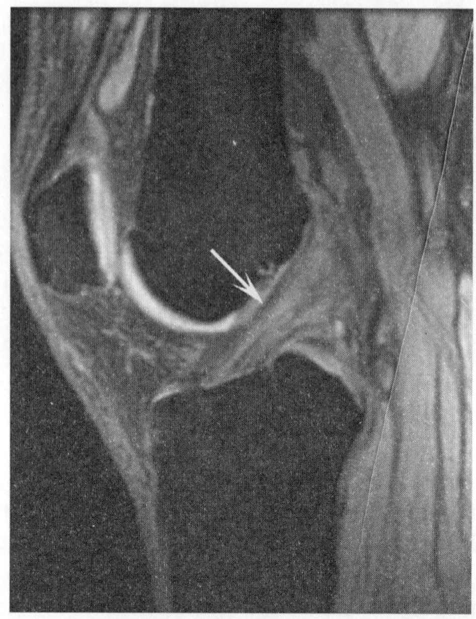

A

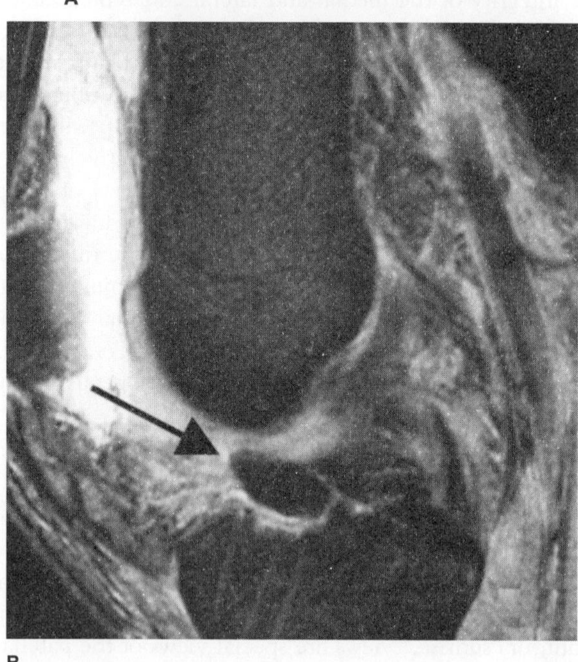

B

Figure 22–2. (**A**) Sagittal T2-weighted fat-saturated MRI of the knee showing a normal ACL (*arrow*). Notice the fascicular arrangement. (Reproduced, with permission, from Chen MYM, Pope TL, Ott DJ. *Basic Radiology*. 2nd ed. New York, NY: McGraw-Hill; 2011:Fig. 7-20.) (**B**) Lateral T1-weighted MRI showing an acute rupture of the anterior cruciate ligament (*arrow*). (Reproduced, with permission, from Doherty GM. *Current Diagnosis & Treatment: Surgery*. 13th ed. New York, NY: McGraw-Hill; 2010:Fig. 40-30.)

TREATMENT

Rationale for Treatment

ACL-deficient patients complain of their affected knees frequently "giving out." This recurrent instability prevents the majority of these patients from reaching their preinjury level of activity and places them at an increased risk for meniscal and chondral injuries. The development of arthritis in ACL-deficient knees compared with those that undergo reconstruction is controversial, as some authors have found that the patients *with* ACL-reconstructed knees have more long-term degenerative changes.

Factors influencing the treatment of ACL-deficient knees include patient age, functional demand, instability, expectations, and associated injuries. Many orthopaedic surgeons also prefer that patients regain knee range of motion before performing a reconstructive procedure. **In general, patients younger than 30 years of age should undergo surgical reconstruction, whereas those older than 30 years of age should undergo an initial period of rehabilitation followed by reevaluation.** In the latter setting, reconstruction is indicated in the presence of recurrent instability. Repair of concurrent meniscus tears, cartilage lesions, and/or associated ligamentous injuries often mandates ACL reconstruction, either at the same time or as a later staged procedure, to attain good outcomes. For example, meniscus repairs in ACL-deficient knees do not heal and therefore should be done in conjunction with ACL reconstruction. Additionally, posterolateral corner (PLC) and posteromedial corner (PMC) injuries that are undiagnosed or untreated in the setting of an ACL tear are common causes of ACL reconstruction failure.

Nonoperative Treatment

Nonoperative treatment of ACL injuries involves activity modification, bracing, and physical therapy. Activities that require cutting and jumping, such as basketball and soccer, should be replaced with straight-ahead activities, such as biking and running. **Braces do not replace a native, intact ACL.** However, there are specific ACL braces that can provide symptomatic comfort. Physical therapy focuses on hamstring strengthening and can have good functional outcomes.

ACL Reconstruction

Early efforts for the treatment of the ACL-deficient knee focused on primary repair of the ligament. However, mid- and long-term outcomes were poor, which led to the development of a variety of intra- and extraarticular autologous soft tissue and synthetic augmentation procedures. These treatments were also found to have poor long-term outcomes and increased complications. There are several theories regarding why primary repair was ineffective and pertain to the ACL's location within the knee joint. As an intraarticular structure, synovial fluid prevents the formation of a fibrin blood clot that bridges the tear. The torn ends of the ligament subsequently fibrose, and end-to-end healing does not occur.

Because primary ACL repair is ineffective, current operative treatment involves arthroscopically assisted reconstruction in which bone tunnels are placed at the ACL's tibial insertion and at the femoral origin. A soft tissue autograft or allograft is ultimately passed through these tunnels. **Classically, a bone-patellar tendon-bone**

autograft has been used for primary reconstructive procedures, with allograft reserved for older patients, multi-ligamentously injured knees, and revision cases. Although autografts are healthy, living tissue, they risk donor site morbidity. Conversely, allografts do not cause donor site morbidity but have variable tissue quality and carry the low risk of disease transmission (ie, hepatitis C and human immunodeficiency virus). More recently, quadrupled hamstring autografts have gained favor with the advancement of fixation techniques. This involves harvesting of the distal gracilis and semitendinosus tendons at their pes anserine insertion and doubling them over themselves to create 4 strands. This technique is inherently stronger than a bone-patellar tendon-bone graft, but its initial fixation to bone is not as strong. Other graft options include Achilles tendon and tibialis anterior tendon allograft. Some surgeons perform a double-bundle reconstruction, as there is thought that this more closely simulates normal knee kinematics. However, double-bundle reconstruction is a significantly more complex procedure, and more clinical data must be presented proving its superiority over the more classic, single-bundle reconstruction techniques before it is deemed the standard of care.

Complications

The goal of ACL reconstruction is restoration of normal knee kinematics. **However, one of the most common complications after ACL reconstruction is loss of motion—specifically, development of a flexion contracture.** The causes of this include arthrofibrosis, cyclops lesions, improper graft tensioning and placement, and inadequate postoperative extension bracing. A **cyclops lesion** is a hypertrophied remnant of the native ACL on the tibia, which results in the inability to attain full extension and may also cause anterior knee pain. These patients often present 4 to 6 months after reconstruction with an inability to achieve full extension. Arthroscopy is diagnostic and the lesion can be excised, which usually resolves the problem. Aberrant graft positioning may lead to loss of motion and early graft failure. A graft placed anteriorly to its normal axis of rotation will make it tight in flexion and thus limit it. A graft placed too posterior will limit terminal extension, as it becomes too tight in extension.

Other complications of ACL reconstruction include infection, graft donor site morbidity, and the development of complex regional pain syndrome, formerly known as reflex sympathetic dystrophy.

Postoperative Care and Rehabilitation

The goal of postoperative rehabilitation is to reduce swelling, maintain patellar mobility to limit anterior knee pain, and regain full range of motion of the knee. Strengthening exercises revolve around the quadriceps, which atrophy quickly after surgery, and the hamstrings. Isometric hamstring and quadriceps contractions are appropriate and do not place excessive stress on the graft. Closed chain exercises (foot planted) should be emphasized. Open chain quadriceps strengthening must be avoided, in addition to isokinetic quadriceps strengthening during early rehabilitation. Joint motion promotes healing, and full passive extension should be allowed early in rehabilitation. Most patients are placed in a knee brace locked in extension postoperatively and are allowed to bear weight on it as tolerated, with crutches for comfort. In general, return to full sporting activities is not advised until at least 5 months after surgery. Pain and swelling must have subsided, full range of motion achieved, and quadriceps and hamstring strength close to that of the normal knee (80% and 90%, respectively). It is important to recognize that specific rehabilitation protocols vary from surgeon to surgeon and that these are only general guidelines.

COMPREHENSION QUESTIONS

22.1 A 22-year-old male basketball player presents with a swollen, painful left knee. He was on a fast break and as he began to jump for an alley-oop, he felt his knee give out and he collapsed to the floor. What is the most likely diagnosis?

A. Patello-femoral dislocation
B. Medial collateral ligament injury
C. Hamstring strain
D. Anterior cruciate ligament injury
E. Posterior cruciate ligament injury

22.2 A 28-year-old female professional skier presents with an exquisitely tender, swollen right knee after a crash during a training run for the alpine downhill. She is unable to bear weight. Knee radiographs reveal an avulsion fracture off of the lateral tibial plateau, but are otherwise unremarkable. What is the most likely positive physical exam finding?

A. Posterior drawer
B. Lachman test
C. McMurray test
D. Patellar apprehension
E. Exam will be unremarkable

22.3 Nonoperative rehabilitation for an ACL-deficient knee should include which of the following?

A. Quadriceps strengthening
B. Straight leg raises
C. Leg presses
D. Short distance sprints
E. Hamstring strengthening

22.4 Where is the primary restraint to anterior translation of the tibia at mid-ranges of knee flexion?

A. Posteromedial bundle of the ACL
B. Posterolateral bundle of the ACL
C. Anteromedial bundle of the ACL
D. Anterolateral bundle of the ACL
E. Both bundles function identically throughout all knee ranges

ANSWERS

22.1 **D.** The history provided describes a noncontact injury to the knee during an acceleration-deceleration/pivoting move with the patient experiencing a feeling of giving way in his knee. The player quickly accumulates a knee effusion and has significant pain. These findings are characteristic descriptions of an ACL injury. The Lachman test is diagnostic for this injury, and an MRI would confirm the diagnosis.

22.2 **B.** Skiing, along with soccer, is strongly associated with ACL injury. The patient presents after a crash with an effusion and inability to bear weight. Knee radiographs demonstrate a lateral capsular avulsion fracture (Segond fracture). This is pathognomonic for an ACL injury. The Lachman test, performed by translating the tibia anteriorly with the knee in 30 degrees of flexion and assessing for a firm end point, is highly sensitive for an ACL injury.

22.3 **E.** When treating a patient with an ACL-deficient knee nonoperatively, rehabilitation should consist of aggressive hamstring strengthening.

22.4 **C.** The ACL is the primary restraint to anterior translation of the tibia with respect to the femur. It consists of 2 bundles, the anteromedial and posterolateral bundles. The anteromedial is the largest of the 2 bundles and functions as the primary restraint to anterior translation in the mid-ranges of knee flexion.

CLINICAL PEARLS

- The ACL originates from the medial wall of the lateral femoral condyle and travels obliquely, inserting on the tibia just anterior to and between the intercondylar eminences of the tibia.
- The primary role of the ACL is restraining anterior translation of the tibia with respect to the femur. It is a secondary restraint to tibial rotation.
- ACL tears are caused by noncontact pivoting injuries with the foot firmly planted on the ground. They are commonly seen in soccer players and skiers.
- Nonoperative treatment is typically reserved for older, sedentary patients and is based on a rehabilitation protocol encouraging aggressive hamstring strengthening, bracing, and activity modifications.
- The goal of ACL reconstruction is restoration of normal knee kinematics.
- ACL reconstruction is the treatment of choice for young, active patients.

REFERENCES

Arnoczky SP. Anatomy of the anterior cruciate ligament. *Clin Orthop*. 1983;172:19-25.

Beynnon BD, Johnson RJ, Abate JA, et al. Treatment of anterior cruciate ligament injuries: Part 1. *Am J Sports Med*. 2005;33:1579-1602.

Beynnon BD, Johnson RJ, Abate JA, et al. Treatment of anterior cruciate ligament injuries: Part 2. *Am J Sports Med*. 2005;33:1751-1767.

Boden BP, Sheehan FT, Torg JS, Hewett, TE. Noncontact anterior cruciate ligament injuries: mechanisms and risk factors. *J Am Acad Orthop Surg*. 2010;18:520-527.

Honkamp NJ, Fu FH, et al. Anterior cruciate ligament injuries. In: DeLee J et al, ed. *DeLee & Drez's Orthopaedic Sports Medicine*. 3rd ed. Philadelphia: Saunders Elsevier; 2010:1644-1676.

CASE 23

A 28-year-old otherwise healthy man presents to the office complaining of pain and swelling in his right knee. He reports that he first noticed pain when he pivoted off of the right leg during a pickup football game 2 days earlier. He was able to finish playing the game. He did not recall an audible "pop" or immediate swelling. The effusion developed later that evening. He denies any sense of instability. The patient denies any other medical or surgical history. On physical exam of the right knee, there are no abrasions or ecchymosis. There is a mild to moderate effusion and tenderness to palpation along the medial joint line. There is no pes anserine, lateral joint line, or other bony tenderness. He has complete, but painful, range of motion. He is stable to varus and valgus stress at 0 and 30 degrees. He has negative Lachman, anterior, and posterior drawer tests. McMurray and Apley tests are positive. He is neurovascularly intact distally.

- ▸ What is your most likely diagnosis?
- ▸ What should be included in the differential diagnosis?
- ▸ What is your next diagnostic step?
- ▸ What is the next step in therapy?

ANSWERS TO CASE 23:

Meniscal Tears

Summary: A 28-year-old healthy man who sustained a right knee twisting injury during a pickup football game presents with right knee pain. His exam is significant for a moderate effusion, medial joint line tenderness, positive McMurray and Apley tests, and a stable ligamentous exam.

- **Most likely diagnosis:** Tear of the medial meniscus.
- **Differential diagnosis:** Osteoarthritis, loose body, patellar subluxation or dislocation, osteochondritis dissecans, articular cartilage lesions, tibial plateau fractures, ligamentous injury, pes anserine bursitis, and fat pad impingement syndrome.
- **Next diagnostic step:** Plain radiographs of the knee, followed by magnetic resonance imaging (MRI).
- **Next step in therapy:** Arthroscopic partial meniscectomy, with resection to a stable, smooth rim of meniscus. Meniscal repair is also a possibility, depending on the location of the tear.

ANALYSIS

Objectives

1. Understand the typical patient demographics and mechanism of injury associated with meniscal tears.
2. Be familiar with the treatment options for meniscal pathology.

Considerations

This is a 28-year-old man who presents after an injury to his right knee sustained during a pickup football game. The history and physical exam are very typical for meniscal pathology. This includes his twisting mechanism of injury, pain, late-onset joint effusion (versus a sudden-onset effusion, which may indicate isolated or concomitant anterior cruciate ligament tear), and medial joint line tenderness. Additionally, 2 meniscus-specific tests, the McMurray and Apley tests, are positive (Figure 23–1). Although the patient's history and examination are consistent with an acute meniscal injury, the orthopaedist must also be familiar with patients presenting with symptoms indicative of the more chronic "degenerative" and "complex" meniscal tears. In the setting of a meniscal tear, radiographs and potentially MRI should be obtained. Treatment, which consists of either operative or more conservative measures, is patient specific, with multiple factors determining the ideal approach.

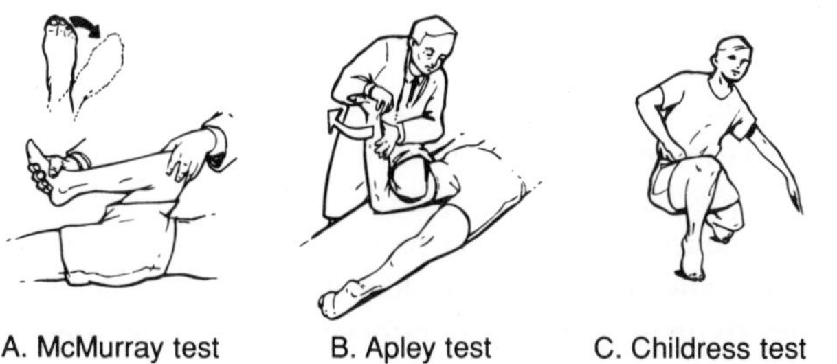

Figure 23–1. Tests for tear of the medial meniscus. (A) McMurray test. (B) Apley test. (C) Childress test. (Reproduced, with permission, from LeBlond RF, DeGowin RL, Brown DD. *DeGowin's Diagnostic Examination.* 9th ed. New York, NY: McGraw-Hill; 2009:Fig. 13-24.)

APPROACH TO: Meniscal Tears

DEFINITIONS

MENISCI (MEDIAL AND LATERAL): Fibrocartilaginous (predominantly type I collagen) structures within the knee joint that increase contact area, distribute load (50%-70% in extension and 85%-90% in flexion), absorb shock, and play a role in joint stability and proprioception. Removing the entire meniscus decreases the overall knee contact area and subsequently results in increased stress throughout the knee, pain, and degenerative joint disease. The medial meniscus is larger and more oblong than the lateral meniscus. It is also an important secondary stabilizer to anterior tibial translation and is thus essential for stability in an anterior cruciate ligament (ACL)-deficient knee.

VASCULAR ZONES: The meniscus is divided into thirds based on vascularity. The peripheral third is the most vascularized and deemed the "red-red" zone. The middle third, referred to as the "red-white" zone, has an intermediate vascularity. The inner third, or the "white-white" zone, is avascular.

MCMURRAY TEST: Flexion and rotation of the knee. To test the medial meniscus, the examiner flexes the knee, places a hand on the medial or posteromedial joint line of the knee, and then brings the knee from flexion to extension while externally rotating the leg. To test the lateral meniscus, the examiner places a hand on the lateral joint line and applies an internal rotation force to the leg. A positive test is found with a palpable "clunk" at the joint line and occurs as the torn meniscus displaces. It is the most specific test (98%) for a meniscal tear but is only 15% sensitive.

APLEY TEST: The patient is prone with the knee flexed to 90 degrees. A downward compressive force is applied by the examiner through the lower leg while laterally rotating the lower leg. Pain during this maneuver is indicative of a meniscal injury.

CLINICAL APPROACH

Etiology

Meniscal tears have an incidence of 60 to 70 cases per 100,000 people per year and occur with a male predominance of approximately 3:1. **Tears can be divided into 2 etiologies: those occurring in younger patients and caused by an acute, twisting, or rotational force and those seen in older patients with menisci vulnerable to injury secondary to underlying degenerative changes of the knee.**

Diagnosis

A thorough history and physical exam is the first step in diagnosis, and patients with meniscal pathology may describe an acute injury or a more indolent onset of symptoms. Patients may have recurring knee effusions, medial or lateral joint line tenderness, posterior knee pain, and/or mechanical symptoms, such as locking and clicking.

The physical exam includes observing the patient's gait, knee alignment, symmetry, and use of assistive devices. Palpation and evaluation of the patella for tenderness and laxity, palpation of the medial and lateral joint lines, the pes anserinus, medial and lateral collateral ligaments, tibial tubercle, and Gerdy tubercle should also be done. Range of motion (both hip and knee) must be assessed and compared with the contralateral side, as should a ligamentous (ACL, posterior cruciate ligament, medial collateral ligament, lateral collateral ligament) exam. **Of note, a torn lateral meniscus is the most commonly associated meniscal injury in the setting of an acute ACL tear, whereas the medial meniscus is most commonly torn in the setting of a knee with a chronic ACL deficiency.** Crepitus or locking should also be noted.

Two tests commonly used for the evaluation of meniscus-specific pathology are the **McMurray and Apley tests** (Figure 23–1). Both have a high specificity but poor sensitivity. Joint line tenderness remains the most sensitive test (74%) for a meniscal injury. **Childress sign (Squat test)** can also be used and is positive when the patient, who attempts to squat and walk like a duck, feels pain, is unable to squat all the way down, and feels a snap or click from the knee (Figure 23–1).

Plain radiographs should be the first imaging obtained. This includes bilateral weightbearing posteroanterior (PA) views, 45-degree flexion PA views, 20 degrees of flexion in patellofemoral view, and a lateral radiograph. MRI is used to confirm the physical exam findings concerning for a meniscal tear and will identify the tear pattern and displacement (Figure 23–2). It has an accuracy of approximately 95% in diagnosing tears.

TREATMENT

Treatment of meniscal tears is patient- and tear-specific and varies from nonsurgical, conservative measures to resection, repair, or transplant. **Nonsurgical treatment includes ice, nonsteroidal anti-inflammatory drugs (NSAIDs), intraarticular corticosteroid injections, and physical therapy.** Indications include asymptomatic, partial-thickness tears less than 5 to 10 mm in length.

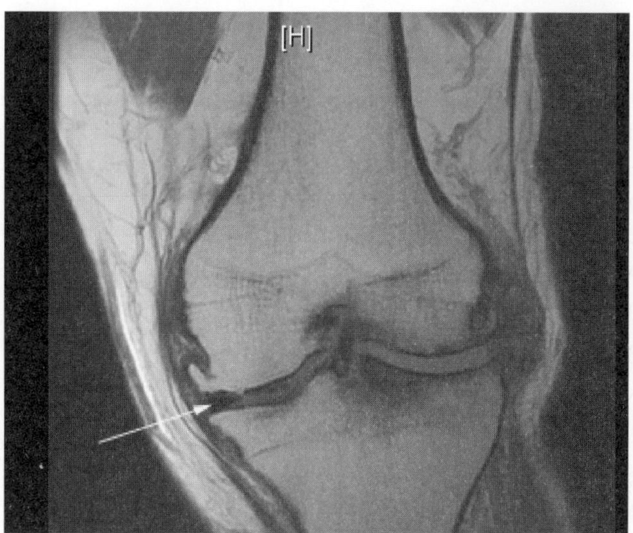

Figure 23–2. Medial meniscal tear on the MRI frontal view, seen as a small white line through the black meniscus. (Courtesy of Heidi Chumley, MD)

Surgical options include meniscal repair, open and arthroscopic partial meniscectomy, and meniscal transplant. **Meniscal repair is reserved for acute tears in the "red-red" zone of a nondegenerative meniscus. Arthroscopic partial meniscectomy is the current standard of care for most tears and can relieve pain and eliminate mechanical blocks to motion while preserving as much healthy tissue as possible.** Indications include symptomatic radial or longitudinal tears, patients who have failed nonoperative management, displaced bucket-handle tears, tears creating a mechanical block, and symptomatic discoid lateral meniscus. Patients with severe degenerative joint disease may be candidates for knee replacement. Meniscal allograft transplant is indicated in a select group of young patients who have failed prior partial or total meniscectomy with minimal degenerative changes.

Complications

Because the meniscus is responsible for the distribution of load and shear forces across the knee, the initial meniscal injury as well as its management (ie, partial or total meniscectomy) can increase the contact pressures between the femur and tibia, accelerating the progression of degenerative joint disease. Additionally, repairs can fail and infections can occur, either postoperatively or after an intraarticular injection.

COMPREHENSION QUESTIONS

23.1 A college football player reports pain along the medial joint line with intermittent locking and an inability to fully extend the knee after a twisting injury to his right knee. He has a negative Lachman exam and a positive McMurray test. What is the most likely diagnosis?

A. Longitudinal vertical lateral meniscus tear
B. ACL injury
C. PCL injury
D. Bucket-handle medial meniscus tear
E. None of the above

23.2 Which of the following physical examination maneuvers is the most sensitive in the diagnosis of a medial meniscus tear?

A. Apley test
B. McMurray test
C. Medial joint line tenderness
D. Lachman test
E. Pain with valgus stress

23.3 A 20-year-old soccer player sustained a twisting injury to his knee approximately 1 month ago. He complains of continued medial-sided knee pain with occasional locking and catching. MRI findings are consistent with a tear of the medial meniscus. What physical exam finding is classically seen with this injury?

A. Positive anterior drawer test
B. No end point with varus stressing of the knee
C. Palpable pop when bringing the flexed knee to extension while internally rotating the leg
D. Palpable pop when bringing the flexed knee to extension while externally rotating the leg

ANSWERS

23.1 **D.** The patient has a bucket-handle medial meniscus tear after an acute injury. Such tears are associated with knee locking and a block to full extension. These tears are more common in young patients, often associated with ACL tears, and are the most commonly missed meniscal tear on MRI.

23.2 **C.** Although the McMurray and Apley grind tests are commonly used to aid in diagnosis, joint line tenderness to palpation has been shown to be the most sensitive physical exam finding for meniscal injury.

23.3 **D.** A positive McMurray test in the setting of a medial meniscus tear is the presence of a palpable pop as the knee is brought from a flexed to extended position while externally rotating the leg. C describes a positive McMurray test for a lateral meniscus tear. A and B do not describe tests for meniscal pathology, but instead the anterior cruciate ligament and the lateral collateral ligament, respectively.

CLINICAL PEARLS

- Meniscal tears are most accurately diagnosed by history and physical exam, with joint line tenderness being the most sensitive indicator of a meniscal tear.
- Two tests commonly used for the evaluation of meniscus-specific pathology are the McMurray and Apley tests, both of which have a high specificity and low sensitivity.
- MRI has an accuracy of approximately 95% in diagnosing tears. Asymptomatic, partial-thickness tears less than 5 to 10 mm in length are typically treated nonoperatively.
- Indications for arthroscopic partial meniscectomy include symptomatic radial or longitudinal tears, patients who have failed nonoperative management, displaced bucket-handle tears, tears creating a mechanical block, and symptomatic discoid lateral meniscus.

REFERENCES

Douglas JA, Sgaglione NA. Meniscal injuries. In: Schepsis AA, Busconi BD, eds. *Orthopaedic Surgery Essentials: Sports Medicine*. Philadelphia, PA: Lippincott Williams & Wilkins; 2006.

Greis PE, Bardana DD, Holmstrom MC, Bruks RT. Meniscal injury: I. Basic science and evaluation. *J Am Acad Orthop Surg*. 2002;10:168-176.

Ryzewicz M, Peterson B, Siparsky PN, Bartz RL. The diagnosis of meniscus tears: the role of MRI and clinical examination. *Clin Orthop Relat Res*. 2007;455:124-133.

CASE 24

A 21-year-old right-hand dominant college baseball pitcher presents to your office with a 1-month history of right elbow pain. He reports that the pain is localized to the medial side of the elbow and that his symptoms are exacerbated by any overhead throwing activities. He has recently noticed a significant change in throwing accuracy and states that his throwing velocity has significantly diminished (98 mph to 86 mph). He denies any associated mechanical symptoms such as locking or catching within the elbow; however, he does report occasional numbness and tingling in his ring and small fingers. Physical examination demonstrates focal tenderness over the medial epicondyle as well as the flexor-pronator mass. He has approximately 5 degrees less elbow extension as compared with the contralateral elbow. He has significant pain with valgus stress applied to the elbow.

- ▶ What is your most likely diagnosis?
- ▶ What is your next diagnostic step?
- ▶ What is the next step in therapy?

ANSWERS TO CASE 24:

Ulnar Collateral Ligament Injury of the Elbow

Summary: A 21-year-old right-hand dominant college baseball pitcher presents with a 1-month history of right elbow pain during overhead throwing activities and complaints of decreased athletic performance. On examination, he has focal tenderness over the medial epicondyle and the flexor pronator mass, as well as reproducible pain with a valgus stress applied to the right elbow.

- **Most likely diagnosis:** Ulnar collateral ligament (UCL) tear.
- **Next diagnostic step:** Standard radiographs with or without "throwers series."
- **Next step in therapy:** UCL reconstruction.

ANALYSIS

Objectives

1. Review relevant elbow anatomy and biomechanics as it pertains to the throwing athlete and recognize common associated pathology in athletes who present with UCL tears.
2. Discuss a diagnostic approach to UCL injury in throwing athletes, including common physical exam findings and the specific role of standard and advanced imaging techniques.
3. Be familiar with the available treatment modalities and the primary principles of nonoperative (physical therapy) and operative management (UCL reconstruction).

Considerations

The UCL is composed of 3 distinct bundles, namely the anterior bundle, the posterior bundle, and the oblique bundle (ie, transverse ligament). The **anterior bundle** serves as the **primary stabilizer to valgus stress** when the elbow is in a flexed position. To understand the contribution of the UCL to elbow stability during throwing, it is important to be familiar with the **6 phases of the baseball pitch.** These highly coordinated phases include the (1) wind-up, (2) early arm-cocking, (3) late arm-cocking, (4) acceleration, (5) deceleration, and (6) follow-through phases. Valgus force generated at the elbow during the throwing motion is **highest during the late cocking and early acceleration phases.**

Throwing athletes place significant functional demands on the UCL, and repetitive overuse can result in chronic injury to the ligament. These injuries were once considered career-ending; however, improved understanding of elbow biomechanics and throwing kinematics has resulted in successful clinical outcomes in the majority of patients who undergo surgical reconstruction of the UCL. The 21-year-old baseball pitcher in this clinical scenario developed a UCL tear from repetitive valgus force placed on the UCL during pitching. Overhead throwing can produce forces that **exceed the ligament's tensile strength,** thus resulting in ligament rupture and debilitating medial elbow pain. UCL reconstruction is the principal procedure to restore valgus stability and relieve medial elbow pain in the setting of UCL injury.

APPROACH TO:
UCL Injury of the Elbow

DEFINITIONS

LIGAMENT: A dense connective tissue structure comprising primarily type I collagen with the primary function of restricting joint motion (ie, stabilize joints).

VALGUS STRESS: Refers to a force at the elbow that is produced with outward angulation (ie, away from the body's midline) of the distal segment of the arm.

TENSILE STRENGTH: A measure of a material's ability to resist a specific force that tends to tear it apart. It is expressed as the maximum stress/force that the material can withstand without disruption.

CLINICAL APPROACH

When obtaining a history from a throwing athlete who presents with medial elbow pain, it is important to obtain specific information regarding the athlete's sport (baseball, softball, javelin, etc.), level of participation, and any recent changes in the athlete's training routine (ie, increase in pitch count, types of pitches thrown). In general, patients can present with an acute tear of the ligament, characterized by the sudden onset of medial elbow pain accompanied by a **"popping"** sensation, or with chronic overuse injuries, which are typically characterized by persistent bouts of pain during pitching and complaints of decreased throwing accuracy, velocity, and stamina. **Most patients report significant pain during the late cocking and early acceleration phases of throwing, as it represents the phase at which the ligament experiences the greatest amount of valgus stress.** Mechanical symptoms such as locking or catching during elbow motion can represent associated pathology, including olecranon osteophytes or intraarticular loose bodies. Ulnar nerve pathology typically manifests as specific neurologic complaints, including numbness and tingling that radiates to the ring and small fingers.

Physical exam should begin with inspection of the elbow to detect the presence of an effusion. If a UCL injury is suspected, the ligament should be palpated along its anatomic course from the medial epicondyle (origin) to the sublime tubercle (insertion) located on the ulna. Any tenderness within this area can represent significant injury to the ligament or the flexor-pronator musculature. Both passive and active range of motion should be compared with the opposite extremity, as it is common to observe slight elbow flexion contractures in the dominant extremity. Several physical examination tests can be used to specifically test the integrity of the UCL. The **valgus stress test** is performed with the arm stabilized against the examiner and the elbow flexed to 30 degrees (Figure 24–1). Valgus stress is then gently applied at the elbow to detect any abnormal widening at the ulnohumeral joint and/or reproduction of painful symptoms. The **"milking maneuver"** is performed with the elbow flexed beyond 90 degrees, as the contralateral arm is used to grasp the thumb and generate a valgus force at the elbow (Figure 24–2). If the patient reports pain with this test, a UCL injury should be suspected. The **moving valgus stress test** is performed with the examiner applying a valgus torque at the elbow in full flexion and

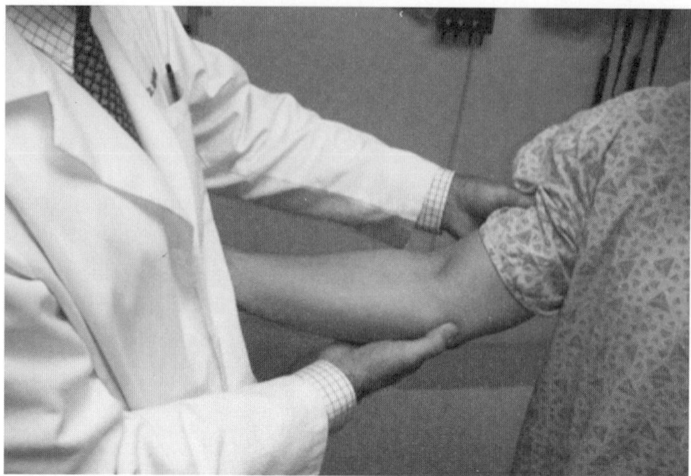

Figure 24–1. The valgus stress test is performed with the arm stabilized against the examiner and the elbow flexed to 30 degrees. Valgus stress is then gently applied at the elbow to detect any abnormal widening at the ulnohumeral joint and/or reproduction of painful symptoms. (Courtesy of Christopher Dodson, MD)

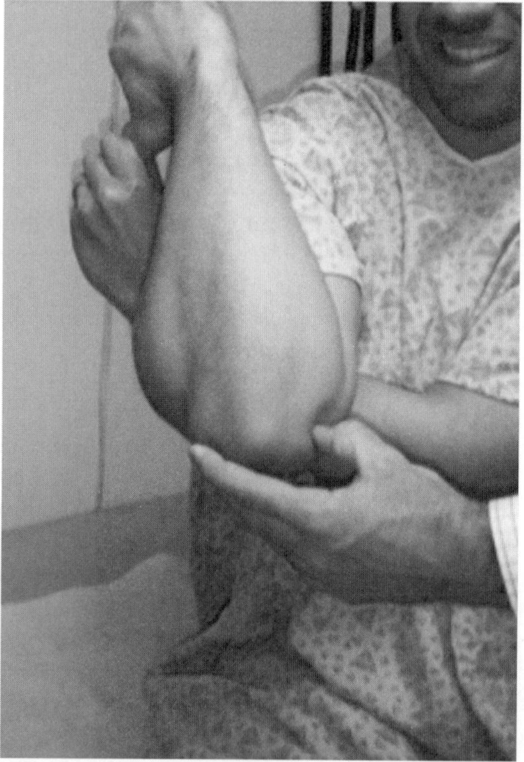

Figure 24–2. The "milking maneuver" is performed with the elbow flexed beyond 90 degrees, as the contralateral arm is used to grasp the thumb and generate a valgus force at the elbow. If the patient reports pain with this test, a UCL injury should be suspected. (Courtesy of Christopher Dodson, MD)

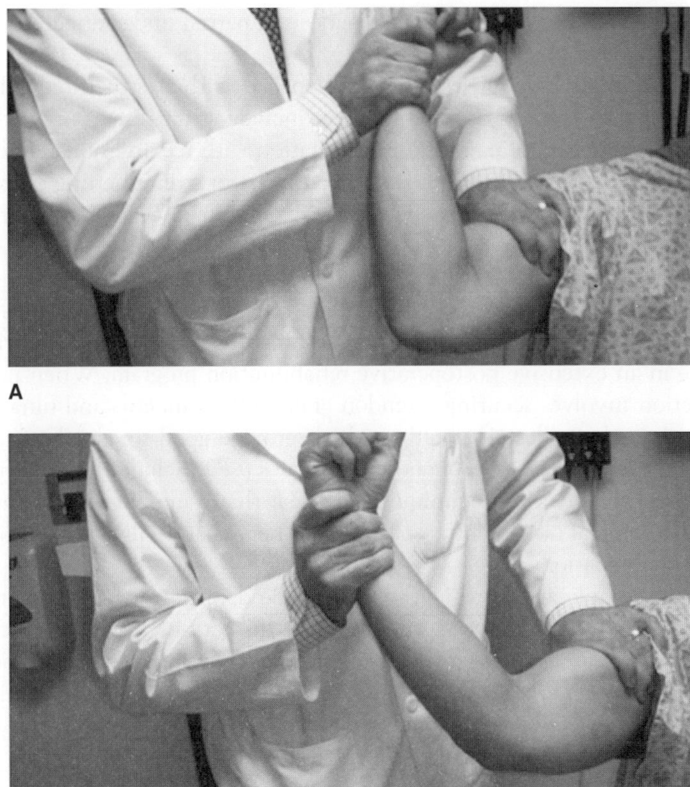

Figure 24–3. The moving valgus stress test is performed with the examiner (**A**) applying a valgus torque at the elbow in full flexion and (**B**) quickly extending the elbow to produce a shear force. This test is highly sensitive (100%) and specific (75%) for UCL injury. (Courtesy of Christopher Dodson, MD)

quickly extending the elbow to produce a shear force (Figures 24–3A and 24–3B). This test is highly sensitive (100%) and specific (75%) for UCL injury.

Several basic and advanced imaging studies can be used to facilitate accurate diagnosis and guide proper treatment in any athlete who presents with a suspected UCL tear. Routine diagnostic imaging should begin with standard AP and lateral radiographs of the elbow. A **"throwers series,"** which includes two oblique radiographic views in internal and external rotation and an oblique axial view with the elbow in 110 degrees of flexion, can also be obtained to look for subtle associated pathology (ie, osteophyte formation, radiocapitellar osteochondritis dissecans, intraarticular loose bodies). Lastly, stress AP radiographs (x-rays obtained with valgus stress applied to the elbow) of both the injured and uninjured elbows can be used to detect any subtle differences in ulnohumeral widening secondary to UCL disruption. Advanced imaging, such as magnetic resonance imaging (MRI), can help identify ligament thickening from chronic overuse injury or more obvious full-thickness tears. Magnetic resonance arthrography obtained with intraarticular injection of gadolinium can aid in the diagnosis of partial undersurface tears of the ligament.

Some UCL tears can successfully be managed with a structured rehabilitation protocol. Early phases of rehabilitation include strict rest from all throwing activities and reduction of pain and inflammation with ice and nonsteroidal anti-inflammatory drugs (NSAID). Gradual flexor-pronator strengthening exercises are incorporated, along with a progressive throwing program once all painful symptoms have resolved.

Surgical reconstruction of the UCL is indicated when patients demonstrate continued symptoms after a trial of structured rehabilitation. UCL reconstruction should only be performed in high-demand, throwing athletes who are willing to participate in an extensive postoperative rehabilitation program. When indicated, reconstruction involves securing a tendon graft to the humerus and ulna. Several techniques have been described, all of which provide good to excellent results in approximately 85% of cases. Common techniques used include the **modified Jobe technique** and the **docking technique.** It is clear that a muscle-splitting approach and minimal surgical manipulation of the ulnar nerve can limit postoperative morbidity and complications.

The main complications to beware of include damage to the ulnar or medial antebrachial cutaneous nerve during surgical dissection, ulnar or epicondylar fracture during tunnel drilling, and postoperative elbow stiffness from inadequate rehabilitation. In general, athletes can expect to return to competitive throwing 12 months after surgery if the shoulder, elbow, and forearm are pain-free and full range of motion has been restored.

COMPREHENSION QUESTIONS

24.1 A 19-year-old college javelin thrower presents with medial elbow pain during overhead throwing. He is diagnosed with a UCL tear after physical examination and MRI. What anatomic structure is the primary stabilizer to valgus stress at the elbow?

A. Anterior bundle of the UCL

B. Transverse ligament

C. Radial head

D. Flexor pronator mass

24.2 A 17-year-old baseball pitcher presents with medial elbow pain during overhead throwing. He is diagnosed with a UCL tear after physical examination and MRI. During what phase of throwing is he most likely to complain of medial elbow pain?

A. Follow-through

B. Deceleration

C. Acceleration

D. Wind-up

24.3 A 21-year-old javelin thrower is diagnosed with a full-thickness UCL tear. On presentation, he complains of numbness and tingling in the ring and small fingers. Which muscle group would he be most likely to have motor weakness in as well?

A. Brachioradialis

B. Extensor carpi ulnaris

C. Abductor digiti minimi

D. Palmaris longus

ANSWERS

24.1 **A.** The anterior bundle of the UCL is the primary stabilizer to valgus stress at the elbow.

24.2 **C.** Throwing athletes typically complain of medial elbow pain during the acceleration phase of throwing. Valgus force generated at the elbow during the throwing motion is highest during the acceleration phase.

24.3 **C.** The patient is experiencing ulnar nerve paresthesias. If the patient had associated motor symptoms, they would manifest as weakness within the abductor digiti minimi. The other answer choices are not muscles innervated by the ulnar nerve.

CLINICAL PEARLS

- The anterior bundle of the UCL is the primary stabilizer to valgus stress at the elbow.
- Patients with UCL injuries typically report medial elbow pain during the acceleration phase of throwing.
- The most sensitive and specific clinical test for UCL injury is the moving valgus stress test.
- A muscle-splitting surgical approach and minimal manipulation of the ulnar nerve can limit postoperative morbidity to the flexor pronator mass and the ulnar nerve.
- Ulnar nerve transposition can be performed in conjunction with UCL reconstruction if patients demonstrate significant pathology related to the nerve (ulnar nerve subluxation or motor weakness).

REFERENCES

Fleisig GS, Andrews JR, Dillma CJ, Escamilla RF. Kinetics of baseball pitching with implications about injury mechanisms. *Am J Sports Med*. 1995;23:233-239.

Hariri S, Safran MR. Ulnar collateral ligament injury in the overhead athlete. *Clin Sports Med*. 2010;29:619-644.

Jobe FW, Stark H, Lombardo SJ. Reconstruction of the ulnar collateral ligament in athletes. *J Bone Joint Surg [Am]*. 1986;68A:1158-1163.

Williams RJ, Urquhart ER, Altchek DW. Medial collateral ligament tears in the throwing athlete. *Instr Course Lect*. 2004;53:579-586.

CASE 25

A 45-year-old musician comes to the office complaining of a 3-month history of neck pain that radiates into his right arm. It is "electric" in nature, spontaneously sending a shooting sensation down his arm. Last week, he noted weakness in his right arm with elbow flexion. His pain is relatively constant and is accompanied by some loss of sensation in his thumb and index finger. He is finding it difficult to play the piano with his right hand. The patient gains some relief by lying down, but states that occasional bouts of "shooting" pain are interfering with his sleep. He denies other systemic complaints, such as fevers and chills. His past medical and surgical history is unremarkable except for a 20-pack-year smoking history.

On physical exam, gait testing demonstrates a fluid, nonataxic, nonantalgic gait. Neck range of motion is decreased with lateral bending and axial rotation to the right side, and neck extension is uncomfortable. Right shoulder range of motion is pain-free. Neurologic testing demonstrates marked weakness with resisted elbow flexion (4/5) and shoulder abduction and forward flexion (4/5) with full strength in all other right upper extremity muscle groups. He has a decreased bicipital reflex as compared with the unaffected side. Capillary refill is brisk. No lesions, ecchymosis, or erythema is present in the arm or hand. Examination of the left upper extremity and both lower extremities are within normal limits. Plain radiographs of the cervical spine and right shoulder are obtained and show no acute pathology, revealing only mild degenerative changes.

- What is the most likely diagnosis?
- What is the next step in therapy?

ANSWERS TO CASE 25:
Herniated Nucleus Pulposus of the Cervical Spine

Summary: A 45-year-old male smoker presents with 3 months of electric-like pains beginning in his neck and radiating down his right arm. He has weakness in his biceps. Radiographs reveal only mild cervical spondylosis.

- **Most likely diagnosis:** Cervical radiculopathy due to a herniated nucleus pulposus (HNP).
- **Next step in therapy:** Nonoperative (conservative) management with over-the-counter medications including acetaminophen and nonsteroidal anti-inflammatory drugs (NSAIDs) and possibly muscle relaxants. Short courses of oral corticosteroids, such as methylprednisolone (Medrol) dose packs, are also an option. Brief courses of low-dose narcotics for breakthrough pain may be prescribed, and recommendations for stretching exercises and application of cold and/or warm compresses may be given. Smoking cessation is indicated, as tobacco and nicotine use has been associated with the pathogenesis of degenerative changes in the disk and HNP.

ANALYSIS

Objectives

1. Develop a diagnostic approach to cervical neck pain.
2. Understand the workup for radiculopathic pain.
3. Be familiar with the natural history of HNP and the indications for surgery.

Considerations

This 45-year-old man developed neck pain insidiously. Although he has slight weakness, he does not have any symptoms requiring urgent intervention. A careful history eliminates the possibilities of radiculopathy as secondary to trauma, infection, or other inflammatory neoplastic processes. The physician must be sure to localize the pathology to the cervical spine, as ipsilateral shoulder and upper-extremity pathologies such as brachial plexus injury or peripheral nerve entrapment may present similarly. On physical exam, strength, sensation, and reflexes are tested in all applicable myotomal and dermatomal distributions of the bilateral upper and lower extremities. This patient exhibits mild weakness consistent with a right-sided C6 nerve root pathology. Special tests, like the Spurling test, help diagnose nerve root compression at the cervical level. Plain radiographs, although not always necessary on first presentation, are relatively inexpensive and painless and are a simple and convenient way to evaluate for processes other than an HNP, such as fracture or facet arthropathy.

Given this patient's history, radiographs consistent with only mild degenerative changes and physical exam findings that include weakness with resisted elbow flexion, positive Spurling test, and blunted biceps reflex, he likely has a C6 radiculopathy due to a C5-6 HNP. There is no clear consensus on whether further imaging is necessary in this patient. Indeed the great majority of patients with spinal radiculopathies experience a spontaneous resolution of symptoms with little more than over-the-counter therapies. Because this patient has yet to try NSAIDs and other conservative treatments, he may be trialed on such therapies before further workup is performed. Should the patient experience a dramatic worsening of symptoms or simply a failure to improve on this regimen, magnetic resonance imaging (MRI) of his cervical spine should be obtained.

APPROACH TO:
Cervical Radiculopathy

DEFINITIONS

RADICULOPATHY: Clinical findings of sensory or motor dysfunction in the distribution of a specific nerve root. Radiculopathies are typically caused by nerve root compression.

HOFFMAN SIGN: A physical exam finding suggestive of upper motor neuron dysfunction in the upper extremity. Hoffman sign is elicited by repeatedly "flicking" the tip of the patient's index or middle finger and observing for reactive flexion of the thumb or fingers. It is analogous to the Babinski sign of the lower extremities.

SPURLING SIGN: A physical exam finding elicited with neck extension and rotation toward the affected side. The test is positive when the pattern of radicular pain into the upper extremity is reproduced. Spurling sign is highly suggestive of a cervical spine etiology for upper-extremity pain and should be negative in situations in which radicular-like symptoms are caused by brachial plexus or peripheral nerve compressive etiologies.

CLINICAL APPROACH

Anatomy and Pathophysiology

The most common disk level of the cervical spine responsible for radiculopathic pain is C6-7, which typically manifests as symptoms attributable to C7 nerve root dysfunction. A disk herniation at the C5-6 level is the second most common location in the cervical spine.

Cervical radiculopathy is thought to result from several mechanisms. Most commonly, acute nerve compression occurs from direct nerve root impingement by herniated soft disc material. Typical locations for HNP in the axial plane are posterolateral to the disc space and medial to the uncovertebral joint. Here, the disc-restraining posterior longitudinal ligament and annulus fibrosis are absent, and there is little to restrain an expanding disc when it is placed under pressure. Herniations here typically impinge on the exiting nerve root (ie, the C7 root at C6-7 and the C6 root at C5-6). A second mechanism for cervical nerve root compression may result from chronic disc height loss and hypertrophy of the uncovertebral joint, which is consistent with aging and degenerative disease. Discal height loss may be accompanied by bulging of the disc material or uncovertebral hypertrophy posteriorly against the spinal canal and nerve roots, leading to compression. Similar height loss and degeneration may cause stenosis within the neuroforamina, leading to compression of the exiting nerve root. At least in the acute setting, herniated disc material is thought to be inflammatory in nature and has been associated with the production of inflammatory mediators including interleukin (IL)-1 and IL-6, substance P, bradykinin, tumor necrosis factor α, and prostaglandins.

History and Physical Exam

A thorough history and physical exam should be performed, with special attention to the origin of the patient's symptoms. A history of traumatic onset may suggest fracture or traumatic disc herniation. A history of neoplastic processes or systemic inflammatory states may be suggestive of nerve compression secondary to tumor growth, pathologic fracture, or epidural abscess. Patients may complain of fever, chills, weight loss, or nocturnal malaise in the setting of radicular pain and neurologic dysfunction. In such cases, workup should include advanced imaging of the cervical spine (typically an MRI) and laboratory studies such as white blood cell count, erythrocyte sedimentation rate, and C-reactive protein. If lesions are suggested or suspected, a more generalized exam for metastatic disease involving computed tomography (CT) or nuclear scanning may be required. Common symptoms consistent with HNP of the cervical spine include complaints of occipital headaches; neck pain, worse with motion; and pain in the neck, shoulder, and arms. Root compression often manifests with paresthesias in the affected extremity. It is important to realize, however, that there is a significant overlap and variance in the dermatomal distributions of nerve roots. Therefore, paresthesias associated with single-nerve root compression may not always follow the textbook dermatomal maps.

On exam, motor strength is graded on a 0 to 5 scale. Sensory testing should evaluate for both dorsal column and spinothalamic tract function by evaluation of positional and pain/temperature sensations, respectively. Evidence of upper motor neuropathy should be ruled out. For detailed instruction on performing the spinal exam, please refer to the "Approach to the Orthopaedic Patient" section, located near the beginning of this text.

Differential Diagnosis

Before a clinical diagnosis of cervical radiculopathy can be made, several other disease processes must be considered and then ruled out. Most notably, brachial plexus injuries and peripheral nerve entrapment syndromes of the upper extremity may closely resemble the sensory and motor symptomatology of nerve root compression. Other sources of radicular-like symptoms include degenerative changes, stenosis, and space-occupying lesions, such as abscesses or tumors. The presence of upper motor neuron signs (suggested by a positive Hoffman sign or gait changes) would point to either a cervical stenosis causing cord compression or other neurologic conditions such as amyotrophic lateral sclerosis.

Imaging

Once fractures and other pathology are ruled out by plain x-ray, MRI may be considered a next step in the further workup of cervical radicular pain. It must be stated again, however, that because the great majority of these patients experience a spontaneous resolution of symptoms, not every patient presenting with radicular symptoms needs to undergo urgent MRI. **In patients with unremitting pain that has failed conservative management, continued or progressive weakness, neurologic decompensation, or bowel or bladder changes, MRI is the gold standard to evaluate spinal cord and root compression in the absence of contraindications.** On T2-weighted MRI, cerebrospinal fluid is bright and clearly distinguishes areas of compression and patency. In patients for whom MRI is contraindicated, most commonly those with pacemakers or interventions for intracerebral aneurysms, CT myelography may offer a clear visualization of the spinal cord and roots.

TREATMENT

Nonoperative Treatment

Acute cervical radiculopathy typically has a self-limited course. In fact, 75% of these patients improve without surgical intervention. **The first line against cervical radiculopathic pain should be NSAIDs and/or acetaminophen.** NSAIDs play a distinct role in attenuating the painful local inflammatory response resulting from disc herniations and their inflammatory effects on nerve roots and may decrease pressure around affected nerve roots. Low-dose narcotic analgesics, although not commonly recommended for chronic treatment, may be necessary to control acute pain that is refractory to NSAIDs and acetaminophen. Adjunctive treatment with muscle relaxants such as cyclobenzaprine may help decrease associated painful muscle spasms and may decrease narcotic requirements in certain patients. **Although current literature fails to demonstrate their clear efficacy, brief courses of oral corticosteroids are sometimes prescribed to decrease inflammatory responses to HNP.** Adjunctive therapies such as physical therapy, massage therapy, and the application of heat or ice packs are not strongly supported by the literature, but may be used if helpful to the patient.

When conservative measures fail, epidural steroid injections may offer some transient relief but have not been shown to alter the natural history of the disease process. Localized steroid injections may have an anti-inflammatory effect on irritated nerve roots and may play a role in the inhibition of pain pathways. The true efficacy of epidural injections is debated and varies greatly between individuals.

Surgical Treatment

When nonsurgical treatment fails to relieve symptoms, or if neurologic deficits progressively worsen, surgical decompression may be necessary. **As a general rule, surgical approaches to the cervical spine should be directed "where the pathology is."** Because herniation originates in the disc space, an anterior surgical approach is preferred in the setting of central and posterolateral anterior compressive pathology. Anterior cervical discectomy and fusion (ACDF) is the most common surgical treatment for cervical HNP. For isolated single-level nerve root compression, posterior approaches to the cervical spine may be used if the pathology is accessible through the neural foramen. Posterior laminoforaminotomy relieves pressure on the nerve root by unroofing the neuroforamen and allowing the root to decompress. This technique preserves motion between vertebral levels because the disc is left intact, and thus fusion of vertebral segments is unnecessary. Surgical outcomes for relief of radicular pain range from 80% to 90% with either anterior or posterior approaches.

Lastly, a relatively new and controversial technique in the treatment of single-level disease is cervical disc arthroplasty (replacement). Although limited in both application and supporting data at this time, this promising procedure may offer the best of both worlds: preserving motion between segments while allowing for a thorough discectomy and decompression.

Complications

Although ACDF procedures typically have good outcomes, they are not without potential complications. The anterior approach to the cervical spine puts several vulnerable neurovascular structures at risk, including the recurrent laryngeal nerve (1% risk of injury with ACDF) and, to a lesser degree, the hypoglossal nerve, vagal nerve, and the carotid arteries. Horner syndrome is "classically" characterized by ptosis, anhidrosis, and miosis and results from injury to the sympathetic chain, located laterally to the longus colli muscles at the C6 level. Finally, pseudarthrosis, or the failure of bony fusion, may occur at rates as high as 5% to 10% for single-level fusions. Rates dramatically increase to 30% to 40% for multiple-level fusions, but few pseudoarthroses are actually symptomatic or require revision work. Tobacco and chronic corticosteroid use is a significant risk factor for the development of pseudoarthrosis.

COMPREHENSION QUESTIONS

25.1 A 56-year-old female bodybuilder presents to your clinic after straining her neck during an overhead clean and jerk contest. She complains of numbness in her middle finger and weakness in her elbow extension. Which of the following findings would most likely be present in this patient?

A. Elbow flexion weakness

B. Finger grip weakness

C. Decreased biceps reflex

D. Decreased sensation over the ring and small fingers

E. Decreased triceps reflex

25.2 A 49-year-old downhill skier "tweaks" his neck while loading heavy ski equipment atop his family SUV. He complains of 3 days of small finger numbness and difficulty gripping his ski poles. Which of the following nerve roots is most likely entrapped?

A. C5
B. C6
C. C7
D. C8
E. T1

25.3 A 42-year-old construction worker has experienced 8 weeks of unremitting left biceps weakness, wrist extensor weakness, and both pain and numbness in his index finger and thumb. His pain is especially bad when turning his head to the left. He has tried oral steroids, opiates, NSAIDs, acetaminophen, acupuncture, and a local steroid injection 3 weeks ago; all have failed to provide adequate relieve. He states his biceps and wrist weakness is getting worse, as he is now unable to lift even a glass of water with his left arm. MRI confirms HNP at the left-sided C5-6 neuro foramen. What is the next best step in the management of this patient?

A. Repeat corticosteroid injection at C5-6 level
B. Anterior cervical discectomy and fusion (ACDF) of C5-6
C. Increasing oral steroid dosing
D. Prescribing a hard collar for neck immobilization
E. CT scan and/or bone scan to rule out fracture or other injury

ANSWERS

25.1 **E.** This patient has a C6-C7 HNP affecting the C7 nerve root, which is classically responsible for elbow extension and wrist flexion. The triceps reflex is most commonly associated with C7 nerve root pathology, making E the correct answer choice.

25.2 **D.** Grip strength and sensation to the small and sometimes ring fingers are classically attributed to the C8 nerve root, most often affected by C7-T1 disc herniations.

25.3 **B.** ACDF of C5-6 disc with fusion is an effective and highly successful procedure for patients with clearly defined symptomatology and imaging consistent with pathology. This patient has progressive neurologic changes consistent with a well-defined dermo/myotomal distribution. He has failed conservative therapy; increasing steroid dosing and even additional steroid injection are unlikely to help. Further imaging is unnecessary given the consistency between his symptoms and MRI and a lack of suspicion for further injury.

CLINICAL PEARLS

- More than 75% of patients with cervical radiculopathic pain improve without surgical intervention.
- NSAIDs and acetaminophen are the mainstays and first line against cervical radiculopathy.
- Beware of treating MRI findings without a careful clinical correlation. MRI has high rate of false positives, with almost 30% of normal, asymptomatic individuals >40 years of age positive for HNP or foraminal stenosis on MRI.

REFERENCES

Nordin M, Carragee EJ, Hogg-Johnson S, et al, for the Bone and Joint Decade 2000-2010 Task Force on Neck Pain and Its Associated Disorders. Assessment of neck pain and its associated disorders: results of the Bone and Joint Decade 2000-2010 Task Force on Neck Pain and Its Associated Disorders. *Spine*. 2008;33(4 suppl):S101-S122.

Rhee JM, Yoon T, Riew D. Cervical radiculopathy. *J Am Acad Orthop Surg*. 2007;15:486-494.

Shelerud RA, Paynter KS. Rarer causes of radiculopathy: spinal tumors, infections, and other unusual causes. *Phys Med Rehabil Clin N Am*. 2002;13:645-696.

Tong HC, Haig AJ, Yamakawa K. The Spurling test and cervical radiculopathy. *Spine*. 2002;27:156-159.

CASE 26

A 43-year-old obese man presents to the emergency department (ED) with complaints of 12 hours of right leg pain and "tingling" in his left foot. Yesterday he was helping his neighbor carry a sofa up a flight of stairs when he experienced sudden "lightning-like" pain in his back that radiated down his legs. He went home and took acetaminophen before bed. This morning, he awoke with worsening back and left leg pain, and he was startled to notice weakness in his left foot and ankle. Now, in the ED, he reports an almost complete inability to move his left foot and a burning, constant pain throughout both legs. Physical exam reveals decreased motor strength in his left lower extremity, notably 2/5 extensor hallucis longus and foot dorsiflexor strength. He is unable to plantar flex this foot. His left hip and knee extensors are 5/5 in strength, as are all major muscular groups of his right lower and bilateral upper extremities. He has normal patellar reflexes bilaterally, but an Achilles reflex is only present on his right side. Sensation testing demonstrates decreased sensitivity to light touch and pin-prick stimulation in the perianal regions, perineum, and posterior thighs, bilaterally. The dorsum and plantar aspects of the left foot are similarly insensate. Digital rectal examination demonstrates decreased tone, and the patient is surprised to learn that his underwear is damp with urine. Bladder scan demonstrates a retained volume of 1100 mL. Vascular examination reveals warm and well-perfused skin with palpable dorsalis pedis pulses bilaterally.

- ▶ What is the most likely diagnosis?
- ▶ What are some of the most common causes of this condition?
- ▶ What are the next steps in the management of this patient?

ANSWERS TO CASE 26:
Cauda Equina Syndrome

Summary: This is a 43-year-old man who presents with a 12-hour history of progressively worsening lumbosacral back and left leg pain, weakness, and sensory loss that began after he tried to lift a heavy object. He is experiencing bilateral lower extremity and perianal paresthesias, with significant weakness in his left lower extremity, diminished left-sided reflexes, decreased rectal tone, and urinary retention.

- **Most likely diagnosis:** Cauda equina syndrome (CES) secondary to herniated nucleus pulposis (HNP), most likely at the L4-5 level.
- **Most common causes:** Compression of the cauda equina secondary to lumbar disc herniation, primary tumors or metastatic disease, infections, stenosis, hematomas, and ischemic insult.
- **Management of CES:** Pain control, placement of urinary catheter, MRI of lumbosacral spine to confirm diagnosis and to identify region of compression, and, if positive, emergency surgical decompression of cauda equina.

ANALYSIS

Objectives

1. Recognize the presentation of cauda equina syndrome (CES).
2. Understand the anatomic and pathophysiologic bases of this condition.
3. Be familiar with the management of CES and understand its outcomes.

Considerations

Low back pain is one of the most common complaints in EDs and primary care offices in the United States. Although back pain is disconcerting, even debilitating, to patients, very few patients presenting with acute-onset pain—0.05% by some estimates—require urgent operative intervention. CES is one such urgent indication. This patient's symptoms, although mild at first, rapidly developed into a syndrome including sciatica, lower-extremity sensorimotor loss, and bowel and bladder dysfunction. This rapid progression of symptoms demands urgent and careful attention by knowledgeable physicians, as **delayed intervention can result in devastating consequences if left untreated for greater than 24 to 48 hours.**

After adequate pain relief, a complete and thorough medical history should assess for factors that make the patient prone to cauda equina, such as a history of symptoms of radicular disease, previous spinal surgery or injections, trauma, infection, the use of anticoagulants, or previous spine pathology. Potential spine fractures should be ruled out, because this patient's symptoms began as he was undergoing significant axial loads that may have caused vertebral fractures with cord compression. Next, a thorough physical exam should be performed and must include the often-neglected assessment of sensation, motor, and reflexive function of the perianal and rectal

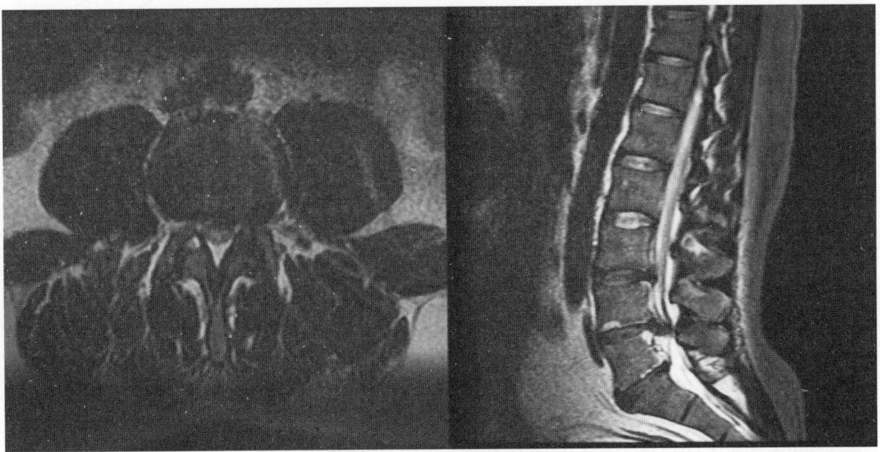

Figure 26–1. Axial (*left*) and sagittal (*right*) slices of T2-weighted spinal MRI of large, centrally herniated disc at L4-5. (Courtesy of Timothy T. Roberts, MD)

regions, including evaluating the presence or absence of normal tone. For detailed instruction on performing the spinal exam, please refer to the "Approach to the Orthopaedic Patient" section, located near the beginning of this text.

The next step in this patient's workup includes urgent acquisition of appropriate imaging, either through magnetic resonance imaging (MRI) of the lumbosacral spine or computed tomography (CT) myelography in the presence of contraindications to MRI. **MRI serves to elucidate the cause and location of the cauda equina compression, as well as to guide the surgical approach (anterior or posterior) and the need for potential arthrodesis (in the setting of instability attributable to trauma, infection, or tumor).** In this case, axial and sagittal T2-weighted images, seen in Figure 26–1, demonstrate a large, posteriorly herniated disc at the L4-5 level extruding paracentrally and laterally on the left side. Roots caudal to this level show varied levels of dysfunction consistent with midline compression of the descending lumbosacral roots. Plans should be made for urgent passage to the operating room, as permanent neurologic damage may result from delayed decompression of the cauda equina.

APPROACH TO:

Cauda Equina Syndrome

DEFINITIONS

SCIATICA: A referred pain syndrome in the buttock, leg, and/or foot distributions of the sciatic nerve, caused by compression of either the sciatic nerve itself, or its individual lumbosacral roots.

ANAL WINK REFLEX: A normal reflex of anal sphincter contraction, elicited by stroking the skin lateral to the anus. Absence of this reflex may suggest dysfunction of the S2-4 nerve roots.

LOWER MOTOR NEURON LESION: Any lesion that disrupts the function of the motor nerve fibers between the anterior horn of the spinal cord and its innervated muscles. Characterized by hypotonia, hypo- or areflexia, flaccid paralysis or weakness, fibrillations, and fasciculations. By contrast, upper motor neuron lesions affect motor nerve pathways between the cerebral motor cortex and the spinal cord and are characterized by hypertonia, hyperreflexia, and spastic paralysis.

CLINICAL APPROACH

CES is an uncommon and relatively rare condition that accounts for fewer than 1 in 2000 patients who present with lower back pain. This condition is associated with a large space-occupying lesion within the lumbosacral spine that impinges on the loose terminal roots of the spinal nerves within the spinal canal. These roots form the cauda equina, or "horse's tail" in Latin, so named for their likeness to the equine appendage. **Diagnostic criteria for CES include 1 or more of the following: (1) bladder and/or bowel dysfunction—typically retention in its early stages, (2) reduced sensation in the saddle area, or (3) sexual dysfunction, with possible motor/sensory/reflex deficit in the lower limb.** Signs and symptoms of CES develop in **less than 24 hours** from a given insult in more than 85% of reported cases. Nerve root compression in CES most commonly results from a herniated lumbar disc, but is thought to represent only 1% to 6% of all operative lumbar HNP cases. Risk factors for HNP include obesity, male sex, age greater than 40 years, and history of spine disorders. Less common etiologies of CES include compression by a tumorous growth, infection and abscess formation, spinal stenosis, hematoma formation, and inflammation.

Anatomy and Pathophysiology

The pathophysiology of CES is complex and not fully understood. In adults, the spinal cord terminates between the L1 and L2 vertebrae body, below which the cauda equina descend as a collection of peripheral nerve roots to the L1 to coccygeal levels. These roots are thought to be especially vulnerable to compression because they are only protected by a single layer of endoneurium, whereas most other peripheral nerves and indeed the spinal cord itself are surrounded by an epineurium, perineurium, and endoneurium. Compression and damage to the cauda equina can lead to diffuse **lower motor neuron lesions,** resulting in uni- or bilateral sciatica, lower extremity weakness, saddle anesthesia (resulting from insult to the S2-4 roots), and bowel and bladder dysfunction (also primarily the S2-4 roots).

Patients presenting with back pain and bowel or bladder dysfunction should raise immediate flags for the possibility of CES. Neurogenic bladder dysfunction, characterized by urinary retention more often than incontinence, is an essential symptom of CES. In normal urinary bladder physiology, the detrusor urinae muscle is responsible for contracting the bladder during voiding and is controlled by the parasympathetic nervous system (PNS) via S2, S3, and S4 nerve roots. During urinary voiding, the PNS directs detrusor contraction with simultaneous relaxation of the internal urinary sphincter. When damage to the S2-4 nerve roots occurs, the bladder cannot contract or release through the sphincter, and thus overflow incontinence develops. Postvoid residual volume should be obtained in patients in whom CES is suspected.

The S2-4 nerve roots also provide sensation to the saddle region, including the perineum, buttocks, and posteromedial thighs. A complete rectal examination, including testing for an **anal wink reflex** and a **bulbocavernosus reflex,** should be performed on CES patients. Patients presenting with both saddle anesthesia and urinary incontinence—suggestive of extensive insult to the sacral roots—have been found to have poor prognosis with regard to long-term bladder function.

Radiologic Evaluation

After a thorough history and physical exam, urgent diagnostic imaging should be performed. Plain radiographs are of limited value in the diagnosis of CES, but may be useful to evaluate for alternate pathology such as a fracture, dislocation or subluxation, tumor, or infection. Diagnosing lumbar disc herniation in CES requires a CT or MRI. **MRI is the gold standard** for evaluating patients because it allows for detailed visualization of the spinal canal, disc spaces, nerve roots, and visualization of any potential space-occupying lesion within the canal or foramina. If MRI is contraindicated or unavailable, CT myelogram is the next best study to evaluate for CES. In addition to confirming the diagnosis, advanced imaging is helpful for preoperative planning for decompression.

TREATMENT AND OUTCOMES

In patients without absolute medical contraindications, CES is treated with emergent surgical exploration and nerve root decompression. A variety of surgical procedures and techniques are performed in the treatment of CES, ranging from minimally invasive micro-discectomies to extensive multiple-level bilateral laminectomies, discectomies, and occasionally arthrodeses. No significant evidence, however, supports the superiority of any one procedure. It is generally thought that surgical decompression should occur within 24 to 48 hours of CES diagnosis to prevent further neurologic decline and to improve chances of recovery. **There is evidence to suggest that patients treated more than 48 hours after diagnosis had significantly decreased odds of recovering complete sensory, motor, sexual, urinary, and rectal function.**

COMPREHENSION QUESTIONS

26.1 A 63-year-old woman with a history of metastatic lung cancer, diabetes, and bradycardia requiring a permanent pacemaker presents with 24 hours of urinary retention and progressive bilateral lower extremity weakness, beginning spontaneously. What is the next step in management?

A. Metastatic workup including CT of chest and preparations for biopsy, if applicable

B. High-dose intravenous methylprednisolone × 24 hours and short-term bedrest

C. Administration of nonsteroidal anti-inflammatory drugs (NSAIDs), acetaminophen, activity modification, physical therapy, and close follow-up

D. Emergency CT myelogram of the lumbosacral spine

E. Emergency MRI of chest with gadolinium contrast

26.2 A 55-year-old man presents with low back pain and right "foot drop" 72 hours after straining his back trying to shovel snow from his driveway. He denies bowel or bladder changes. Sensation is intact throughout his bilateral lower extremities and perianal region, with the exception of some numbness to light touch across the dorsum of his right foot. He has a weak extensor hallucis longus and tibialis anterior (3/5) on his right side, but otherwise full strength in his bilateral low extremities. Straight leg raise is positive on his right side, sending "electric shock" sciatic pain down to his foot. He takes warfarin for atrial fibrillation, and his international normalized ratio (INR) is 2.5. He has no additional symptoms, nor medical history. What is the next step in the management of this patient?

A. High-dose intravenous methylprednisolone for 24 hours
B. Emergency MRI, if not contraindicated, of lumbosacral spine
C. NSAIDs, acetaminophen, activity modification, and physical therapy
D. Urgent reversal of INR with vitamin K and/or fresh-frozen plasma and preoperative planning including making the patient nothing by mouth (NPO), acquiring preoperative laboratory studies, chest x-ray, and electrocardiogram (ECG)
E. Epidural steroid injection

26.3 A 44-year-old woman suffers a fall while rock climbing, landing on her buttocks and falling forward. Despite prolonged airlift to the ED, she is hemodynamically stable. She complains of bilateral pain in her legs, distal to her knees. She has profound weakness in her bilaterally extensor hallucis longi and gastrocsoleus complexes and has marked saddle anesthesia. MRI shows a large, midline herniated disc, compressing each of the traversing nerve roots and entire cauda equina below its level, but sparing the exiting nerve roots. Which disc is most likely involved in this injury?

A. L2-3
B. L3-4
C. L4-5
D. L5-S1
E. S1-2

ANSWERS

26.1 **B.** This patient has acute symptoms of CES. Although MRI of the lumbosacral spine is the ideal study to confirm this diagnosis, this patient's pacemaker may be a contraindication to MRI. In such situations, CT myelography is the next best option. When performed for CES evaluation, MRIs should focus on the lumbosacral spine, not the chest and abdomen, and gadolinium contrast is usually unnecessary. Although steroids and/or NSAIDs and physical may play a role in treatment of acute HNP, they are not the first line in the treatment of CES. Likewise, this patient may require metastatic workup, but this is not the priority in the acute management of CES.

26.2 **C.** This patient's history and presentation is consistent with an isolated, acutely HNP at L4-5. Although his motor and sensory deficits are concerning, the majority of patients will experience resolution of symptoms with nonoperative conservative management including NSAIDs, acetaminophen, physical therapy, and activity modification. Although an MRI may be helpful in making this diagnosis, it is not emergently indicated, as this patient does not have evidence of CES or other pathology that would require emergency, extensive workup, or surgical intervention. Epidural steroid injection is not the first line of treatment for an acute HNP, but may offer some relief in patients with refractory symptoms. Generally, epidural injection should not be performed with a significantly elevated INR.

26.3 **C.** This patient has weak extensor hallucis longi (L5 nerve root), weak gastrocsoleus complexes (S1), and saddle anesthesia (S2-4). She has normal function above this level, suggesting that the L5 nerve roots and those below are affected. An injury at L4-5 that spares the exiting roots (L4) but affects the traversing roots (L5) and those below (S1-5) would be most consistent with these symptoms. Remember the sacral spine does not have interbody discs, as it is fused.

CLINICAL PEARLS

- CES is defined by a characteristic cluster of symptoms, including low back pain, sciatica, lower extremity sensorimotor loss, and bowel and bladder dysfunction.
- CES is treated with urgent surgical decompression, unless there is an absolute contraindication to surgery.
- CES is a surgical emergency! Preparations for urgent operative intervention should begin as soon as the diagnosis is suspected.

REFERENCES

Flynn, JM, ed. Lumbar degenerative disease. In: *Orthopaedic Knowledge Update: Ten*. Rosemont, IL: American Academy of Orthopaedic Surgeons; 2011:599-610.

Spector LR, Madigan L, Rhyne A, Darden B, Kim D. Cauda equina syndrome. *J Am Acad Orthop Surg*. 2008;16:471-479.

CASE 27

A 34-year-old male construction worker arrives in the emergency department (ED) after a 25-foot fall at a construction site 3 hours ago. The patient landed on his feet and then fell backwards and was unable to stand after the accident. He is complaining of right ankle and low back pain, as well as numbness and tingling in both legs. He has no prior medical history. On exam, the patient is hemodynamically stable with vital signs within normal limits. His right heel is swollen and tender, but the skin is intact. He has midline tenderness in the upper lumbar spine and substantially decreased sensation to light touch in his bilateral proximal thighs and extending distally. Rectal exam demonstrates decreased rectal tone, as well as decreased but intact perianal sensation. Bulbocavernosus reflex is absent, as are his bilateral patella and Achilles reflexes. Plain films and a computed tomography (CT) are acquired by the ED and are shown in Figure 27–1.

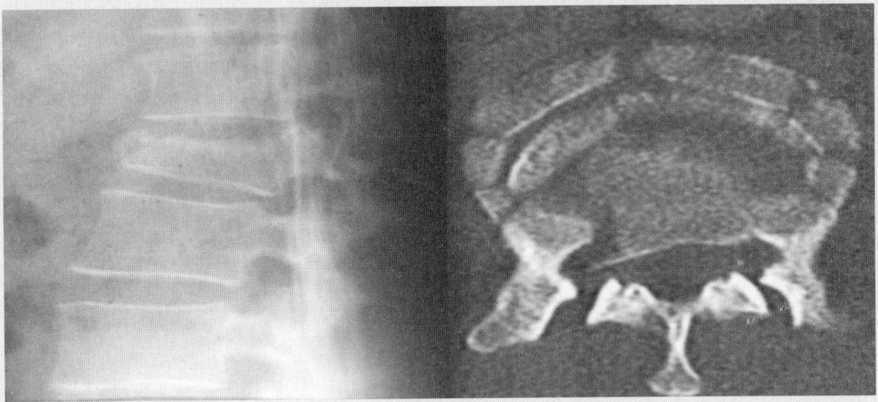

Figure 27–1. Lateral plain radiographs (*left*) of the lumbar spine and an axial CT cut (*right*) of the L1 vertebral body. (Courtesy of Timothy T. Roberts, MD)

- What type of fracture is seen in Figure 27–1?
- What is the most likely mechanism of injury for this fracture?
- What is the next diagnostic step?

ANSWERS TO CASE 27: Lumbar Burst Fracture

Summary: A 34-year-old healthy male construction worker presents to the ED with apparent injuries to his right heel and lower back after a fall from 25 feet. He landed in an upright, standing position. Furthermore, he has evidence of loss of sensation and tingling in his legs and perineal region and substantial weakness in both legs. The lack of a bulbocavernosus reflex (ie, the reflexive contraction of the anal sphincter when the glans penis is pinched or a Foley catheter is pulled) means that the patient is in spinal shock. He was unable to walk after his injury, which may be secondary to spinal cord injury and/or an additional injury to his heel.

- **Spine fracture:** This patient has a lumbar spine burst fracture.
- **Common mechanism of injury:** Lumbar spine burst fractures are commonly the result of high-energy axial loading, most often from a fall from a height or a motor vehicle collision.
- **Next diagnostic step:** Neurologic changes in the setting of spinal fracture should warrant magnetic resonance imaging (MRI) to evaluate involvement of the spinal cord and/or roots. Given the high-energy fall, this patient will also need a minimum of an anteroposterior (AP) or posteroanterior (PA) chest x-ray, an AP pelvis x-ray, C-spine imaging (x-rays and/or CT scans), and x-rays of the right ankle, given the heel tenderness and swelling on examination.

ANALYSIS

Objectives

1. Learn how to grade spinal cord injury with regard to sensation and muscle strength.
2. Understand the definition, diagnosis, and prognosis of spinal shock, and understand its role in the management of patients with acute neurologic injuries.
3. Know the diagnostic approach to acute injuries of the lumbar spine, and identify "red flags" for serious injuries requiring immediate surgical intervention.

Considerations

This 34-year-old male sustained an injury to his lumbar spine, based on both the presence of tenderness in the lumbar region and his motor and sensory examination. Additional injuries must be excluded through imaging of the entire spinal axis. Although there are multiple types of spine injuries that could result in the neurologic deficits seen in this patient, the type of mechanism (axial load) and level of neurologic deficit suggest that he has sustained lumbar burst fracture at or around the region of L1. This is confirmed by the lateral radiograph and axial CT shown in Figure 27–1.

The presence of a neurologic deficit suggests that fracture fragments or displaced soft tissues have compressed or directly injured the spinal cord and/or its roots.

This patient's injury is at the L1 level; the spinal cord typically ends somewhere between the top of L1 and bottom of L2, so this patient could have an injury either to the end of his spinal cord (known as the conus medullaris) or to the nerve roots traveling to the legs from the conus medullaris (known as the cauda equina). Because the patient demonstrates evidence of spinal shock, however, we can reason that he has likely suffered injury to his conus medullaris. Spinal shock does not occur at injury levels distal to the cord.

Several other orthopaedic injuries are characteristic of high-energy axial loading mechanisms, including calcaneus fractures, femoral shaft and neck fractures, vertical shear pelvis fractures, and lumbar spine injuries. This patient has a swollen and tender heel, likely consistent with a calcaneus fracture. Further workup and management of this extremity injury is also required.

APPROACH TO: Lumbar Spine Fracture

DEFINITIONS

CONUS MEDULLARIS: The caudal end of the spinal cord, beneath which nerves to the lower extremities and pelvis travel in their individual roots. The conus medullaris is typically located between L1 and L2, although substantial variation in its location emphasizes the importance of locating this structure for every patient undergoing surgery on the upper lumbar spine to verify its location.

CAUDA EQUINA: The collection of nerve roots beneath the conus medullaris that transmit signals from the spinal cord to the lower extremities and pelvis. The nerve roots making up the cauda equina are independently mobile and can thus tolerate a greater degree of spinal canal compression before injury when compared with spinal levels adjacent to the spinal cord itself.

BURST FRACTURE: A type of vertebral fracture characterized by injuries to 2 or 3 "columns" of the vertebrae: the **anterior column,** including the anterior two thirds of the vertebral body and the anterior longitudinal ligament; the **middle column,** including the posterior third of the vertebral body and the posterior longitudinal ligament; and the **posterior column,** including the facet joints, lamina, spinous processes, and interspinous ligaments. Burst fractures may injure the neural elements if the posterior aspect of the vertebral body is pushed backward into the spinal canal. This is known as **retropulsion.**

COMPRESSION FRACTURE: Similar to burst fractures, these axial loading injuries involve fracture of the vertebral body; however, compression fractures only involve the anterior column or anterior portion of the vertebral body. They are inherently more stable than burst fractures and do not typically result in neurologic deficit, as the fracture does not propagate into the spinal canal.

CHANCE FRACTURE: A spinal injury in which a flexion-distraction mechanism results in injury to all 3 spinal columns. Injuries may propagate through the vertebral bony elements or result in partial or complete ligamentous disruption, with forces instead tearing through the interspinous ligaments and disc space. These injuries have a high incidence of both intra-abdominal and neurologic injuries and are associated with seatbelt restraints during violent deceleration.

SPINAL SHOCK: A temporary state of paralysis, sensory loss, and complete absence of reflexes below the level of a spinal cord injury. Spinal shock typically lasts 24 to 48 hours and ends when cord-mediated reflexes return, specifically the bulbocavernosus reflex.

CLINICAL APPROACH

History and Physical Exam

Lumbar spine trauma is often the result of high-energy mechanisms, and thus all patients should undergo a complete and thorough trauma evaluation. After the patient has been stabilized—both hemodynamically and physically—a complete history must be obtained, including the timing and mechanism of injury, symptoms immediately after the injury and on arrival to the ED, and whether the patient was moved after the initial injury. The practitioner should be wary of progressive neurologic changes, both since the initial injury and throughout the workup period in the ED. Serial examinations are essential.

After an efficient history is obtained, physical exam should be performed. With the patient supine, motor strength, graded 0 through 5, is tested in the upper and lower extremities. A sensory exam is then performed to define sensory deficits according to nerve root dermatomes. Instructions on how to perform a complete motor, sensory, and reflex testing on patients with suspected spinal injuries are found in the first section of this text, "The Approach to the Orthopaedic Patient."

After neurovascular examination of the extremities, the patient is then rolled onto his or her side so that the entire spine can be palpated for regions of tenderness, crepitus, or step-off, and a rectal exam is performed. Log-roll precautions are employed to prevent further injury to a potentially unstable spine. During the rectal exam, the patient is asked whether they can sense that an exam is being performed, rectal tone is evaluated (absent, decreased, or intact), and the patient is asked to bear down as if he or she is having a bowel movement to test volitional contraction of the external sphincter. Finally, the bulbocavernosus reflex is tested by either pinching the glans penis or pulling on the Foley catheter and noting whether the anal sphincter contracts. **If a patient has a spinal cord-level injury, has an absent bulbocavernosus reflex, and is less than 48 hours from injury, he or she is considered to be in spinal shock.** In such situations, recognize that neurologic deficits *may* improve or resolve completely. Patients who have a return of this reflex or patients who are more than 48 hours from injury and have complete loss of neurologic function below the level of injury are considered to have a complete spinal cord injury. They are thus unlikely to regain any function below this level. Note that the bulbocavernosus reflex is only relevant for spinal cord-level injuries and not for injuries that affect the cauda equina.

Imaging

After plain radiographs of the entire spine are obtained, areas of potential injury should undergo further imaging. CT is helpful to define bony injury and plays an essential role in surgical planning. MRI is useful for evaluating spinal cord compression or edema, individual nerve roots, and intervertebral discs and assessing for ligamentous and other soft-tissue injuries. MRI is also helpful in evaluating sequelae from direct injuries such as hematoma formation, which may result in cord compression and neurologic injury.

TREATMENT

Initial treatment consists of stabilization, immobilization, pain and spasm control, and possibly administration of steroids. Although its true efficacy is controversial, high-dose intravenous (IV) methylprednisolone may be indicated for patients with nonpenetrating spinal cord injury who have presented within 8 hours of injury. Theoretically, steroids attenuate the deleterious inflammatory processes that lead to secondary nervous injury after primary spinal cord trauma.

The treatment of lumbar fractures depends on the **stability of the fracture.** Although the exact definition is disputed, **unstable fractures** generally include those with **marked neurologic compromise or complete 3-column disruption** (whether bony or ligamentous) or those **at risk of significant progression to deformity.**

Nonoperative Treatment

Patients with compression fractures or burst fractures without neurologic injury and with anatomic or near anatomic alignment may be definitely treated in a well-fitted brace. Compression fractures do not generally need surgical stabilization if they have less than 30 degrees of kyphosis or less than 40% to 50% loss of height anteriorly. Stable burst fractures may be treated with the same criteria and should have no greater than 40% of spinal canal compromise by retropulsed bony fragments. Chance fractures may be treated nonoperatively if they are bony in nature and are without significant deformity (ie, result in <15 degrees of kyphosis). Purely bony, minimally displaced Chance fractures are amenable to nonoperative treatment because the large surface area of cancellous bone involved in the fracture has a significantly greater chance of healing than their equivalent ligamentous ruptures.

Operative Treatment

Generally, patients with unstable burst fractures must undergo surgical decompression and stabilization. Patients with evidence of a neurologic injury with preservation of some function should undergo urgent decompression of compressed neural elements and stabilization of fractured vertebral levels, preferably within 12 hours of the injury to maximize chance of neurologic recovery. Patients without a neurologic injury may require surgical stabilization if imaging demonstrates unsatisfactory alignment or evidence of instability, as defined previously. Chance fractures are inherently unstable and require surgical stabilization if they are ligamentous in nature, accompanied by neurologic compromise, or result in deformity of greater than 15 degrees of kyphosis. All patients with unstable injuries must be immobilized in a brace until they are able to undergo surgery.

COMPREHENSION QUESTIONS

27.1 A 44-year-old cab driver is involved in a high-speed, head-on collision. In the ED, he is hemodynamically stable and has full neurologic function of his lower extremities. He is complaining of severe lower back pain. Radiographs and CT imaging are acquired of his lumbar spine. Which of the following findings is indicative of an unstable lumbar burst fracture that may need surgical stabilization?

A. 50% loss of vertebral height at the level of injury
B. 20 degrees of kyphosis at the level of injury
C. 30% of canal compromise
D. Injury to the anterior and middle spinal columns only
E. Injury to the posterior column only

27.2 A 43-year-old woman who fell from a third-floor balcony presents to the ED with bilateral foot numbness as well as 2/5 bilateral extensor hallucis longus (EHL) function and absent plantar flexion. Radiographs demonstrate an L5 burst fracture with 40% retropulsion and 30% loss of height. On further history, the patient states she fell 4 days ago and finally sought care because she was experiencing decreasing sensation in her groin and can no longer void. What is the next most appropriate step in management?

A. IV high-dose corticosteroids
B. Epidural steroid injection
C. Nonsteroidal anti-inflammatory drugs (NSAIDs), bedrest, and appropriate bracing
D. Surgical anterior decompression with fusion
E. Surgical posterior decompressive lumbar laminectomy without fusion

27.3 A 56-year-old male rock climber falls 8 feet from a ledge and lands on his buttocks. He arrives 6 hours later in the ED and complains of lower back pain. He is completely neurologically intact. Imaging of his lumbar spine shows an L3 burst fracture involving both anterior and middle columns with 30% loss of height anteriorly and minimal retropulsion. He has no other injuries. What is the most appropriate treatment for this patient?

A. IV steroids and appropriate bracing
B. Low-dose narcotics, NSAIDs, and appropriate bracing
C. Surgical decompression with fusion
D. Further imaging must be obtained, including an MRI to rule out spinal cord injury
E. Reassurance and activity modification

ANSWERS

27.1 **A.** Lumbar burst fractures are considered unstable and indicate surgical stabilization if they involve all 3 columns, result in >40% to 50% loss of height or >30 degrees of kyphosis, or have >40% canal compromise. Burst fractures by definition are not exclusive to the posterior elements.

27.2 **D.** Although there are details suggesting that this patient's burst fracture may be stable (ie, only 40% retropulsion and only 30% loss of height), her progressive neurologic symptoms are indication for surgical intervention. E is incorrect because it does not address the fracture or provide stabilization, as would an anterior decompression and fusion. Local epidural steroids do not address the fracture. IV steroids are controversial; however, they are not indicated greater than 8 hours from injury.

27.3 **B.** This patient has a stable burst fracture involving only the anterior and middle columns without significant loss of height or angulation. The appropriate treatment is pain control (narcotics are appropriate given his acute painful injury) and brace immobilization. Because the injury is stable and because he has no neurologic disruption, he does not necessarily need surgical stabilization, nor does he need extensive, expensive imaging such as an MRI. The patient may be reassured and should certainly refrain periodically from rock climbing, but requires a minimum of brace immobilization until the fracture has healed.

CLINICAL PEARLS

- Patients with injuries secondary to axial-loading mechanisms should be evaluated for additional associated injuries, such as calcaneus fractures and lumbar burst fractures.
- A careful physical exam, including testing of the bulbocavernosus reflex, gives valuable information about whether neurologic injury has occurred and whether or not the patient is in spinal shock.
- Patients with incomplete neurologic injuries (preservation of motor or sensory function below the level of the injury) should undergo urgent decompression and stabilization of the injury to maximize the likelihood of neurologic improvement or preservation.

REFERENCES

Egol KE, Koval KJ, Zukerman JD, eds. Thoracolumbar spine. In: *Handbook of Fractures*. 4th ed. Philadelphia: Lippincott Williams & Wilkins; 2010:123-140.

Mikles MR, Stchur RP, Graziano GP. Posterior instrumentation for thoracolumbar fractures. *J Am Acad Orthop Surg*. 2004;12:424-435.

Singh K, Kim D, Vaccaro AR. Thoracic and lumbar spinal injuries. In: Herkowitz HG, Garfin SR, Eismont FF, Bell GR, Balderson RA, eds. *Rothman-Simeone: The Spine*. Philadelphia: Saunders Elsevier; 2006:1132-1156.

CASE 28

A 12-year-old girl is referred to your clinic for concerns of shoulder asymmetry. She states that her friends first noticed that her back was not symmetric when she was changing clothes for basketball practice. She notices occasional back pain that she attributes to carrying a heavy backpack. The review of systems is otherwise unremarkable. Her past medical and developmental history are also noncontributory. She is in the seventh grade and is active in athletics and gymnastics. She experienced menarche 4 months prior and her menses have been regular. On examination, her right shoulder is 2 cm higher than the left, but her posterior iliac wings are of equal and symmetric heights. She has mild tenderness to palpation and slight spasms of the paraspinal musculature of her right-sided thoracic spine. There are no cutaneous lesions in the midline of her back. On forward bending, she has a 7-degree angle of trunk rotation in the thoracic spine, with the right side higher than the left. She has 5/5 strength in bilateral lower extremities throughout all muscle groups and no sensory abnormalities. Knee and ankle jerk reflexes are 2+ and symmetric. She has no sustained clonus or pathologic reflexes.

- What is the most likely diagnosis?
- What is your next diagnostic step?
- What are the treatment options?

ANSWERS TO CASE 28:
Adolescent Idiopathic Scoliosis

Summary: A healthy 12-year-old girl presents with mild back pain, shoulder asymmetry, and a 7-degree rotational deformity of her thoracic spine. She has recently experienced menarche and has no other complaints. Neurologic exam is unremarkable.

- **Most likely diagnosis:** Adolescent idiopathic scoliosis (AIS).
- **Next diagnostic step:** Standing 36-in posteroanterior (PA) and lateral spine radiographs.
- **Treatment options:** Observation, brace treatment, surgical spinal fusion.

ANALYSIS

Objectives

1. Understand the common presentation and characteristics of patients with AIS.
2. Recognize pertinent negatives that distinguish idiopathic scoliosis from scoliosis caused by other etiologies.
3. Consider the factors that lead to the decision making in the treatment algorithm of scoliosis.

Considerations

This 12-year-old girl depicts a classic presentation of a patient with AIS, a disease characterized by both abnormal curvature and rotation of the spine from an unknown cause. This is an otherwise healthy adolescent, like most patients with idiopathic scoliosis. This patient is also female, representing the 8:1 female-to-male ratio of patients with scoliosis large enough in magnitude to require treatment. Often, concerns of both patients and parents are not of pain or dysfunction, but of cosmetic appearance. Shoulder, trunk, and flank asymmetry can be very noticeable and can significantly harm the self-image of the patient. The goals of treatment are to prevent long-term complications of cardiovascular and pulmonary dysfunction, which tend to present later with curve progression in adulthood. Surgical intervention in adults carries greater risk of morbidity.

In addition to her deformity, the patient's complaints of back pain should not be ignored. Although rare, physicians must first rule out potential pathologic causes of scoliosis, as AIS is a **diagnosis of exclusion.** Both the history and physical exam, with judicious use of radiologic and laboratory studies, should be used to evaluate for other potential causes of back pain, including osteomyelitis, discitis, spondylolysis, disc herniation, or even skeletal and mesenchymal-derived tumors.

Several red flags may arise in the workup of a patient with scoliosis that warrant further evaluation, including history of fever or constitutional symptoms, unexplained weight loss, neurologic abnormalities, pain unrelated to activity, and/or pain at night. Idiopathic scoliosis is typically characterized by **thoracic dextroscoliosis,** or a right-sided thoracic curve. Particular attention should be paid to **atypical curve patterns** such as **levoscoliosis** (left-sided curve), juvenile-onset deformities (<10 years of age at time of diagnosis), **hyperkyphosis** (a sharp posterior-facing or "hunchback" curve), and large curves without rotational deformities. Spinal deformity can be the initial presenting complaint for patients with central nervous system anomalies such as Arnold-Chiari malformations, syringomyelia, diastematomyelia, tethered cords, or central nervous system tumors. **Neuromuscular scoliosis is the second most common type of scoliosis,** following AIS, and often occurs in patients with cerebral palsy, muscular dystrophy, and other neurologic disorders. Scoliosis may also occur secondary to underlying genetic diseases such as neurofibromatosis, Marfan syndrome, Ehlers-Danlos syndrome, osteogenesis imperfecta, or as secondary to previous spine trauma. On occasion, subclinical neuromuscular diseases such as mild cerebral palsy and Charcot Marie Tooth disease can remain unrecognized into adolescence but be an underlying cause of scoliosis. Alterations in the neurologic exam, unexplained pain, and atypical curve patterns should raise suspicion that the spinal deformity is **not** idiopathic. In such situations, the physician must obtain further diagnostic imaging such as magnetic resonance imaging (MRI) of the entire spine and/or ultrasound exams to evaluate for common congenital correlates to malformed vertebrae (ie, renal ultrasound, cardiac echocardiogram).

APPROACH TO: Scoliosis

DEFINITIONS

SCOLIOSIS: Defined by greater than 10 degrees of curvature of the spine in the coronal plane. Although measured on a 2-dimensional x-ray, scoliosis is typically a 3-dimensional process with rotational deformities. It is commonly measured using the Cobb method.

KYPHOSIS: A deformity in the sagittal plane characterized by apex-posterior curvature of the spine. A small degree of kyphosis is normal and should measure between 20 and 40 degrees in the thoracic spine.

COBB ANGLE: The angle subtended by lines drawn through vertebral endplates at each point of curve inflection. Cobb angles are typically measured on standing full-length spine x-rays.

PEAK GROWTH VELOCITY: The skeletal growth spurt usually seen early in the second decade of life. Progression of scoliosis curves is at highest risk during this time.

RISSER SIGN: The ossification of the iliac apophysis, seen on coronal radiographs. Graded from 0 through 5, based on quartiles of the total length of the iliac crest with ossified from lateral to medial. Ossification is a marker of skeletal maturity and can thus be used to determine the likelihood of curve progression.

CLINICAL APPROACH

Etiologies

Scoliosis is defined by greater than 10 degrees of spinal curvature in the coronal plane; less than 10 degrees of curvature is termed **spinal asymmetry.** Although it is typically observed on 2-dimensional x-rays, scoliosis is actually a **3-dimensional rotational deformity** of the vertebral column. Although adolescent idiopathic scoliosis is the most commonly seen presentation of scoliosis, it is a **diagnosis of exclusion.** To diagnose scoliosis, less common, but more insidious, causes must be investigated.

The etiology of scoliosis is best described as multifactorial. Hereditary studies have shown an increased incidence of scoliosis within families, but penetrance is variable. Several genes have been implicated in the etiology for scoliosis, but clinical results are inconclusive for a single gene responsible for the condition. Similarly, hormonal and neuromuscular etiologies have been implicated, but current research has failed to demonstrate conclusive independent causation.

Clinical Presentation of Scoliosis

The majority of patients with AIS present with complaints of cosmesis. Only in cases of severe curve magnitude (≥80 degrees) is evidence of cardiovascular or pulmonary dysfunction seen in adolescents. Often, patients' curves have first been observed by classmates, physical education teachers, school nurses, or found incidentally on routine exams by pediatricians. Pain associated with scoliosis is common in adulthood but is rare in adolescence. Complete gestational and birth history as well as neurologic developmental milestone achievement should be reviewed, along with a detailed physical and neurologic exam at the initial visit. Radiographic imaging should be performed at regular intervals to monitor for progression of the curve with consideration given to the cumulative radiation dose to which the patient will be exposed.

TREATMENT

Treatment is defined by the likelihood of curve progression during both adolescence and adulthood. Most AIS patients are healthy and active despite sometimes pronounced deformities. When discussing the natural history of scoliosis with patients and their families, the consequences of curve progression into adulthood and its effects on cardiopulmonary health must be discussed. Such dysfunctions are often absent in the asymptomatic adolescent, but may manifest later in life with significant morbidity.

Generally, AIS patients with curves of less than 20 degrees are managed with clinical observation and intermittent radiographic follow-up if the curve is at high risk of progression. Brace treatment is indicated for AIS patients with curve magnitudes of 25 to 40 degrees and who are still growing. Patients most likely to benefit from bracing include premenarchal girls, girls or boys in or before their peak height velocity, or girls or boys with less than 50% of iliac apophysis ossification (ie, Risser stage of 0, 1, or 2). As stated, curve magnitude increases at the greatest rate during the period of **peak growth velocity.** Remember to discuss with patients that the realistic

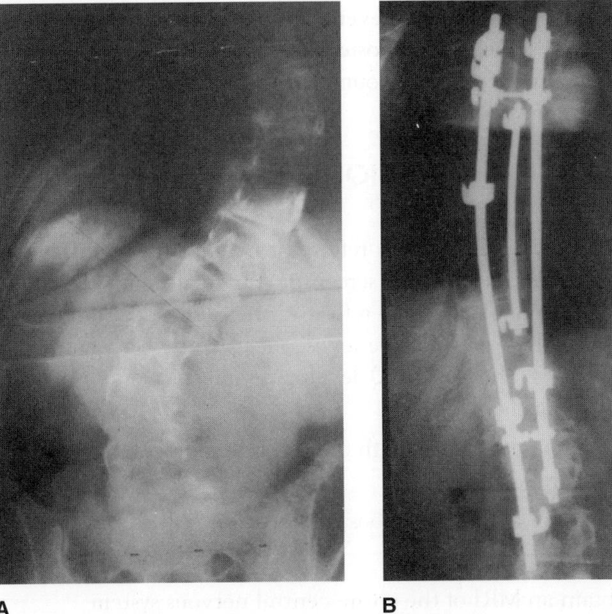

Figure 28–1. Treatment of a scoliotic curve by instrumentation and fusion. (A) Preoperative view and (B) postoperative view. (Reproduced, with permission, from Skinner HB. *Current Diagnosis & Treatment in Orthopedics.* 4th ed. New York, NY: McGraw-Hill; 2006:Fig. 11-36.)

goal for brace treatment is not to correct the spinal curvature, but to prevent it from increasing in magnitude. The best prognostic indicator for successful scoliosis bracing is the ability to immediately improve the prebracing radiographic curve by 50% when the first brace is applied. Braces must be worn at a minimum of 16 to 23 hours per day, and, not surprisingly, patient compliance is a considerable issue.

AIS curves greater than 50 degrees are a potential indication for spinal fusion surgery. Natural history studies of AIS suggest the greatest increased risk of progression into adulthood when curves are beyond 50 degrees. The primary goal of AIS surgical treatment is to halt the progression of deformity by achieving a solid fusion of the spine. Additional surgical goals include the sparing of spinal motion segments wherever possible, obtaining a pain-free spine, and correcting as much of the curvature as is safely possible. Surgical spinal fusion typically involves a combination of bone grafting and instrumentation to fix the curved spine into a rigid structure. Surgical approaches may be posterior, anterior, or combined in cases of severe disease. Instrumentation used to hold the fusion may include rods, pedicle screws, hooks, wires, and other implants (Figure 28–1).

Complications

Spinal fusion procedures are often long, painful, and highly morbid procedures with significant blood loss, requiring transfusion and/or the use of intraoperative blood salvage techniques. Early wound infection (1%-2%), pseudoarthrosis (1%-2%), painful prominent hardware, and hardware breakage are described complications. The most devastating but rare complication is iatrogenic neurologic injury. Intraoperative neurologic monitoring may help prevent this. A **crankshaft phenomenon** may occur when an immature spine is fused posteriorly, but continues to grow anteriorly, causing the expanding spine to spiral around the posterior fusion. This may be prevented with concomitant anterior fusion.

COMPREHENSION QUESTIONS

28.1 A 10-year-old healthy girl is referred to your office after testing positive for scoliosis during a schoolwide screening. Physical exam is unremarkable except for absence of her abdominal reflex on the right side. Standing 36-in scoliosis radiographs show a 25-degree levoscoliosis curve with minimal rotation and hyperkyphosis. She is Risser 0 developmental stage on x-ray. What is the next step in management?

A. Reassure and observe with clinical and radiographic examination in 3 to 4 months

B. Fitting for a thoracolumbosacral orthosis (TLSO)

C. Obtain a bone scan

D. Obtain an MRI of the entire central nervous system

E. Book patient for spinal fusion after obtaining appropriate consent

28.2 A 15-year-old male athlete presents for evaluation of shoulder asymmetry pointed out by his football teammates. His mother had never noticed the discrepancy until now but is very concerned. The boy has a 15-degree right-sided trunk rotation on the Adam forward-bending test. His neurologic examination is unremarkable. Thirty-six inch PA standing scoliosis radiographs show a 60-degree right thoracic curve and shoulder elevation 2 cm greater on the right than left. What is the next step in management?

A. Trial nonoperative treatment with a thoracolumbosacral orthosis (TLSO)

B. Reassure and observe patient with repeat clinical and radiographic evaluation in 3 to 4 months

C. Obtain an MRI of the entire central nervous system

D. Obtain a bone scan and laboratory studies for evidence of underlying pathology including erythrocyte sedimentation rate, C-reactive protein, and complete blood count

E. Book patient for spinal fusion after obtaining appropriate consent

28.3 A 15-year-old girl has asymptomatic adolescent idiopathic scoliosis. Her parents ask you how debilitated she might be compared with her peers who do not have scoliosis. Which of the following is true regarding the natural history of idiopathic scoliosis?

A. Difficulty with pregnancy

B. Increased risk of developing cancer

C. Acute or chronic back pain

D. Athletic limitations

ANSWERS

28.1 **D.** Atypical curve patterns require MRI evaluation of the spine and central nervous system for workup of underlying pathology. Bone scans, although useful for diagnosing infection or subacute bony injury, are not sensitive to other potential pathology etiologies. Bracing and observation are inappropriate without first ruling out a pathologic etiology.

28.2 **E.** Spinal fusion is indicated in curves measuring greater than 50 degrees. Although workup with MRI or laboratory studies is necessary when patients have evidence of pathologic etiology for scoliosis, patients without concerning symptoms do not require such an extensive workup. This patient's curve is too great in magnitude to be managed with observation or with bracing.

28.3 **C.** Scoliotic patients have been found to have more acute or chronic back pain, as well as cosmetic concerns. Pregnancy complications, athletic limitations, and an increased cancer risk are not associated with AIS.

CLINICAL PEARLS

- ▶ Adolescent idiopathic scoliosis is a diagnosis of exclusion, meaning physicians must rule out potential congenital, neuromuscular, traumatic, or syndromic etiologies before making the diagnosis.
- ▶ The risk of scoliosis curve progression is greatest during early adolescence when the peak growth velocity occurs.
- ▶ Among many non-AIS causes of back pain in adolescents are discitis, herniated disks, osteoid osteoma, lymphoma, and spondylolysis.
- ▶ Scoliosis bracing is indicated for adolescents in their peak height velocity or those who have not yet reached their peak height velocity, as well as patients with significant curve magnitudes (>25-40 degrees) and those in Risser 0 through 2 stages of skeletal maturity.
- ▶ Spinal fusion surgery is generally indicated for patients with progressive curves greater than 50 degrees.

REFERENCES

Cobb JR. Outline for the study of scoliosis. In: Thomson JEM, Boount WP, eds. *The American Academy of Orthopaedic Surgeons. Instructional Course Lectures*. Ann Arbor, MI: JW Edwards; 1948;5:261-275.

Miller MD, ed. Pediatric orthopaedics. In: *Review of Orthopaedics*. 5th ed. Philadelphia: Saunders Elsevier; 2008:198-244.

Sanders JO, Browne RH, Cooney TE, Finegold DN, McConnell SJ, Margraf SA. Correlates of the peak height velocity in girls with idiopathic scoliosis. *Spine*. 2006;31:2289-2295.

Song KM, Little DG. Peak height velocity as a maturity indicator for males with idiopathic scoliosis. *J Pediatr Orthop*. 2000;20:286-288.

CASE 29

A 47-year-old right-hand dominant female presents to the clinic with a 2-month history of intermittent numbness and tingling in her right hand, specifically the index and middle fingers. She often finds the symptoms worst when using her computer and when driving home. Her symptoms are significantly affecting her career as a journalist. She also complains of pain in the same distribution that wakes her up almost nightly. She denies any history of trauma. Her past medical history is significant only for type 2 diabetes mellitus (DM), which is well controlled with oral agents. She does not smoke and drinks 1 or 2 glasses of wine on occasion, and her body mass index is 32 kg/m^2. Physical examination reveals a slightly overweight but otherwise healthy-appearing female. Both of her upper extremities appear normal, with no obvious signs of trauma. On her right hand, there is a palpable 2+ radial pulse and a normal Allen test. Two-point discrimination is measured at 8 mm on both the radial and ulnar borders of the index and middle fingers as well as the radial border of the ring finger. There is normal (<5 mm) 2-point discrimination on the ulnar border of the ring finger and on both sides of the small finger. Sensation in the palm is normal.

- What is the most likely diagnosis?
- How would you confirm the diagnosis?
- What is the initial treatment for this condition?

ANSWERS TO CASE 29: Carpel Tunnel Syndrome

Summary: A 47-year-old woman with a history of well-controlled type 2 DM has complaints of worsening numbness and tingling in her right hand for 2 months. She works as a journalist, spending much of her time on a computer. She has no history of trauma and is otherwise healthy. Vital signs are normal, and physical exam is remarkable for decreased 2-point discrimination on her index and middle fingers, as well as the radial side of her ring finger.

- **Most likely diagnosis:** Carpal tunnel syndrome (CTS).
- **Diagnostic testing:** An electromyogram (EMG) and nerve conduction studies may help confirm the diagnosis. EMG studies may show an increase in motor and/or sensory latency across the wrist. Up to 10% of patients with clinical symptomatology, however, have normal EMG studies.
- **Initial management:** Nonsteroidal anti-inflammatory drugs (NSAIDs), if not contraindicated, and night splinting are the best initial management strategy.

ANALYSIS

Objectives

1. Understand the pathoanatomy responsible for carpal tunnel syndrome.
2. Describe the physical exam findings of carpal tunnel syndrome.
3. Recognize underlying conditions (both physiologic and pathologic) that may predispose one to carpal tunnel syndrome.
4. Distinguish carpal tunnel syndrome from other diseases or conditions that may mimic its presentation.
5. Understand the conservative and surgical treatment options for carpal tunnel syndrome and their indications.

Considerations

For any patient with acute neurologic complaints isolated to an extremity, it is important to first rule out trauma as an underlying cause. This patient denies a history of trauma, is without significant medical comorbidities, and appears reliable, so further imaging is unlikely to aid the diagnosis. In patients with complicated, unclear, or unreliable histories, radiographs may help eliminate several causes of neurologic symptoms such as fractures, deformities, congenital abnormalities, masses, and other lesions.

There are other conditions that may mimic carpal tunnel syndrome, but can often be distinguished with a thorough physical exam and history. Traumatic conditions such as a distal radius fracture or scaphoid fracture may present with some symptoms that overlap with those of carpal tunnel syndrome, but would likely be discovered with adequate workup. More proximal nerve pathologies such as cervical radiculopathy or proximal median nerve compression should have additional findings not found in isolated carpal tunnel syndrome, such as paresthesias in the thenar distribution, and would not have positive test findings on provocative tests aimed at eliciting symptoms within the carpal canal (ie, Phalen, Tinel, and Durkan signs). Cubital tunnel syndrome has similar pathology and presentation to carpal tunnel syndrome, but in a different nerve distribution. If the patient fails conservative management, carpal tunnel release surgery is very effective at alleviating symptoms of carpal tunnel syndrome. If performed early, surgical decompression can prevent permanent denervation of the thenar muscles and halt further deterioration of symptoms. In many operative cases, sensation is restored and symptoms resolve. With regard to operative technique, the results from open and endoscopic surgery are comparable.

APPROACH TO:
Carpal Tunnel Syndrome

DEFINITIONS

CARPAL TUNNEL: A narrow canal in the volar (palmar) wrist that typically contains the median nerve, superficial and deep finger flexor tendons, and the long flexor tendon of the thumb.

GUYON CANAL: Also known as the ulnar tunnel, this volar wrist canal is located just ulnar (medial) to the carpal tunnel and contains the ulnar artery and ulnar nerve. Compression within this tunnel can lead to a similar syndrome to carpal tunnel, with symptoms instead found in an ulnar nerve distribution.

MEDIAN NERVE COMPRESSION SYNDROME: A spectrum of compression neuropathies of the median nerve with varying names and symptoms, depending on the location of pathology. When the nerve is compressed proximally, most commonly between the two heads of the pronator teres muscle, it is called pronator teres syndrome, and is characterized by volar hand and forearm numbness as well as potential weaknesses in the thumb flexors and distal flexors of the index and middle fingers. The median nerve can be compressed in several key locations, the most distal of which is in the carpal tunnel.

CLINICAL APPROACH

Relevant Anatomy

The carpal tunnel can be described exactly as it is named—as a tunnel (or canal) passing through the wrist. Understanding the anatomy of the canal, including its borders and its contents, is key to understanding the basis of carpal tunnel syndrome. The carpal canal is formed by the **transverse carpal ligament volarly** (palmar), **the scaphoid and trapezium radially,** and the **hamate and triquetrum ulnarly.** Within the canal passes the **median nerve** and 9 flexor tendons: **4 tendons of the** flexor digitorum profundus (**FDP**), **4 tendons of the** flexor digitorum superficialis (**FDS**), and the single tendon of the flexor pollicis longus (**FPL**).

The median nerve is responsible for sensation to the volar (palmar) surface of the thumb, index finger, long finger, and the radial (lateral) half of the ring finger. The **sensation of the palm and thenar eminence is normal** in carpal tunnel syndrome because the palmar cutaneous branch of the median nerve arises proximal to the carpal tunnel and crosses the wrist superficial to the transverse carpal ligament to give sensation to the palm. In most instances, the recurrent motor branch of the median nerve comes off the median nerve distal to the nerves coursing within the canal, so that compressive effects on the median nerve may also affect the recurrent motor branch.

Decreasing the effective size of the canal (ie, prolonged or repetitive wrist flexion/extension, etc) or increasing the relative size of the canal's contents (ie, flexor tendon inflammation/swelling) can lead to carpal tunnel syndrome. This explains why many patients with carpal tunnel syndrome complain of worsened symptoms at night, as it is thought that most people sleep with their wrists in a flexed position.

Diagnosis

Carpal tunnel syndrome is a **clinical diagnosis,** meaning the diagnosis is based primarily on history and physical exam findings, with adjunctive tests such as EMG studies used to confirm—but never make—the diagnosis. Physical exam findings such as **decreased sensation and 2-point discrimination in the distribution of the median nerve** at the fingers with **sparing of sensation of the thenar eminence and palm** are pathognomic for carpal tunnel syndrome. **Tinel sign** involves **percussion over the median nerve at the wrist,** and **Phalen sign** involves **holding the wrist in flexion for 1 minute.** Both **tests are positive if they result in reproduction of symptoms.** The **Durkan test,** or carpal tunnel compression test, is performed with the examiner holding pressure over the patient's carpal tunnel, while distracting the patient. Reproduction of symptoms within 30 seconds of compression is considered positive. Although the patient in this case does not describe weakness or atrophy of the thenar musculature, a decrease in pinch/grip strength may occur in more advanced stages of carpal tunnel syndrome.

EMG studies may help clarify the diagnosis of CTS. Such studies may demonstrate a latency and/or asymmetry between the affected and nonaffected hands. Many normal physiologic and/or pathologic conditions may promote the onset of carpal tunnel syndrome. These include, but are not limited to, pregnancy, type 2 DM, gout, rheumatoid arthritis, and hypothyroidism. The mechanisms by which these conditions cause carpal tunnel syndrome are not fully understood. However, each condition is thought to promote a state of inflammation and thus elevated pressure within the carpal canal. Patients should be evaluated for potential underlying causes of carpal tunnel syndrome. Underlying etiologies, if present, must be addressed prior to operative treatment.

TREATMENT

When carpal tunnel syndrome is diagnosed, the most conservative mode of treatment is attempted first. Nighttime symptoms are often the result of the naturally-flexed position of the resting wrist. Removable splints that hold the wrist in neutral, the position in which the carpal tunnel is least compressed, are usually effective at reducing symptoms. Additionally, anti-inflammatories (NSAIDs) are an effective treatment option. In patients whose symptoms are not sufficiently relieved by these options, corticosteroid injections directly into the carpal tunnel may be an option. Local steroid therapy may provide transient relief; however, symptoms often return. Note that there is prognostic value to such therapies, as patients who respond well to steroid injections have a greater chance of successful relief from surgery.

The definitive treatment for carpal tunnel syndrome refractory to conservative management is a carpal tunnel release. This involves releasing the transverse carpal ligament using either a direct open or endoscopic technique. Carpal tunnel release is a relatively fast outpatient procedure with generally low complication rates and excellent outcomes.

COMPREHENSION QUESTIONS

29.1 A 43-year-old health care worker complains of nocturnal wrist pain and has significant pain when pressure is applied to her volar wrist for more than 10 seconds. Which of the following structures is *not* usually contained within the carpal tunnel?

A. Tendon(s) of FDP

B. Tendon(s) of FPL

C. Palmar cutaneous branch of the median nerve

D. Tendon(s) of FDS

E. Motor fibers of the median nerve

29.2 A 52-year-old retired woman is referred to your clinic with complaints of numbness and tingling in her left (dominant) hand worse at night for the past 3 months. She also complains of significant fatigue and 10-lb weight gain over the same period of time. She denies any medical history and takes no medications. On exam, she is overweight and appears somewhat lethargic, but appears healthy otherwise. On her left hand she has decreased 2-point discrimination on her index and middle fingers. Her grip strength is normal, and she has no thenar atrophy. What is the next best step in management of this patient?

A. Left hand carpal tunnel release

B. EMG/nerve conduction velocity studies of left upper extremity

C. Cervical spine magnetic resonance imaging (MRI)

D. Lab studies including complete blood count, basic metabolic panel, thyroid-stimulating hormone, T3, and free T4

E. Referral for counseling regarding recent changes in her lifestyle

29.3 A 56-year-old postmenopausal woman is seen in the clinic with complaints of mild numbness and tingling in her right hand, most notably in the index and middle fingers. She takes medication for osteoporosis but is otherwise healthy. Her history is unremarkable except for a wrist fracture after a fall onto her right hand 2 years ago that was fixed with open reduction internal fixation. Her postoperative course was uncomplicated. Physical examination in the office reveals a well-healed surgical incision on the volar aspect of her wrist, normal grip strength, and no sensory deficits. X-rays reveal hardware in adequate alignment, with evidence of bony union at a previous distal radius fracture site. What is the next best step in her management?

A. Provision cast immobilization and follow-up x-ray for occult refracture
B. MRI of right wrist
C. Emergency surgical release of transverse carpal ligament
D. NSAID administration with close follow-up
E. Serum erythrocyte sedimentation rate, C-reactive protein, complete blood count, and wrist aspiration, with cytologic analysis, Gram stain, and culture of aspirate

ANSWERS

29.1 **C.** The palmar cutaneous branch of the median nerve is given off approximately 5 cm proximally to the carpal tunnel in most patients. This explains why patients with carpal tunnel syndrome typically have sparing of sensation of the thenar/palmar aspect of the affected hand. The motor fibers of the median nerve branch off distally to the tunnel, and as a result, patients may exhibit weakness and/or atrophy of the thenar musculature. The 9 flexor tendons of FDP, FDS, and FPL are all contained within the carpal tunnel.

29.2 **D.** The patient in this question does exhibit symptoms of carpal tunnel syndrome. However, her history and physical exam also point strongly to undiagnosed hypothyroidism. Further workup and treatment of her metabolic condition should be performed before intervention of her carpal tunnel symptoms.

29.3 **D.** Distal radius fractures and subsequent fixation are associated with a number of potential complications, including iatrogenic carpal tunnel syndrome of variable severity. In this case, the patient does have postoperative symptoms that are consistent with carpal tunnel syndrome, but they are mild and intermittent. Acute or emergency carpal tunnel release is not indicated. There are no signs of infection or refracture, and cast immobilization may exacerbate her symptoms. MRI of the wrist would not likely provide any new information. The correct choice would be conservative management with close follow-up to monitor for change in symptoms.

CLINICAL PEARLS

- The carpal tunnel is an effectively closed space, containing the median nerve, among other structures. Any reduction in volume of this finite space can lead to increased pressure upon, and thus dysfunction of, the median nerve. This results in carpal tunnel syndrome.
- Carpal tunnel syndrome is a clinical diagnosis, made by history and physical exam findings; adjunctive tests such as EMG studies may be used to confirm, but never make, the diagnosis.
- Other neurologic conditions or injuries may be differentiated from carpal tunnel syndrome by thorough history and physical exam, including exact localization of motor and sensory symptoms.
- Conservative management should always be attempted before operative treatment of CTS. If conservative management fails, surgical carpal tunnel release is performed with either open or endoscopic techniques. Both methods are associated with excellent outcomes.

REFERENCES

American Academy of Orthopaedic Surgeons. Clinical guideline on diagnosis of carpal tunnel syndrome. 2007. www.aaos.org/Research/guidelines/CTSdiagnosisguide.asp.

American Academy of Orthopaedic Surgeons. Clinical practice guideline on the treatment of carpal tunnel syndrome. 2008. www.aaos.org/Research/guidelines/CTStreatmentguide.asp.

Bednar MS, Light TR. Disorders of the nerves of the hand. In: HB Skinner, ed. *Current Diagnosis and Treatment in Orthopedics*. 4th ed. New York: McGraw-Hill; 2006:559-567.

Bienek T, Kusz D, Cielinski L. Peripheral nerve compression neuropathy after fractures of the distal radius. *J Hand Surg Br*. 2006;31:256-260.

Fuller DA, Barrett M, Marburger RK, Hirsch R. Carpal canal pressures after volar plating of distal radius fractures. *J Hand Surg Br*. 2006;31:236-239.

CASE 30

A 45-year-old right-hand dominant woman presents to the orthopaedic hand clinic with a 6-month history of right hand numbness and tingling. She denies any trauma or inciting incident but reports that she noticed the numbness and tingling after waking up one morning. The symptoms come and go throughout the day and are worse in the night time, waking her up 3 to 4 times a week. Over the past month, her symptoms have gotten progressively worse, with some days of constant numbness. She denies any symptoms in her neck, shoulder, or arm. She denies any pain. She reports feeling weaker in her right hand, especially with opening a bottle or buttoning her shirt. Over the last few months, her right hand has fatigued faster than her left.

On physical exam, she has full active range of motion of her neck, right shoulder, elbow, wrist, and fingers. Focused exam of her right upper extremity reveals no gross deformity or muscle atrophy. She has ulnar deviation of her small ringer. There is no erythema, ecchymosis, or effusions. She localizes her numbness to her ring and small fingers and cannot discern whether the symptoms are dorsal or volar. On strength testing, she has 5/5 strength of her biceps, triceps, wrist extensors/flexors, thumb extensors/flexors, and flexors of her index and middle finger. She has 3/5 strength of her hand intrinsics and the flexors of her ring and small finger. She has normal sensation to light touch but decreased sensation to pinprick over the volar and dorsal ulnar aspect of her hand. She has a 2+ radial pulse and normal Allen test. Elbow, wrist, and hand radiographs are negative for any pathology.

- What is the most likely diagnosis?
- What muscles does this disease process affect?
- What is your next diagnostic step?
- What are the treatment options?

ANSWERS TO CASE 30:
Cubital Tunnel Syndrome

Summary: A 45-year-old right-hand dominant woman presents with 6 months of right hand numbness, tingling, and now weakness. She denies any history of trauma or specific inciting event and states that her symptoms have worsened over the last month. On exam there is no gross deformity or muscle atrophy of her right upper extremity, but weakness of her intrinsics and ring and small finger flexors is observed. She also has decreased sensation to pinprick over the volar and dorsal ulnar aspect of her hand.

- **Most likely diagnosis:** Cubital tunnel syndrome.
- **Affected muscles:** Flexor carpi ulnaris (FCU), hand intrinsics (lumbricals for ring and small finger, dorsal interossei, palmar interossei), hypothenar muscles (palmaris brevis, abductor digiti minimi, opponens digiti minimi, flexor digiti minimi), flexor digitorum profundus (FDP) for ring and small finger, adductor pollicis, deep head of flexor pollicis brevis.
- **Next diagnostic step:** Electrodiagnostic testing.
- **Treatment options:** Nonsurgical options include bracing, activity modifications, and physical therapy, whereas surgery involves ulnar nerve decompression at the cubital tunnel.

ANALYSIS

Objectives

1. Understand the anatomy of the ulnar nerve and the potential sites of compression.
2. Understand the physical exam findings and electromyelogram (EMG) analysis associated with ulnar nerve entrapment.
3. Know the treatment options for cubital tunnel syndrome.

Considerations

This 45-year-old woman presents complaining of symptoms concerning for an entrapment neuropathy. The first priority is to perform a thorough history, which will help in narrowing down the possible diagnoses. This patient denies any trauma or inciting event, and her symptoms (right hand numbness, tingling, and weakness), which have become more constant over the last month, typically wax and wane throughout the day and are most severe at night. Given this history, the practitioner must consider the entrapment neuropathies of the upper extremity in the differential diagnosis. This includes carpal tunnel and cubital tunnel syndromes. A focused physical exam of the right upper extremity will further aid the clinician in determining the diagnosis. This includes ruling out cervical spine pathology that can cause similar symptoms, as well as a brachial plexopathy. In this specific case, for which ulnar nerve entrapment is likely, plain radiographs should be obtained and electrodiagnostic testing performed. Treatment options can then be discussed pending confirmation of the diagnosis of cubital tunnel syndrome.

APPROACH TO:
Cubital Tunnel Syndrome

DEFINITIONS

TINEL TEST: A way to detect irritated nerves. It is performed by lightly tapping or percussing over a given nerve to elicit a sensation of "tingling" or "pins and needles" in the distribution of the nerve.

FROMENT SIGN: A test for ulnar nerve palsy that specifically assesses the action of the adductor pollicis (ulnar nerve innervated). The patient is asked to hold a piece of paper between the thumb and index finger. Normally, as the examiner attempts to pull the paper away, an individual will be able to maintain a hold on the paper with little or no difficulty. However, the patient with ulnar nerve palsy will flex the thumb via the flexor pollicis longus (innervated by the anterior interosseous branch of the median nerve) to try to maintain a hold on the paper.

WARTENBERG SIGN: A sign noting the position of abduction and extension assumed by the small finger in the setting of cubital tunnel syndrome.

CLINICAL APPROACH

Anatomy

Cubital tunnel syndrome, the second most common upper-extremity compressive neuropathy after carpal tunnel syndrome, is a term used to describe symptoms related to ulnar nerve compression and/or traction around the elbow. Cubital tunnel syndrome includes any ulnar neuropathy in the mid-arm to mid-forearm.

The ulnar nerve is the terminal branch of the medial cord of the brachial plexus (C8-T1). The nerve courses between the medial head of the triceps and the brachialis muscle before coursing posterior to the medial epicondyle and entering the cubital tunnel. The tunnel's anatomic borders are as follows: **Anterior, medial epicondyle; posterior, olecranon; floor, medial collateral ligament; roof, arcuate ligament.** After leaving the cubital tunnel, the ulnar nerve passes into the forearm between the 2 heads of the FCU and exits under the deep flexor pronator aponeurosis. At this point it lies deep to the FDS and FCU and superficial to the FDP. There are several major sites at which the ulnar nerve often becomes compressed (Figure 30–1):

1. Arcade of Struthers: Band of fascia connecting the medial head of the triceps with the medial intermuscular septum, approximately 7 to 10 cm proximal to the medial epicondyle
2. Medial intermuscular septum
3. Medial head of triceps: Can become hypertrophied in bodybuilders

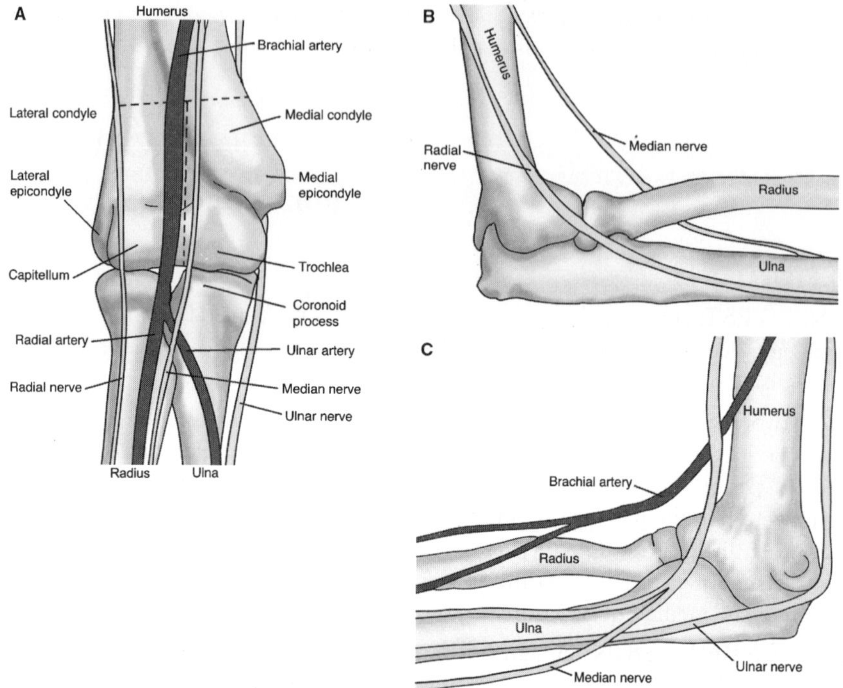

Figure 30–1. Elbow anatomy. (**A**) Anterior view, (**B**) lateral view, and (**C**) medial view. (Reproduced, with permission, from Tintinalli J, et al. *Tintinalli's Emergency Medicine: A Comprehensive Study Guide.* 7th ed. New York, NY: McGraw-Hill; 2010:Fig. 267-1.)

4. Medial epicondyle: Can cause compressive or traction forces via deformity from a prior supracondylar fracture (Tardy ulnar nerve palsy owing to development of progressive valgus deformity associated with these fractures) or osteophytes in an arthritic elbow
5. Arcuate ligament: The roof of the cubital tunnel
6. Osborne fascia: This is the proximal fibrous edge of the FCU and most common site of ulnar nerve compression
7. Epicondylar groove: A shallow groove increasing risk of ulnar nerve subluxation; a site where external compression can occur from leaning on a flexed elbow for prolonged period of time
8. Anconeus epitrochlearis: Accessory muscle arising from medial olecranon and triceps and inserting on the medial epicondyle; seen in 10% of patients undergoing cubital tunnel release
9. Deep flexor pronator aponeurosis

Physical Exam

Patients often present with poorly localized numbness and tingling in their hand. At times they are able to localize the symptoms in an ulnar nerve distribution.

The symptoms can be occasional or constant and exacerbated by elbow flexion. With longstanding ulnar nerve compression, patients may have wasting of their intrinsic muscles and hand weakness. An intrinsic minus or claw hand (hyperextension of the metacarpal phalangeal joints and flexion of the proximal and distal interphalangeal joints) may result from longstanding compression. Look for a **Wartenberg sign** (ulnar deviation of the small finger)—patients complain of inability to put their hand in their pocket or their small finger getting caught on things. Patients may have weakness of their pinch and compensate by flexing the thumb interphalangeal joint during pinching (**Froment sign**).

Patients may complain of medial elbow pain and have a positive Tinel test (exacerbation of the ulnar hand numbness by tapping on the ulnar nerve). It is important to do a thorough neck and shoulder exam to rule out nerve compression proximal to the elbow. This includes cervical range of motion to evaluate for associated pain and/or radiculopathy. Range the elbow and evaluate for ulnar nerve subluxation. **The functional range of motion of the elbow is 30 to 130 degrees.** The normal carrying angle is 7 to 15 degrees. Sensation in the hand should also be examined.

Radiographs of the elbow should be evaluated for osseous causes of compression (ie, osteophytes). Magnetic resonance imaging (MRI), although not typically indicated, can identify space-occupying lesions or edema within the nerve. Electrodiagnostic testing, which includes EMG and nerve conduction studies, is the gold standard to evaluate for ulnar neuropathy. Nerve conduction studies are considered positive if the motor conduction velocity across the elbow is less than 52 m/s, increased distal sensory latency of greater than 3.2 ms, and motor latencies of greater than 5.3 ms. Of note, abnormal EMG results are associated with poor surgical outcomes.

TREATMENT

To determine the appropriate treatment for a patient with cubital tunnel syndrome, the following considerations must be taken into account: patient compliance, worker's compensation, occupation, age, comorbidities, duration of symptoms, and severity of symptoms. Additionally, the orthopaedist must be certain that other causes of the patient's symptoms have been ruled out and that concurrent carpal tunnel syndrome (present in 40% of patients with cubital tunnel syndrome) is not present, which often requires simultaneous release.

For patients with mild cubital tunnel syndrome, nonsurgical options can alleviate symptoms and help prevent long-term nerve damage. A splint that keeps the elbow at approximately 70 degrees of flexion, especially when worn at night, can alleviate symptom exacerbation. Physical therapy (PT) that works on nerve mobilization and gliding, in addition to activity modification, can also aid in symptom relief. Nonsteroidal anti-inflammatory drugs (NSAIDs) as well as soft elbow padding can also be used.

For patients with constant numbness/tingling, muscle atrophy, muscle weakness, or severe slowing of conduction velocity, surgical intervention is recommended. **Surgery includes decompressing the nerve with or without transposition.** This is achieved via in situ decompression (decompressing the nerve and leaving it where it is), subcutaneous transposition (moving the nerve anterior to the medial epicondyle), intramuscular transposition (moving the nerve into an area surrounded by the flexor-pronator muscles), submuscular transposition (moving the nerve under the flexor-pronator muscles), and medial epicondylectomy (removing part of the medial epicondyle). The cubital tunnel can also be released endoscopically.

Most cases of cubital tunnel syndrome requiring surgical intervention can be treated with in situ decompression. There are inherent risks with nerve transposition, including compromised blood supply, nerve scarring, injury to adjacent structures, and a longer incision. Studies have shown that in situ decompression is adequate for most patients and has equivalent outcomes to decompression with transposition. Patients with a hypermobile nerve will likely benefit from moving the nerve to a new location.

COMPREHENSION QUESTIONS

30.1 A 40-year-old left-hand dominant man presents with an 8-month history of left hand numbness, tingling, and now weakness. On exam, you note a positive Froment sign. The patient subsequently undergoes electrodiagnostic testing, which is consistent with cubital tunnel syndrome. The cubital tunnel is formed by which structures?

A. Anterior, lateral epicondyle; posterior, olecranon; floor, medial collateral ligament; roof, arcuate ligament

B. Anterior, medial epicondyle; posterior, olecranon; floor, medial collateral ligament; roof, arcuate ligament

C. Anterior, lateral epicondyle; posterior, olecranon; floor, lateral collateral ligament; roof, arcuate ligament

D. Anterior, medial epicondyle; posterior, humerus; floor, medial collateral ligament; roof, arcuate ligament

30.2 A 50-year-old man complains of numbness and tingling along his right small finger. Elbow flexion reproduces the numbness and tingling. Physical therapy and splinting have failed to relieve the symptoms over the last 3 months. Which of the following is the most appropriate intervention?

A. In situ ulnar nerve decompression at the cubital tunnel

B. Ulnar nerve decompression at the cubital tunnel with anterior submuscular transposition

C. Ulnar nerve decompression at the cubital tunnel with anterior subcutaneous transposition

D. Continued physical therapy, splinting, and conservative management

30.3 An amateur bodybuilder presents with physical examination findings concerning for an ulnar nerve compression neuropathy. Which of the following anatomic locations is more commonly associated with ulnar nerve compression in bodybuilders as compared with the regular population?

A. Osborne fascia

B. Arcuate ligament

C. Medial epicondyle

D. Medial head of the triceps

ANSWERS

30.1 **B.** The cubital tunnel is formed by the medial epicondyle anteriorly and the olecranon posteriorly. The medial collateral ligament forms the floor, and the roof consists of the arcuate ligament.

30.2 **A.** The patient has cubital tunnel syndrome that has failed conservative management. In situ decompression of the ulnar nerve is less invasive and has clinical outcomes equivalent to that of decompression with transposition. Decompression with transposition has also been shown to have higher complication rates.

30.3 **D.** All of the choices are possible sites of ulnar nerve compression, even in bodybuilders. However, hypertrophy of the medial head of the triceps in this population can cause ulnar neuropathy. This is an uncommon site of compression in the general population.

CLINICAL PEARLS

- Cubital tunnel syndrome includes any ulnar neuropathy in the mid-arm to mid-forearm.
- The anatomic borders of the cubital tunnel are as follows: Anterior, medial epicondyle; posterior, olecranon; floor, medial collateral ligament; roof, arcuate ligament.
- Nerve conduction studies are considered positive if the motor conduction velocity across the elbow is less than 52 m/s, increased distal sensory latency of greater than 3.2 ms, and motor latencies of greater than 5.3 ms.
- Conservative management of cubital tunnel includes splinting, NSAIDs, elbow padding, and PT.
- Operative interventions include ulnar nerve decompression with or without transposition and/or medial epicondylectomy.

REFERENCES

Grana W. Medial epicondylitis and cubital tunnel syndrome in the throwing athlete. *Clin Sports Med.* 2001;20:541-548. Review.

Palmer BA, Hughes TB. Cubital tunnel syndrome. *J Hand Surg Am.* 2010;35:153-163.

CASE 31

A 64-year-old, right-hand dominant male is referred to your office with complaints of progressive hand stiffness and deformity over the past 2 years. The small finger of the right hand is most affected. The left hand is also affected, but not as severe. He denies any history of trauma or previous hand problems, and he has no complaints of pain, nor finger locking or clicking. His father had similar problems with his hands.

The patient's past medical history includes high cholesterol and blood pressure. More than 5 years ago, he underwent surgery for early-stage colon cancer, and since then has been cancer-free. He currently does not drink alcohol, although he drank heavily during his younger years. He is of English-Irish decent.

Examination of both hands reveals nodules and skin thickening in the palm along the small finger ray. The right small finger metacarpophalangeal (MCP) joint is fixed at 45 degrees of flexion, and the proximal interphalangeal (PIP) joint is fixed at 20 degrees. There is no redness, tenderness, edema, or pain with passive flexion. The left hand has a nodule and cord with a resting flexion contracture of the small finger of 20 degrees that is improved with passive extension. Additionally, examination of his left foot reveals nontender nodules along the first ray proximal to the metatarsal head.

- ▶ What is the most likely diagnosis?
- ▶ What is the most appropriate treatment for this patient?

ANSWERS TO CASE 31:

Dupuytren Disease

Summary: This right-hand dominant, 64-year-old male patient has a progressive soft tissue condition leading to digital flexion deformity or contracture. The stiffness is associated with decreased functionality. The contracture in the right hand is not passively correctible.

- **Most likely diagnosis:** Dupuytren disease.
- **Most appropriate treatment:** Collagenase injection(s), needle aponeurotomy, or surgical fasciotomies, depending on the extent of disease and surgeon preference.

ANALYSIS

Objectives

1. Understand the clinical presentation, etiology, risk factors, anatomic features, and pathoanatomy of Dupuytren disease.
2. Be familiar with basic treatment options and associated complications.
3. Identify criteria to guide choice of treatment.
4. Recognize prognostic factors for recurrence and poor outcome.

Considerations

This patient presents with progressive right small finger stiffness and deformity. His MCP joint is fixed in 45 degrees of flexion and his PIP joint is fixed in 20 degrees of flexion. His deformity (see Figure 31–1) is most obvious as he tries to extend all his fingers. Furthermore, the patient denies any locking symptoms, and there is no redness, tenderness, edema, or pain with passive flexion. The differential diagnosis for digital flexion contractures includes Dupuytren disease, trigger finger(s), stenosing tenosynovitis, ganglion cysts, soft-tissue masses, hyperkeratosis, intrinsic joint disease, and traumatic scarring. Despite this broad differential, there are several components of this patient's presentation that favor a diagnosis of Dupuytren disease. These include a family history of similar pathology, a history of heavy alcohol use, being of Northern European decent, and presence of similar, nontender nodules in his left foot. After the **clinical diagnosis** of Dupuytren disease is made, treatment options can be considered, including nonoperative and operative modalities.

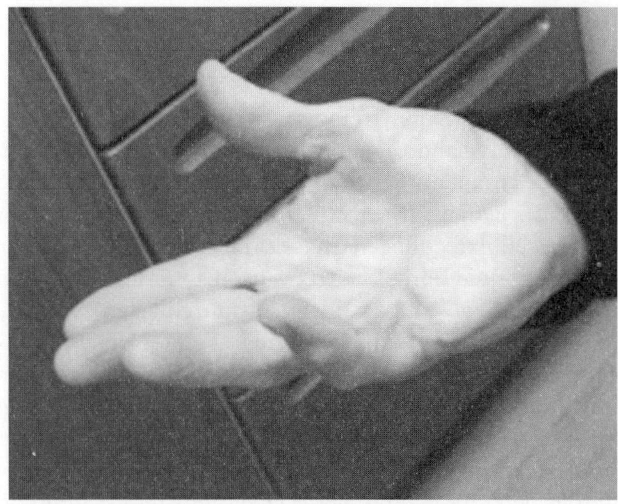

Figure 31–1. Dupuytren disease of the small finger. Note the **MCP and PIP flexion contracture** as the patient attempts to extend his fingers.

APPROACH TO: Dupuytren Disease

DEFINITIONS

DUPUYTREN DISEASE: A benign fibroproliferative disorder involving the palmar and digital fascia.

SPIRAL CORD: An arrangement of abnormal fibrous tissue associated with PIP joint flexion contractures. Spiral cords can displace digital neurovascular bundles centrally and volarly (palmar superficially), making them especially prone to injury during surgical release.

DUPUYTREN DIATHESIS: Refers to patients with an aggressive form of the disease, manifesting with early onset, rapid progression, frequent bilaterality, and/or involvement of the radial digits.

CLINICAL APPROACH

Etiology and Anatomic Features

Dupuytren disease is a benign fibroproliferative disorder involving the fascia of the hand and fingers, **most commonly involving the ring and small fingers.** It can present locally as a nodule in the palm or a dimple in the skin crease. Dupuytrens may then progress distally to involve the joints of the fingers.

The exact etiology remains unclear, although a strong genetic predisposition exists. It occurs more commonly in males of northern European descent. Dupuytren disease has been associated with tobacco and alcohol use, diabetes, epilepsy, chronic pulmonary disease, prior myocardial infarction, human immunodeficiency virus (HIV) infection, trauma, and tuberculosis. However, idiopathic presentation is most common.

The pathophysiology of Dupuytren disease is not completely understood, but has been found to involve **abnormal proliferations of myofibroblasts,** cells normally responsible for producing contractile scar tissue when the body attempts to close a wound. In Dupuytrens, hyperactive myofibroblasts deposit disproportionate quantities of extracellular collagen that form collections of fibrous bundles. Additionally, the deposited fibrous matrix is itself abnormal, consisting of greater concentrations of relatively thick and immature collagen type III, versus the mature collagen type I that is found in normal fascia. Dupuytren disease develops in 3 distinct stages: **(1) the proliferative stage,** in which abnormal numbers of oversized myofibroblasts are produced, **(2) the involutional stage,** in which abnormal concentrations and quantities of collagen type III are deposited, and **(3) the residual stage,** in which the myofibroblasts disappear, leaving behind their dense fibrous deposits. Simply put, Dupuytrens results from a pathological triggering of tissue healing in the absence of inciting trauma. Thick scar-like deposits of abnormal collagen coalesce into the characteristic Dupuytren nodules and cords.

Structural anomalies result from contraction of the collagenous palmar fascia and overlying skin and fingers. Normal structures involved in the disease process include the pretendinous band, natatory band, spiral band, Grayson ligament, retrovascular band, and lateral digital sheet. These normal structures, or bands, when diseased, become cords and are thereafter referred to as the pretendinous cord, central cord, lateral cord, spiral cord, abductor digiti minimi cord, and intercommissural cord of the first web space. Spiral cords lead to PIP contractures and receive special attention for putting the neurovascular bundle at risk by displacing it more centrally and volarly as the PIP joint contracture increases.

The natural history and risk for progression for a single individual remain indeterminable. Patients with Dupuytren diathesis have a more aggressive form of the disease that is associated with onset before age 40 years, bilateral hand involvement, thumb and index finger contractures, and fibrotic disease of the feet and penis. Patients need to be informed that recurrence is as high as 40% to 50%. When the fibroproliferative disease results in permanent curvature of the penis, it is known as **Peyronie disease;** similarly, if it involves the plantar foot, it is known as **Ledderhose disease.**

Clinical Presentation and Evaluation

Patients may present early or with mild forms that manifest as a tender palmar nodule (arising over a pretendinous band), skin dimpling, or a palpable cord. **Classic features include fixed finger flexion deformities that impair function of daily living or work and indicate more advanced disease.** There can be fixed flexion of either or both the MCP and PIP joints. (The distal interphalangeal joints are rarely involved and, when they are, are believed to result from formation of the retrovascular cord.) Disease involvement occurs most often in the ring and little fingers, with decreasing order of frequency in the long, thumb, and index digits. It is bilateral in 45% of patients.

Dupuytren disease is diagnosed clinically. Flexion contractures are rarely subtle. MCP flexion may result from a pretendinous cord or a spiral cord. Limitation in finger abduction is frequently present and results from involvement of the web space and the presence of a natatory cord. Fixed flexion of the PIP joint may arise from contracture of the central cord that continues from a pretendinous cord in the palm that extends into the finger. Involvement of the thumb may manifest as contracture of the web space in addition to a fixed flexion contracture.

TREATMENT

The indications for surgery include functional impairment such as inability to wear a glove, reach into pockets, or securely hold or grasp objects. Physical exam criteria include a positive tabletop test (the inability to place the hand flat on a tabletop), **MCP flexion contracture of greater than 30 degrees,** and **any PIP flexion contracture.**

Different surgical techniques have been described. These include percutaneous needle aponeurotomy, limited fasciectomy, and total palmar fasciectomy. Total palmar fasciectomy has recently fallen from favor because recurrence rates after surgery were no better than those of less extensive procedures and it was associated with higher rates of wound complications. The open-palm technique of McCash leaves the wounds open after surgery, resulting in diminished edema and hematoma formation and allowing for early postoperative motion. This historic technique was once preferred for older patients at increased risk for stiffness; but because of wound complications and poor acceptance on the part of the patient, this technique has since been abandoned. Skin coverage deficits are not uncommon after surgical treatment and may be addressed with skin grafting, Z-plasty, or healing by secondary intention.

Nonoperative treatment of Dupuytren disease is evolving. In early stages, corticosteroid injections may provide some relief by softening and flattening prominent or painful nodules. For more advanced disease, an injectable collagenase (clostridial collagenase histolyticum or Xiaflex, which was approved by the US Food and Drug Administration in 2010) is receiving increasing popularity. This drug has been shown to chemically dissolve the Dupuytren's cord, allowing for the subsequent manipulation necessary to mechanically disrupt the contracted tissue and correct the flexion deformity.

Outcomes and Complications

The most common complications after collagenase injection include edema, bruising, and redness localized to the site of injection. More serious but less frequent complications include flexor tendon rupture or neurovascular injury.

The most common complication after operative treatment is recurrence, with long-term rates as high as 40% to 50%. Attention to postoperative therapy with active range of motion and splinting is a major determinant of improved outcomes. Potential complications include infection, digital neurovascular injury, complex regional pain syndrome, hematoma, skin loss, and amputation.

COMPREHENSION QUESTIONS

31.1 A right-hand dominant 48-year-old woman presents with worsening hand stiffness and deformity. On exam, you note nodules and skin thickening in the palm along the small finger ray. You ultimately diagnose the patient with Dupuytren disease and begin discussing the specifics of this condition with her. Which of the following statements regarding Dupuytren disease is true?

A. Dupuytren disease is rarely bilateral.

B. Dupuytren disease is associated with pain.

C. Females are at greater risk than males.

D. Recurrence after surgery is as high as 50%.

E. Rapidly progressive disease suggests malignancy.

31.2 Which of the following patients with Dupuytren contracture would benefit the most from total palmar fasciectomy?

A. 50-year-old police officer with ring and small finger involvement of only the MCP joints

B. 70-year-old sedentary male with small finger involvement including the MCP and PIP joints

C. 45-year-old female tennis player with ring and small finger involvement including MCP and PIP joints

D. None of the above, as total palmar fasciectomy has fallen out of popularity due to its associated recurrence rates and complications, as opposed to regional, or limited fasciectomy

31.3 A 40-year-old man presents to your hand clinic with a diagnosis of Dupuytren disease involving his left small finger. The patient was given this diagnosis last week while at a routine follow-up appointment with your partner for his right total hip arthroplasty. Your partner felt that you, a hand surgeon, would be best equipped to manage the Dupuytren. After receiving this diagnosis, the patient did an internet search on this condition and comes in today inquiring about treatment with Xiaflex. Which of the following statements regarding Xiaflex is most accurate?

A. This drug has been shown to chemically dissolve the Dupuytren cord.

B. Xiaflex is a time-tested and effective means of treating Dupuytren disease.

C. Xiaflex is great because it has no known side effects.

D. Xiaflex can be purchased as an over-the-counter medication.

ANSWERS

31.1 **D.** Patients with Dupuytren disease should be counseled about the high risk for recurrence after surgery. Disease is frequently bilateral, most common in middle-aged men of northern European descent, and not histologically malignant, although patients with Dupuytren diathesis or with a genetic predisposition may have a more clinically aggressive form with rapid progression and high recurrence.

31.2 **D.** As stated in D, total palmar fasciectomy has fallen out of popularity as a result of its associated recurrence rates and complications, as opposed to regional, or limited fasciectomy.

31.3 **A.** Xiaflex has been shown to chemically dissolve the Dupuytren cord, allowing for the subsequent manipulation necessary to mechanically disrupt the contracted tissue and correct the flexion deformity. Although data are promising, Xiaflex was only approved by the US Food and Drug Administration in 2010. Serious side effects include tendon rupture, ligament damage, nerve injury, and allergic reactions. Common side effects include swelling, bleeding, bruising, pain, and/or tenderness at the injection site or hand.

CLINICAL PEARLS

- Dupuytren disease is a clinical diagnosis, and imaging or laboratory tests are needed only to assess or rule out other incidental conditions.
- Treatment is indicated when the fixed contractures interfere with hand function; standard criteria to provide treatment include the contractures of the MCP of 30 degrees and any degree of fixed PIP flexion, but decision to treat should be tailored to the patient.
- Patients with aggressive disease should be warned that there is high recurrence after treatment.
- Patients should be informed of irreversible complications from treatment including flexor tendon rupture, wound complications (eg, hematoma, infection), and injury to neurovascular structures.

REFERENCES

Desai SS, Hentz VR. The treatment of Dupuytren's disease. *J Hand Surg Am*. 2011;36:936-942.

Hurst LC, Badalamente MA, Hentz VR, et al; CORD I Study Group. Injectable collagenase clostridium histolyticum for Dupuytren's contracture. *N Engl J Med*. 2009;361:968-979.

Miller MD. *Review of Orthopaedics*. 5th ed. Philadelphia: Saunders Elsevier; 2008.

Terek RM, Jiranek WA, Goldberg MJ, Wolfe HJ, Alman BA. The expression of platelet-derived growth-factor gene in Dupuytren's contracture. *J Bone Joint Surg Am*. 1995;77:1-9.

CASE 32

A 60-year-old right-hand dominant woman presents complaining of 12 weeks of right ring finger pain. She is an avid gardener but denies any injury. She notes a clicking sensation when she moves her finger. She occasionally experiences the finger "getting stuck" when she bends it and she has to use her other hand to force the finger back into extension. She reports minimal pain at rest. The pain does not awaken her at night, but she does note ring finger stiffness in the morning. She denies swelling or redness. She has tried resting and limiting her gardening, and she has been taking ibuprofen. Her medical history includes diabetes. On examination, the skin is intact and appears normal. There is no atrophy, swelling, ecchymosis, or erythema. She has a full range of passive and active motion of her fingers and wrist. There is tenderness over the palmar aspect of the ring finger metacarpophalangeal (MCP) joint and palpable popping with active finger flexion and extension. Strength is 5/5 in finger flexion, extension, and abduction/adduction. Sensation is intact to light touch. She has 2+ pulses and capillary refill is less than 2 seconds. Compression testing at the carpal tunnel is negative, as is Phalen and Tinel testing. Hand radiographs show intact joint spaces and normal alignment.

- What is the most likely diagnosis?
- What is the next diagnostic step?
- What is the next step in therapy?

ANSWERS TO CASE 32: Trigger Finger

Summary: A 60-year-old diabetic woman presents to the office with 6 weeks of right ring finger pain, popping, and locking with no history of injury. There is tenderness to palpation over the flexor tendons overlying the MCP joint and palpable triggering. There is full range of motion and good strength.

- **Most likely diagnosis:** Trigger finger.
- **Next diagnostic step:** Physical exam is usually sufficient to diagnose this condition. Further confirmation may be achieved with an injection of local anesthetic into the flexor tendon sheath. This results in a temporary resolution of pain so that triggering, if present, can be readily elicited.
- **Next step in therapy:** This patient has a 12-week history of symptoms and has not seen improvement after rest, activity modification, and NSAIDs. The next step is steroid injection into the flexor tendon sheath.

ANALYSIS

Objectives

1. Understand the pathoanatomy of trigger finger.
2. Appreciate the functions of the flexor tendons and the flexor pulley system and how they relate to trigger finger.
3. Be familiar with the treatment options for trigger finger.

Considerations

This 60-year-old woman with finger pain and popping has tendon entrapment, also known as trigger finger. The diagnosis can generally be made with a thorough history and physical examination. It is important to rule out more serious causes for finger pain, including infection or fracture. Infection would have associated swelling, erythema, and possibly constitutional symptoms such as fever and chills. Fractures result from an injury and initially will have swelling and ecchymosis. These conditions can easily be ruled out in this case by the history and exam. If doubt exists, plain radiographs can be used to rule out fracture, arthritis, or underlying bony deformity. Other common conditions should also be ruled out, including arthritis and carpal tunnel syndrome. Arthritis is a common cause of joint pain and stiffness in the hand. Examination will reveal tenderness over the joint. In this patient's case, the tenderness is over the palmar aspect of the MCP joint. Anatomically, this region of the joint is covered by the flexor tendons and pulley system. The radial and ulnar sides of the MCP joint are more accessible to palpation and are nontender in this patient.

The severity of the mechanical symptoms in a patient with trigger finger should be determined. Early on, some patients may complain of pain alone, whereas in more advanced cases, patients may have significant popping and locking to the point that the finger becomes fixed in a flexed position. This can lead to permanent loss of motion in the finger if untreated.

APPROACH TO:
Trigger Finger

DEFINITIONS

TENOSYNOVIUM: Thin synovial lining surrounding tendons that provides lubricating fluid and nutrition to the tendons.

PULLEY: Fibrous sheath through which the flexor tendon glides. The flexor tendon sheath functions to improve mechanics and maintain the tendon against the metacarpal and phalanges. In each finger, there are 4 to 5 annular (circular) pulleys and 3 cruciate (crossing) pulleys that make up the tendon sheath (Figure 32–1).

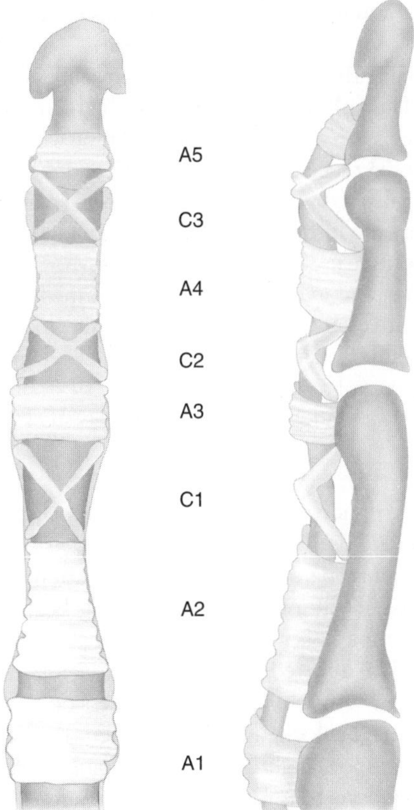

Figure 32–1. Finger flexor tendon pulley system. The pulleys are attached to the palmar surface of each finger metacarpal (MC), proximal phalanx (PP), middle pharynx (MP), and distal pharynx (DP). There are 5 annular pulleys, A1 through A5, and 3 cruciate pulleys (C1-3). **Triggering occurs when there is narrowing at the A1 pulley.** (Reproduced, with permission, from Brunicardi FC, Andersen DK, Billiar TR, et al. *Schwartz's Principles of Surgery.* 9th ed. New York, NY: McGraw-Hill; 2010:Fig. 44-4.)

TRIGGER FINGER (ie, tendon entrapment): Inflammation of the tenosynovium and narrowing of the first pulley, resulting in pain and popping with finger movement.

FINGER FLEXOR TENDONS: Each finger has 1 tendon from the flexor digitorum profundus, which attaches to the distal phalanx and flexes the distal interphalangeal joint (DIP), and 2 slips (derived from a single tendon) from the flexor digitorum superficialis (FDS), which attach to the middle phalanx and flex the proximal interphalangeal joint (PIP). The thumb pulley system contains the flexor pollicis longus and attaches to the distal phalanx, flexing the thumb interphalangeal joint.

CLINICAL APPROACH

Etiologies

Tendon entrapment can occur in any finger or the thumb. It is also common to see patients with multiple fingers affected. Trigger finger is most common in patients 55 to 60 years of age and is at least twice as common in women as in men. It is generally thought to be a degenerative condition resulting from long-term repetitive use of the hand, especially with repeated gripping or pinching. It is more commonly seen in the dominant hand. Systemic factors that can cause or exacerbate tendon entrapment include diabetes, gout, and rheumatoid arthritis.

The flexor tendons glide through a series of fibrous pulleys (Figure 32–1) that make up the tendon sheath. The pulleys act to constrain the tendons against the bone. This increases the force transmission and allows tendon gliding with finger motion. There are 4 to 5 annular pulleys and 3 cruciate pulleys. **The A2 and A4 pulleys are most critical for function.** The first pulley (A1) may become narrowed over time, leading to tendon entrapment. The tendons are lined with a thin tenosynovium that provides lubrication and nutrition. With repetitive use of the hand, the tenosynovium may become inflamed, resulting in pain over the tendon aggravated by use (termed *tenosynovitis*). As the condition worsens, degenerative changes in the fibrous pulley occur, resulting in thickening and inflammatory cell infiltration. As the A1 pulley becomes more hypertrophied, stenosis or narrowing occurs. This leads to a popping or catching sensation with finger flexion and extension as the tendon bunches up and gets stuck in the pulley.

Clinical Presentation

In the early stages of the condition, pain is the primary complaint. Pain is reported with activities that involve use of the hand, especially gripping or holding objects. Most patients report minimal pain at rest but may experience sharp pain with aggravating activities. As the condition worsens, popping begins to occur with active finger motion. The finger may begin to "catch" or temporarily get stuck and, in more advanced cases, may lock in a flexed position, requiring assistance to force the finger back in extension. Patients often complain of stiffness upon waking in the morning and may note that the finger is locked in flexion when they wake up. There is generally no swelling, numbness, or tingling. However, some patients can feel a bump or a nodule in the flexor tendons that is tender to the touch.

Physical examination usually confirms the diagnosis. The A1 pulley, which overlies the metacarpal head and can be felt as a bump at the base of each finger in the distal aspect of the palm, is palpated and is very tender to touch in the setting of trigger finger. There is generally no tenderness elsewhere. Next, range of motion should be examined and is usually normal. In severe cases with chronic locking, some patients may develop a flexion contracture where they cannot fully extend the finger. The examiner should then palpate over the A1 pulley while the patient actively flexes and extends the finger to check for popping. One may also note a nodularity in the tendon as it glides with finger motion. A complete examination of the hand and wrist should be performed to rule out other conditions.

Radiographs are routinely obtained to rule out other conditions including arthritis and fracture. There are no radiographic abnormalities associated with trigger finger. **The diagnosis can be confirmed with an injection of local anesthetic into the flexor tendon sheath. This will result in complete pain resolution.**

TREATMENT

Conservative treatment is effective in most patients with a trigger finger. In early cases with mild symptoms, simple activity modification, rest, and oral anti-inflammatories may be effective. With more significant pain and popping and in more chronic cases, the next step is usually a steroid injection into the flexor tendon sheath. **Injections have been reported to result in complete symptom resolution in 57% of cases, but some patients may require more than one injection.** Patients with systemic causes for trigger finger such as diabetes have worse results with conservative treatment, with success seen in less than 50%.

In cases that do not respond to conservative treatment, surgery is an option. This involves surgically dividing the A1 pulley to relieve the tendon entrapment. The A2 and other distal pulleys remain intact, and no function is compromised. **The success rate of surgery is very high (>90% by most reports).**

COMPREHENSION QUESTIONS

32.1 A 55-year-old woman presents with sudden catching and locking of her ring finger when trying to extend it. She experiences severe pain and notes tenderness in her distal palm. You suspect that this is a trigger finger. What is the best test for confirming this diagnosis?

A. X-rays
B. Computed tomography scan
C. Magnetic resonance imaging
D. Lidocaine injection
E. Ultrasound of the hand

32.2 A 45-year-old woman whom you have recently diagnosed with trigger finger asks you to explain in greater detail why her ring finger locks with flexion. Which of the following statements is most accurate regarding the mechanism for triggering?

A. Trigger finger is caused by entrapment of the flexor tendons at the level of the A1 pulley.
B. The mechanism that causes the finger to trigger is unknown.
C. Trigger finger is due to a vascular anomaly.
D. Trigger finger is caused by a traumatic rupture of the A1 pulley.

32.3 A diabetic patient with a chronic trigger finger has locking of the finger with flexion and has failed 2 prior steroid injections. What is the most effective treatment option for this patient?

A. Surgery
B. Repeat steroid injection
C. Physical therapy
D. Finger splinting
E. Oral anti-inflammatories

ANSWERS

32.1 **D.** A lidocaine injection into the flexor tendon sheath resulting in complete pain relief confirms the diagnosis. However, history and physical exam are usually adequate for the diagnosis, and further confirmation is not required in most cases.

32.2 **A.** The flexor tendons glide through a series of fibrous pulleys that make up the tendon sheath. The first pulley (A1) may become narrowed over time, and as it becomes more hypertrophied, stenosis or narrowing occurs. This leads to a popping or catching sensation with finger flexion and extension as the tendon bunches up and gets stuck in the pulley.

32.3 **A.** This patient has failed 2 injections, and other conservative treatments are unlikely to be effective because of the associated diabetes. Surgical release of the A1 pulley has a success rate of greater than 90%.

CLINICAL PEARLS

- Trigger finger is caused by flexor tendon entrapment in a narrowed A1 pulley.
- Trigger finger usually responds to conservative treatment.
- A steroid injection into the tendon sheath is an effective treatment in most cases and usually should be attempted before considering surgery.
- Surgical release of the A1 pulley is very effective in most cases that do not respond to conservative treatment.

REFERENCES

Fleisch SB, Spindler KP, Lee DH. Corticosteroid injections in the treatment of trigger finger: a level I and II systematic review. *J Am Acad Orthop Surg*. 2007;15:166-171.

Saldana MJ. Trigger digits: diagnosis and treatment. *J Am Acad Orthop Surg*. 2001;9:246-252.

Wolfe SW, et al. *Green's Operative Hand Surgery*. 6th ed. Philadelphia: Elsevier; 2011:2071-2079.

CASE 33

A 43-year-old dentist presents to the clinic with debilitating left elbow pain and stiffness. He states that his left elbow has been bothering him on and off for several weeks but has recently been getting worse. He states that he has been having trouble grasping and gripping objects and feels as if his hand is not working properly. The patient is concerned because the pain and stiffness are beginning to limit him in what he can do in his practice. On physical exam, he is found to have pain on palpation of his lateral elbow and pain with resisted wrist extension and radial deviation. There is minimal swelling present. All motor and sensory findings are normal. His past medical history and review of systems are otherwise unremarkable.

- ▶ What is the most likely diagnosis?
- ▶ What is the initial treatment?
- ▶ Should the patient receive a steroid injection?

ANSWERS TO CASE 33: Lateral Epicondylitis

Summary: A 43-year-old otherwise healthy dentist presents with left elbow pain localized to its lateral aspect. The pain has progressively worsened over the last several weeks, and he now reports stiffness and difficulty with grasping objects. The patient is found to have tenderness with palpation of the lateral epicondyle, specifically at the origin of the forearm extensors, as well as pain with resisted wrist extension and pain with resisted radial deviation. All motor and sensory findings are normal. Radiographs of the elbow are negative for any pathology.

- **Most likely diagnosis:** Lateral epicondylitis (tennis elbow).
- **Initial treatment:** Rest and activity modifications designed to avoid repetitive movements that stress the wrist and forearm extensor tendons. Nonsteroidal anti-inflammatory medications (NSAIDs) can be prescribed, and icing may provide symptomatic relief. A forearm band or "counterforce brace" that is worn distal to the origin of the extensor group could be worn. Once pain has subsided, stretching and strengthening of the forearm extensors should be performed to prevent recurrence of symptoms.
- **Utility of a steroid injection:** Corticosteroids, usually administered concurrently with a local anesthetic, into the area of maximal tenderness, have been shown to be beneficial in achieving transient pain relief. However, multiple corticosteroid injections may be associated with rupture of the extensor tendon origin and/or lateral collateral ligament, both devastating complications.

ANALYSIS

Objectives

1. Know the causes of lateral epicondylitis and the populations most affected.
2. Be familiar with the differential diagnosis for lateral epicondylitis.
3. Know the treatment options for lateral epicondylitis.

Considerations

This 43-year-old dentist presents with left elbow pain localized to the extensor origin at the lateral elbow. His history and physical exam are concerning for lateral epicondylitis, more commonly known as tennis elbow. However, this diagnosis is one of exclusion, and it is essential to rule out other possible injuries, such as a radial and posterior interosseous nerve (PIN) entrapment syndromes, occult fractures, radial head arthritis, C6 and C7 nerve root compression, posterolateral plica, and osteochondral loose bodies. Plain radiographs and physical exam are effective at evaluating for such pathology. In this patient, exam findings that make the diagnosis of lateral epicondylitis more likely include localized elbow tenderness at the origin of the forearm extensors, pain with resisted wrist extension, and pain with resisted radial deviation.

APPROACH TO: Lateral Epicondylitis

DEFINITIONS

LATERAL EPICONDYLITIS: An overuse syndrome or tendinosis affecting the lateral humeral epicondyle. It most commonly involves the extensor carpi radialis brevis (ECRB) but may also involve the extensor digitorum communis (EDC). Lateral epicondylitis is more commonly referred to as **tennis elbow.**

MAUDSLEY TEST: A test used to evaluate for tennis elbow. It is positive when the patient experiences pain in the region of the lateral epicondyle during resisted extension of the middle finger.

CLINICAL APPROACH

Etiology

Lateral epicondylitis is a condition that typically affects middle-aged men and women, resulting in mild to severe discomfort and functional impairment. Although it is also known as tennis elbow because of the vulnerability of tennis players to this injury, javelin throwers, bowlers, swimmers, golfers, and pitchers are also susceptible because of the stress that is placed on the forearm and wrist extensor tendons in those sports. Individuals whose vocational demands include repetitious upper extremity movements, such as carpenters, plumbers, shoemakers, surgeons, and musicians (ie, violinists), are also at risk of developing lateral epicondylitis. The ECRB is most often implicated, but EDC involvement also occurs.

Although epicondylitis is commonly thought of as an inflammatory process, this is a misconception; histology reveals neither acute nor chronic inflammatory changes, but instead hyaline degeneration and vascular proliferation, typically at the ECRB origin (Figure 33–1). These histologic findings have been termed ***angiofibroblastic dysplasia.*** One proposed mechanism by which this occurs involves repetitive microtrauma to the ECRB with an incomplete healing and regenerative response.

Clinical Presentation and Diagnosis

On presentation, patients complain of pain and sometimes stiffness around the lateral aspect of the elbow. They may also describe subjective feelings of tightness in the forearm. It is usually the dominant arm that is affected, and it is rarely seen bilaterally. Physical exam should include evaluation of range of motion at the wrist and elbow, motor strength of the forearm extensor muscles, and palpation of the radial head. Tenderness localized to the lateral epicondyle, where the extensor muscles originate, is present on palpation, especially when the elbow is held in

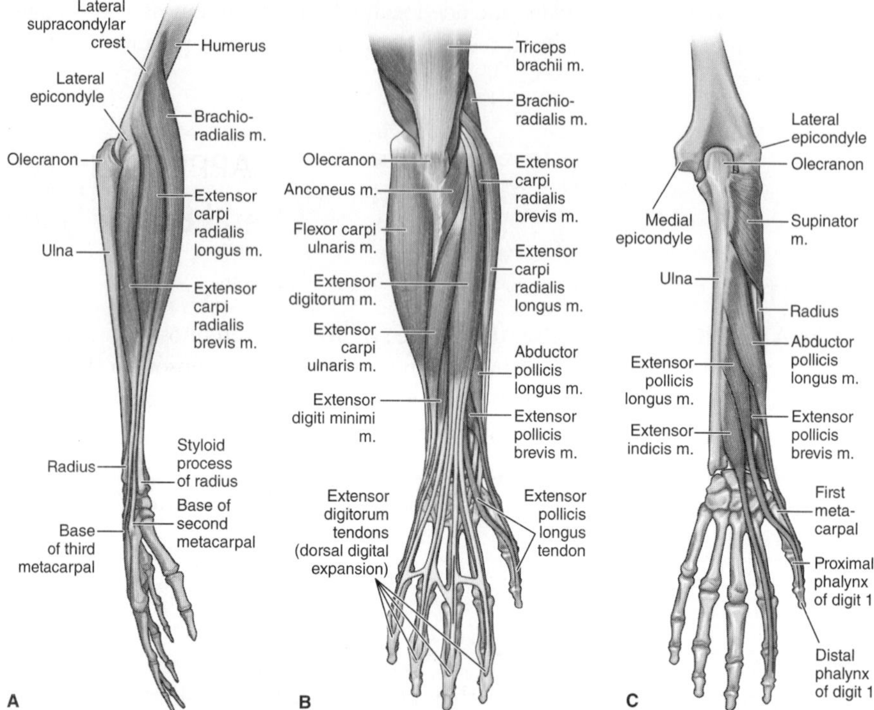

Figure 33–1. (**A**) Lateral view of the forearm. (**B**) Superficial and (**C**) deep muscles of the posterior forearm. (Reproduced, with permission, from Morton DA, Foreman KB, Albertine KH. *The Big Picture: Gross Anatomy.* New York, NY: McGraw-Hill; 2011:Fig. 32-2.)

extension, the forearm held in pronation, and the wrist held in flexion. Additionally, both resisted wrist extension and resisted radial deviation may cause pain in the region of the lateral epicondyle. The **Maudsley test** should also be performed and is positive when the patient complains of pain in the region of the lateral epicondyle during resisted extension of the middle finger. A lidocaine injection test can be used to differentiate between tennis elbow and posterior interosseous nerve (PIN) syndrome, an entrapment neuropathy that is commonly misdiagnosed as lateral epicondylitis as a result of a similar constellation of symptoms. In the case of radial tunnel syndrome, an injection given 4 fingerbreadths distal to the lateral epicondyle will result in a temporary PIN palsy and in the setting of radial tunnel syndrome, a temporary relief in pain. If the injection fails to provide relief, the diagnosis of lateral epicondylitis is more likely and can be confirmed with transient pain relief from a lidocaine injection at the origin of the ECRB tendon.

Imaging has limited utility in the diagnosis of lateral epicondylitis and is most beneficial for ruling out other processes, such as arthritis or fractures. Plain radiographs only rarely show soft-tissue calcification near the lateral epicondyle, which if present would be suggestive of tennis elbow. Ultrasound and magnetic resonance imaging can be used to visualize the extensor tendons and elbow joint, but are only indicated if the patient's symptoms fail to improve after 3 months of conservative treatment.

TREATMENT

Conservative, nonoperative treatment modalities are always attempted first, with operative interventions reserved for refractory cases. Pain reduction is the first treatment goal, and NASIDs, rest, and splinting are often trialled. Patients should be advised to attempt to reduce performing strenuous activities that exacerbate their symptoms for at least 6 weeks. Wrist splints are particularly useful if the elbow tenderness is exacerbated by resisted wrist extension. A counterforce brace can also be used and functions as an inelastic cuff around the proximal forearm against the extensor compartment that reduces the forces generated by the muscles. Other conservative measures that may relieve pain include corticosteroid injections adjacent to the ECRB tendon and extracorporeal shock wave therapy. More recently, injection of platelet-rich plasma has also shown some promise in providing symptomatic relief. Once pain relief is achieved, extensor compartment stretching and strengthening exercises should commence and will help to prevent symptom recurrence.

Cases in which symptoms fail to resolve with 6 to 12 months of conservative treatment can be treated with operative intervention, in which any degenerative, angiofibrotic tissue is debrided, and the ERCB, common extensor tendon, and its aponeurosis are repaired if torn. Both open and arthroscopic techniques have been described. Surgery is followed by a period of rest followed by progressive rehabilitation and strengthening. The major complication following this procedure is posterolateral elbow instability, which results from excessive debridement of collateral ligament and extensor muscle origins on the lateral epicondyle.

COMPREHENSION QUESTIONS

33.1 A 45-year-old carpenter has chronic pain and stiffness over the lateral aspect of the elbow, especially when using a hammer. On exam, Maudsley test is positive. Which muscle attachment is likely to be involved?

A. Extensor carpi radialis longus

B. Brachioradialis

C. Extensor carpi radialis brevis

D. Supinator

33.2 A 65-year-old tennis player presents to your office complaining of pain localized over the insertion of the extensor carpi radialis brevis. On exam, you also note pain with resisted wrist extension and subsequently diagnosis the patient with lateral epicondylitis. What is the histologic term used to describe tennis elbow?

A. Reactive hyperemia

B. Lateral epicondylitis

C. Angiofibroblastic dysplasia

D. Apoptosis

33.3 A 40-year-old woman who you have recently diagnosed with lateral epicondylitis wants to know her treatment options. Which of the following are considered first-line interventions?

A. NSAIDs

B. Wrist splinting

C. ECRB debridement

D. Counterforce brace

E. A, B, D

ANSWERS

33.1 **C.** The extensor carpi radialis brevis is the most common forearm extensor associated with lateral epicondylitis. The extensor digitorum communis has also been implicated. The extensor carpi radialis longus and extensor carpi ulnaris can also be involved, but it is very rare.

33.2 **C.** The histologic term used to describe tennis elbow is angiofibroblastic dysplasia. This is because tennis elbow results from hyaline degeneration and vascular proliferation at the ECRB origin. Microscopic evaluation shows fibroblast hypertrophy, disorganized collagen, and vascular hyperplasia. Although tennis elbow is named lateral epicondylitis, it is not due to inflammatory processes.

33.3 **E.** Conservative measures used in the treatment of lateral epicondylitis include rest, ice, NSAIDs, physical therapy, bracing, steroid injections, extracorporeal shock wave therapy, and platelet-rich plasma. ECRB debridement with possible tendon repair is only performed after 6 to 12 months of failed conservative treatment.

CLINICAL PEARLS

- Lateral epicondylitis, or tennis elbow, is a diagnosis of exclusion.
- The ECRB is most often implicated, but EDC involvement also occurs in tennis elbow.
- Exam findings consistent with lateral epicondylitis include point tenderness at the forearm extensor origin on the lateral epicondyle, pain with resisted wrist extension, pain with resisted radial deviation, and a positive Maudsley test.
- Imaging rarely has a role in the diagnosis of tennis elbow.
- Conservative treatment modalities should always be tried first, with operative intervention reserved for refractory cases.
- Despite its name, lateral epicondylitis is not technically the result of an inflammatory response, but rather a pathological process of hyaline degeneration and vascular proliferation termed *angiofibroblastic dysplasia*.

REFERENCES

De Smedt T, et al. Lateral epicondylitis in tennis: update on aetiology, biomechanics and treatment. *Br J Sports Med.* 2007;41:816-819.

Faro F, Wolf JM. Lateral epicondylitis: review and current concepts. *J Hand Surg Am.* 2007;32:1271-1279.

CASE 34

A 35-year-old man is brought to the emergency department (ED) by his basketball teammates for evaluation of his right leg. The patient was playing a pick-up game at the local gym earlier in the day, at which time he planted his right foot for a jump shot and suddenly felt as though someone kicked him in the back of his leg, although when he looked back no one was close by. The patient reports feeling a "snap" in his calf, experiencing intense pain, and falling to the ground. In the ED, his vital signs are within normal limits. Examination of his left lower extremity reveals a palpable, tender "bulging" mass over his calf and a soft depression on the posterior aspect of his heel. There is no bony tenderness of the left lower extremity. On passive range of motion, there is increased dorsiflexion in the left foot compared with the right foot. The patient cannot actively plantarflex his left foot.

- ▶ What is the most likely diagnosis?
- ▶ What is the next step in workup?
- ▶ What is the best treatment?

ANSWERS TO CASE 34:

Achilles Tendon Rupture

Summary: A 35-year-old man presents with left lower extremity pain after hearing a "snap" in the back of his leg while planting his foot to take a shot during a basketball game. He states that it felt like someone kicked him. Immediately afterward he noticed significant posterior heel swelling. He is unable to actively plantarflex his foot. On exam, you note increased passive range of dorsiflexion on his left side when compared with his right as well as a palpable defect in his Achilles tendon.

- **Most likely diagnosis:** Achilles tendon rupture.
- **Next step in workup:** Pain control, plain radiographs and magnetic resonance imaging (MRI) of the left distal tibia and fibula and ankle if the diagnosis is unclear. Ultrasound is an effective alternative modality for diagnosing an Achilles tendon rupture if MRI is unavailable or contraindicated.
- **Best treatment:** Primary surgical repair.

ANALYSIS

Objectives

1. Understand how to clinically diagnose an acute Achilles tendon rupture using history and specific physical exam maneuvers.
2. Be familiar with treatment options, both nonoperative and operative, for managing Achilles tendon ruptures.
3. Recognize the indications for various treatment options and understand their respective advantages and disadvantages.

Considerations

Initial treatment for this 35-year-old man with a presumed Achilles tendon rupture should focus on pain relief and placing the affected leg in a splint that ensures immobilization in a plantarflexed position. The goal of this initial stabilization is to restore the natural length of the musculotendinous unit disrupted by the injury. The primary goal of treatment is to alleviate pain and restore function. There is debate in the orthopaedic community regarding the best treatment modality for acute Achilles tendon ruptures. Nonoperative treatment includes a period of 6 to 8 weeks of splint or cast immobilization. Operative surgical treatments include open tendon repair and minimally invasive suturing techniques to restore the length and integrity of the torn tendon.

APPROACH TO:
Achilles Tendon Rupture

DEFINITIONS

THOMPSON TEST: With the patient in the prone position, the examiner, squeezes the posterior calf musculature (Figure 34–1). A positive Thompson test occurs when there is an absence of plantarflexion in the affected extremity. The disrupted musculotendinous unit is no longer able to plantarflex the foot on the affected side. This is compared with the unaffected side.

ECCENTRIC CONTRACTION: A muscular contraction during which muscle fibers actually elongate while firing due to overwhelming antagonistic forces. This occurs because the forces that the muscle is trying to overcome are greater than the force generated by the muscle body. Conversely, **concentric contractions** occur when the muscle body shortens with contraction. In concentric contractions, the force generated by the muscle is greater than the antagonistic forces applied to it.

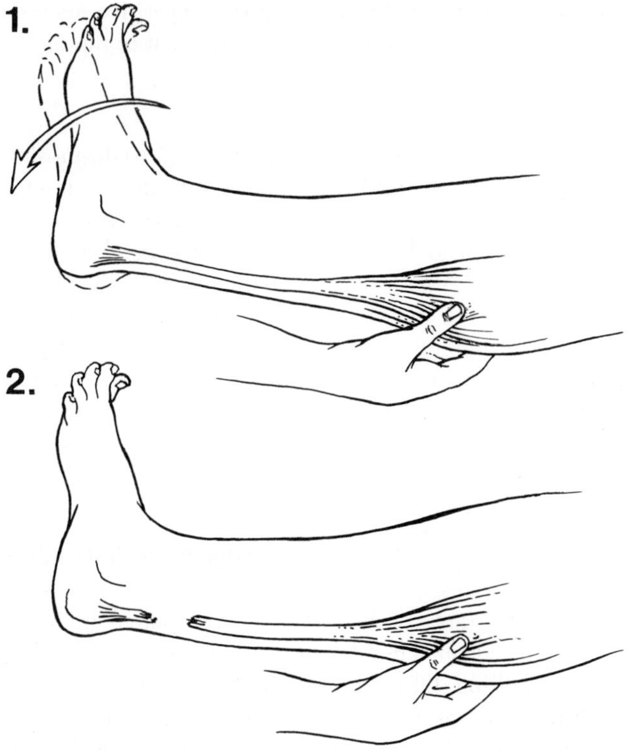

Figure 34–1. Thompson test, in which compression of the gastrocnemius-soleus complex normally produces plantarflexion of the foot (**1**). If the tendon is completely ruptured, this will not occur (**2**). (Reproduced, with permission, from Knoop KJ, Stack LB, Storrow AB, et al. *Atlas of Emergency Medicine.* 3rd ed. New York, NY: McGraw-Hill; 2009:Fig. 11-77.)

CLINICAL APPROACH

Etiologies

Diagnosis of Achilles tendon ruptures are increasing in incidence as more "weekend warrior" athletes are pushing the limits of their typically sedentary and deconditioned bodies. Additionally, the medical community is becoming more aware of and skilled at diagnosing the injury. This injury is commonly observed in men in their fourth through sixth decades of life.

Pathoanatomy

The gastrocnemius and soleus muscle bodies are contained within the superficial posterior compartment of the leg. These muscle bodies converge to form a common Achilles tendon, which inserts on the posterior tuberosity of the calcaneus. This musculotendinous unit acts to plantarflex the foot. The Achilles tendon most commonly ruptures when the gastrocnemius-soleus complex undergoes eccentric loading with the ankle dorsiflexed and the knee extended. Patients are usually able to describe the incident in which they were pushing off or landing on a plantarflexed foot. Most Achilles tendon injuries occur in a hypovascular watershed area located approximately 2 to 6 cm proximal to its insertion. Repetitive microtrauma to this vulnerable hypovascular region is thought to predispose it to rupture.

Physical Exam

Along with the clinical history, the physical exam is key to diagnosing an Achilles tendon rupture. Despite increasing awareness in the medical community, approximately 25% of Achilles tendon ruptures are initially misdiagnosed as ankle sprains. Visual inspection of the affected extremities will likely reveal significant soft tissue swelling in the heel region. A palpable gap, erythema, and/or a bulging muscle mass may be noted after an acute rupture. The Thompson test (Figure 34–1) will aid the clinician in establishing the diagnosis of an Achilles tendon rupture. Although plantarflexion is frequently compromised, be aware that the patient may still exhibit active plantarflexion due to the functions of the unaffected toe flexor and posterior tibialis muscles.

Imaging

The diagnosis of an Achilles tendon rupture is primarily a **clinical diagnosis.** Imaging studies are generally reserved for situations in which the physical exam is inconclusive. Plain radiographs of the lower leg have limited use in diagnosing soft tissues injuries but can adequately rule out any bony injuries and sometimes demonstrate soft tissue swelling. Ultrasound is another imaging modality that can be useful. Although inexpensive, its utility is greatly operator dependent. MRI is the gold standard imaging modality but is not necessary in a clinically obvious diagnosis of Achilles tendon rupture (Figure 34–2). It may, however, be useful in discerning subtleties of partial or chronic Achilles tendon injuries. Of note, the American Academy of Orthopaedic Surgeons Clinical Practice Guideline Summary for acute Achilles tendon rupture states that "We are unable to recommend for or against the

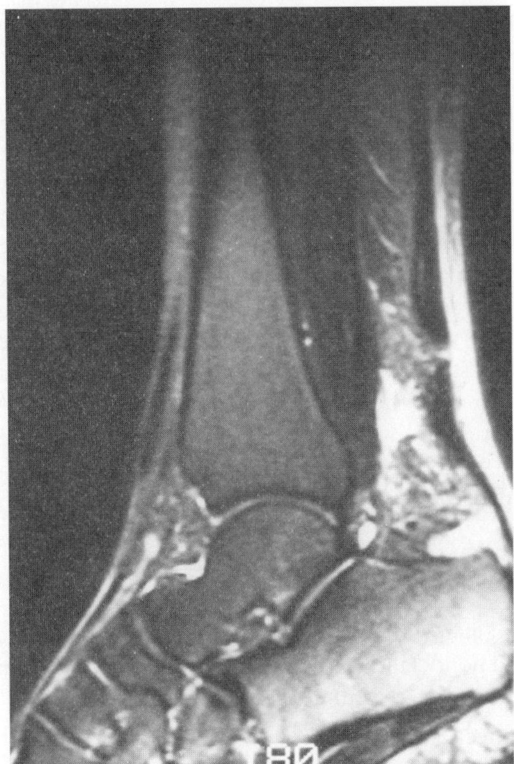

Figure 34–2. Sagittal T2-weighted MRI image of an Achilles tendon rupture. Note the hyperintensity surrounding its calcaneal insertion that is indicative of edema and an absence of tendinous attachment. (Reproduced, with permission, from Skinner HB. *Current Diagnosis & Treatment in Orthopedics.* 4th ed. New York, NY: McGraw-Hill; 2006:Fig. 9-58.)

routine use of MRI, ultrasonography, and radiography to confirm the diagnosis of acute Achilles tendon rupture." In other words, it remains a clinical diagnosis.

TREATMENT

The treatment for an Achilles tendon rupture is controversial and should be individualized to each patient. The primary goal is to reestablish the normal anatomy of the muscle and tendon, in turn restoring function to the musculotendinous unit. If the tendon is left to heal in either extreme of dorsiflexion or plantarflexion, the mechanical functioning of the gastrocnemius-soleus complex with the tendon could be compromised.

Nonoperative treatment is reserved for older, sedentary individuals with multiple medical comorbidities that may compromise wound healing. It focuses on immobilizing the affected leg in a gravity equinus position that maximizes apposition of the 2 ends of the ruptured tendon. Posterior splints, removable boots and short leg casts for 6 to 8 weeks can all stabilize the foot in this manner. Gradual range of motion and resistance exercises begin at 8 to 10 weeks. Such management lacks the risks of surgery, which include infection, wound breakdown, and nerve injury.

However, the limitations of conservative management include suboptimal tendon length after healing and diminished muscle function. Patients must be warned that they will likely have residual weakness and that it can take up to 1 year before maximal plantarflexion is achieved. Furthermore, some studies have shown an increased re-rupture rate with nonoperative management.

Common indications for operative treatment include acute ruptures in young, healthy, active individuals, and following re-rupture of previously immobilization-treated Achilles ruptures. It can be accomplished via open and percutaneous techniques. The surgical approach is on the medial side of the Achilles tendon sheath. The frayed edges are debrided, and the foot is positioned in equinus. Two heavy nonabsorbable sutures are then woven through 3 to 4 cm of each tendon edge, using a Bunnell or Kessler stitch technique. The repair can be augmented with lighter, absorbable sutures or with the plantaris tendon if it is present. Although surgical repair decreases re-rupture rate and increases maximal plantarflexion strength, it does have risks and complications, including infection, skin sloughing and necrosis, and sural nerve damage.

COMPREHENSION QUESTIONS

34.1 A 28-year-old man with an acute Achilles tendon rupture is deciding between operative and nonoperative treatment for his condition. Which of the following statements is true regarding operative treatment?

A. Lower infection rate

B. Lower incidence of tendon re-rupture

C. Decreased muscle strength

D. Increased sensation over the skin of the posterior calf

34.2 A 45-year-old man presents with severe ankle pain and an inability to bear weight after tripping into a sand trap while golfing. Which initial diagnostic test is most appropriate?

A. MRI

B. X-ray

C. Bone scan

D. Ultrasound

34.3 Achilles tendon rupture typically occurs during which type of muscle contraction?

A. Eccentric muscle contraction

B. Isometric muscle contraction

C. Concentric muscle contraction

D. Rhythmic muscle contraction

ANSWERS

34.1 **B.** Surgical repair is associated with a significantly reduced risk of re-rupture when compared with nonsurgical treatment.

34.2 **B.** In a patient with ankle pain and an inability to bear weight, potential fracture must first be ruled out. Although MRI is the gold standard for diagnosing Achilles tendon ruptures, MRI, and similarly ultrasound, should be considered only after other potential injuries are excluded. Bone scans are effective at diagnosing occult bony abnormalities but rarely play a role in diagnosing acute injuries about the ankle.

34.3 **A.** The Achilles tendon most commonly ruptures when the gastrocnemius-soleus complex is undergoing eccentric loading with the ankle dorsiflexed and the knee extended.

CLINICAL PEARLS

- ▶ Approximately 25% of Achilles tendon ruptures are initially misdiagnosed as ankle sprains.
- ▶ Signs and symptoms of an acute rupture include pain, swelling, and ecchymosis around the heel, and a palpable gap in the tendon. Patients classically recall a "popping" sensation during injury or describe the false sensation of being struck on the heel with a blunt object.
- ▶ The Thompson test is an effective physical exam maneuver used to diagnose Achilles ruptures.
- ▶ While Achilles tendon rupture is a predominantly clinical diagnosis, imaging may be necessary in the setting of chronic symptomatology, potential concomitant injuries, or unclear exam findings.

REFERENCES

Azar FM. Traumatic disorders. In: Canale ST, Beaty JH, eds. *Campbell's Operative Orthopaedics*. 11th ed. Philadelphia: Mosby Elsevier; 2008:2737-2788.

Casillas MM, Mann RA. Tendon disorders of the foot and ankle. In: Chapman MW, Szabo RM, Marder R, et al, eds. *Chapman's Orthopaedic Surgery*. 3rd ed. Philadelphia: Lippincott Williams & Wilkins; 2001:3123-3136.

Chiodo CP, et al. AAOS Clinical practice guideline summary: diagnosis and treatment of acute Achilles tendon rupture. *J Am Acad Orthop Surg*. 2010;18:503-510.

Chiodo CP, Wilson MG. Current concepts review: acute ruptures of the Achilles tendon. *Foot Ankle Int*. 2006;27:305-313.

Nilsson-Helander K, et al. Acute Achilles tendon rupture: a randomized, controlled study comparing surgical and nonsurgical treatments using validated outcome measures. *Am J Sports Med*. 2010;38: 2186-2193.

CASE 35

A 47-year-old woman complains of pain at the medial side of her ankle. She works constantly on her feet as real estate agent. She says that she has had a relatively flatfoot her whole life, but it has worsened over the last 3.5 years and believes that the arch is collapsing. She says when she is in the shower it feels like the foot cups the floor. She also has a bunion that seems to have progressed over time. It is dramatically affecting her ability to walk and work. She has tried conservative care in the form of an orthotic and an ankle brace, but the condition continues to worsen her quality of life. On her exam, she has good ankle and subtalar range of motion. She has obvious increased heel valgus on the left side compared with the right. There is a sense of fullness and pain to palpation over the medial aspect of the ankle. On sitting, she can invert, evert, plantar flex, and dorsiflex the ankle with normal strength. However, on standing, she has increased foot abduction, and the arch appears to be collapsed. She cannot perform a single heel raise on the left side but can do so normally on the right side. She also has gastrocnemius tightness. The first ray is hypermobile.

- What is the most likely diagnosis?
- What imaging will help confirm the diagnosis?
- What is the surgical treatment of this condition?

ANSWERS TO CASE 35:
Adult Acquired Flatfoot Deformity

Summary: A 47-year-old woman presents with medial ankle pain and worsening flat foot over the last 3.5 years. The patient has tried orthotics and an ankle brace. On exam, she has increased heel valgus, decreased arch, and inability to single heel raise, with pain over the medial aspect of the ankle.

- **Most likely diagnosis:** Adult acquired flatfoot deformity (AAFD; originally known as posterior tibial tendon insufficiency).
- **Imaging:** Initial plain radiographs of the foot should be obtained in a weight-bearing stance, including an anteroposterior (AP) view to evaluate the talonavicular coverage angle and a lateral view to evaluate the first tarsometatarsal angle (Meary angle), the calcaneal pitch, and the alignment of the hindfoot. Additionally, radiographs of the ankle should be obtained to evaluate for the presence of a valgus tilt.
- **Surgical treatment:** Medializing calcaneal osteotomy with a flexor digitorum longus transfer to the navicular. Other accessory procedures depend on the nature of the deformity.

ANALYSIS

Objectives

1. Understand the pathophysiology behind the development of AAFD, and appreciate the bony, tendinous, and ligamentous anatomy implicated in its development.
2. Understand the nonoperative approach to patients with AAFD.
3. Appreciate the indications and purpose of each step in the algorithm for surgically treating AAFD.

Considerations

This 47-year-old woman has a history of a flatfoot that has worsened over time. The medial arch pain is most likely caused by inflammation and tenderness of the posterior tibial tendon. She has already failed a number of conservative treatments designed to maintain the foot in a more anatomic position. This includes the orthotic, which gives arch support and also tilts the heel out of the valgus position. Figures 35–1, 35–2, 35–3, and 35–4 comprise a standard radiographic workup for AAFD. These radiographs demonstrate collapse at the medial arch (lateral view), a forefoot abduction deformity (AP view), and increased heel valgus (ankle AP and mortise views). An MRI is also very helpful and will show thickening of the posterior tibial tendon and failure of the ligaments of the medial arch. Surgical treatment can be performed after failure of conservative treatment. This consists of a variety of corrective osteotomies and tendon transfers in patients with flexible deformity as present in this patient. Patients with rigid deformity are better served with selective fusions of the hindfoot.

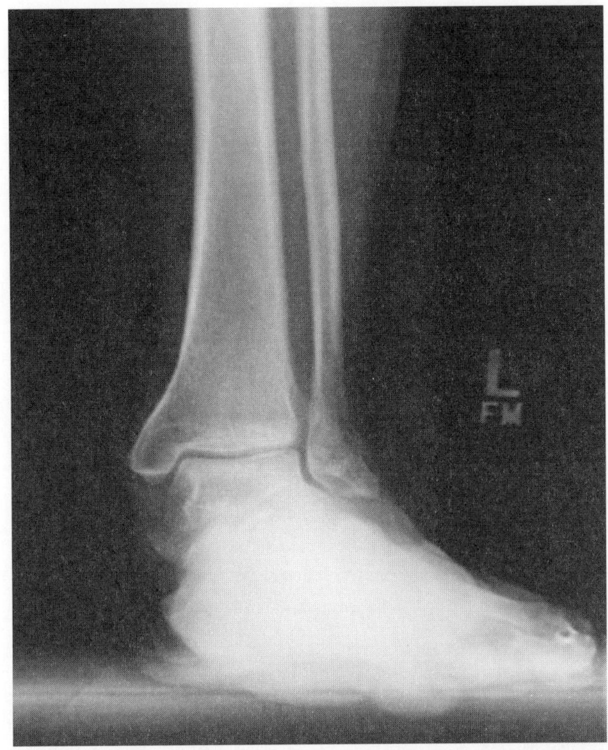

Figure 35–1. Mortise view plain radiograph of the left ankle. (Courtesy of Scott Ellis, MD)

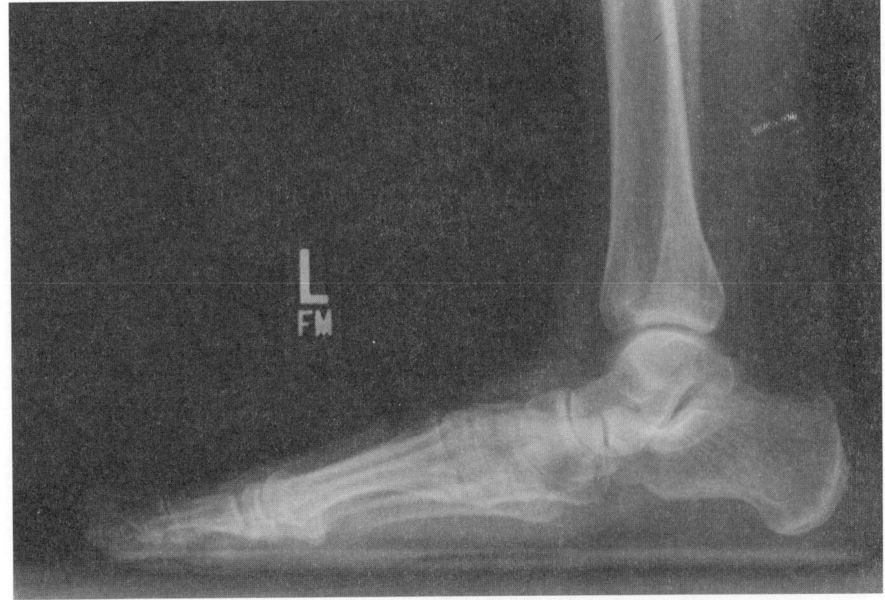

Figure 35–2. Lateral foot plain radiograph showing a decreased pitch at the calcaneus and a decreased first tarsometatarsal angle. (Courtesy of Scott Ellis, MD)

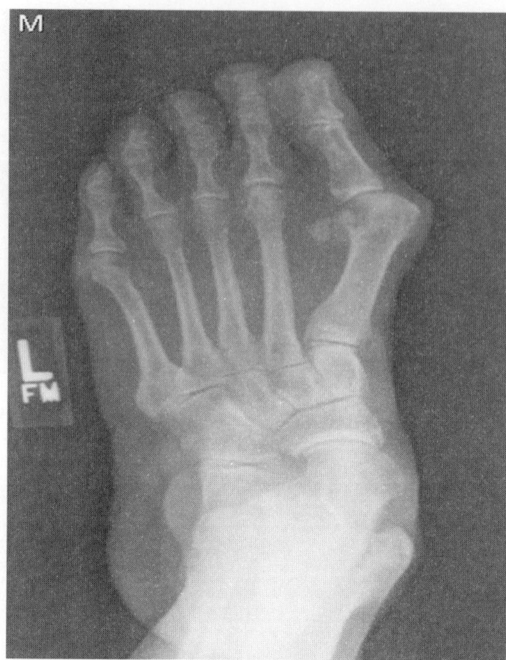

Figure 35–3. Anteroposterior plain radiograph of the left foot demonstrating increased forefoot abduction through the talonavicular joint and the presence of a severe bunion (hallux valgus deformity). (Courtesy of Scott Ellis, MD)

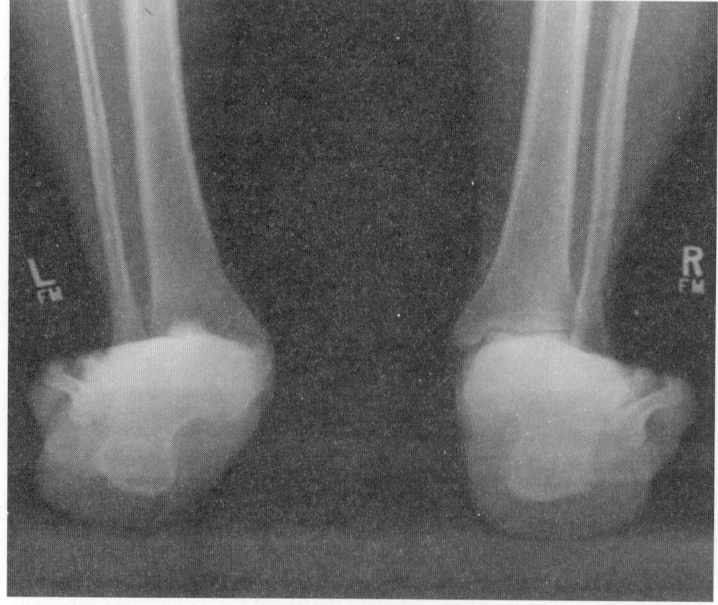

Figure 35–4. Hindfoot alignment view shows increased hindfoot valgus. (Courtesy of Scott Ellis, MD)

APPROACH TO:
Adult Acquired Flatfoot Deformity

DEFINITIONS

POSTERIOR TIBIAL TENDON: The major invertor of the hindfoot, which has its origin along the posterior aspect of the leg and its insertion on the navicular.

MEDIALIZING CALCANEAL OSTEOTOMY: Surgically cutting the calcaneal bone from the lateral side, which is used to translate the posterior portion of the bone attached to the Achilles in a medial fashion. The osteotomy is fixed by 2 screws passed axially up the long axis of the heel bone or calcaneus.

FLEXOR DIGITORUM LONGUS TRANSFER: A surgical rerouting of the tendon, which normally attaches to the plantar surface of the base of the distal phalanges of the 4 lesser toes, to the navicular to replace or enhance the action of the posterior tibial tendon.

GASTROCNEMIUS RECESSION: This is a selective lengthening of the fascia just distal to the muscle body of the gastrocnemius that does not compromise the soleus muscle and therefore lengthens the Achilles complex in a modest fashion.

LATERAL COLUMN LENGTHENING: A surgical cut of the anterior/lateral aspect of the calcaneus that is used to place a graft and move the forefoot out of relative abduction.

SPRING LIGAMENT: The calcaneonavicular ligament, which is a sleeve of tissue that extends from the calcaneus to the navicular and helps support the talar head.

DELTOID LIGAMENT: The ligament connecting the medial malleolus to the talus and calcaneus that helps to prevent the ankle joint from tilting into valgus.

ARIZONA BRACE: A brace that incorporates a custom-made orthotic with a lace-up ankle brace used to help control adult acquired flatfoot deformity.

HINDFOOT VALGUS: A malalignment of the heel with its base displaced laterally when viewed from behind.

FOREFOOT ABDUCTION: A relative position of the toes further away from the midline of the body than normal.

CLINICAL APPROACH

Etiologies

The true cause of the AAFD is not known. Generally, however, it is thought to occur more commonly in women, particularly those who are ligamentously lax and in those who are overweight, which places more strain on the posterior tibial tendon. This tendon goes on to stretch and fail along with the ligaments that support the arch, including the spring ligament. Patients generally complain of having a flatfoot their whole life, which worsens over time. It is thought that the **hypovascular** nature of the tendon in the area of failure is a leading cause. This generally occurs in women beginning in their fifties.

Clinical Presentation

Most patients present first with pain in the medial arch area. This corresponds with the area of the posterior tibial tendon. They also note a decrease in the arch and the position of their heel in more valgus. The foot generally begins to feel weaker. As the disease progresses, pain may shift laterally. This is commonly because the heel begins to impinge underneath the fibula.

The physical exam shows the patient to have a **decreased arch** with the **heel positioned in valgus.** Patients commonly have an **abducted forefoot.** A helpful diagnostic test is the single heel raise. **Patients with posterior tibial tendon insufficiency are unable to raise their heel from the ground or, if they can do so, are not able to fully invert the heel.** Patients also commonly present with a bunion and a tight gastrocnemius muscle, which occurs as the heel moves in the more relative position of valgus and shortens the Achilles.

Diagnosis

The diagnosis is commonly made based on the history. The inability to perform a single heel raise is very suggestive as well. Radiographs indicate the location and amount of deformity (Figures 35–1, 35–2, 35–3, and 35–4). On a lateral x-ray, patients have a decreased first tarsometatarsal angle showing collapse on the inside arch. The hindfoot alignment view generally shows that the heel is in relative position of valgus. AP x-rays show that the navicular bone moves lateral relative to the talus, which suggests that there is forefoot abduction. An MRI can be helpful as well, which shows not only enlargement and degeneration of the posterior tibial tendon, but also failure of the spring ligament complex.

Once the diagnosis of AAFD is made, it can be classified. Classification into 4 stages of severity helps guide treatment and prognosis. In stage I, the foot and ankle are without deformity, however there maybe pain from posterior tibial tendinosis. In stage II, the flatfoot deformity is apparent, but it is flexible throughout, meaning, the examiner can pull it into appropriate alignment. In stage III, the flatfoot deformity becomes rigid and is uncorrectable by manipulation. Finally, by stage IV, there is an additional rigid valgus tilt to the ankle due to compromise of the deltoid ligament.

TREATMENT

Treatment depends on the stage of the deformity. In general, those with **stage I** or no deformity can be treated conservatively with an orthotic and relative rest. Patients with **stage II** deformity generally are first approached with an orthotic, which gives arch support, and a medial post, which is used to raise the inside aspect of the heel and tilt the heel out of valgus. An ankle brace that is usually a lace-up or velcro brace can be used to help stabilize the hindfoot. Commonly, patients must go on to try an Arizona brace, which is a custom-made orthotic built in with an ankle brace. Patients with **stage III** AAFD respond less favorably to orthotics and bracing given that the deformity is rigid and not correctible. **Stage IV** generally also requires more aggressive treatment, given the collapse that is occurring through the ankle unless the patient is relatively asymptomatic.

Surgical treatment also depends on the stage. Surgery is rarely indicated for patients without deformity or stage I. In stage II, a medializing heel slide is commonly performed, along with a transfer of the flexor digitorum longus tendon to the navicular. If the posterior tibial tendon is very diseased, it can be resected. A gastrocnemius resection, lateral column lengthening, and medial column procedures such as first tarsometatarsal fusion or osteotomy to the medial cuneiform (Cotton osteotomy) can be also used. For stage III deformity, a fusion of the triple joint complex, which includes the subtalar, talonavicular, and calcaneal cuboid joint, must be performed. In stage IV, the ankle must be addressed concomitantly with the foot either through trying to reconstruct the deltoid, performing an ankle fusion, or performing ankle replacement.

COMPREHENSION QUESTIONS

35.1 Which of the following best defines the "spring ligament"?

A. Talocalcaneal ligament
B. Calcaneonavicular ligament
C. Talonavicular ligament
D. Calcaneofibular ligament

35.2 Which of the following best describes the action of the posterior tibial tendon?

A. Evert the hindfoot
B. Dorsiflex the ankle
C. Plantar flex the ankle
D. Invert the hindfoot

35.3 A 55-year-old woman presents with a severe flatfoot deformity with arthritis in the subtalar joint. On exam, she has increased hindfoot valgus and forefoot abduction, which is not correctable on physical exam. Which stage is this flatfoot deformity?

A. Stage I
B. Stage II
C. Stage III
D. Stage IV

35.4 A 60-year-old man presents with a 2-year history of medial ankle pain and a severe flatfoot deformity, which is correctable on physical exam. Which of the following best describes the orthotic that may be used to help treat this deformity?

A. Lateral posting and a first metatarsal well
B. Lateral posting with a metatarsal pad
C. Medial heel posting with arch support
D. A carbon-graphite insert with an extension to protect the great toe

35.5 A 52-year-old woman who is moderately obese and who has had flatfoot deformity her whole life is now presenting with worsening hindfoot pain, particularly around the medial aspect of her ankle. She has increased heel valgus on exam with forefoot abduction and a decreased arch. She cannot perform a single heel raise. MRI confirms a decreased arch and posterior tibial tendinosis. Which of the following best describes the surgical treatment?

A. Lateralizing heel slide and a flexor digitorum longus transfer to the navicular
B. Lateralizing heel slide and a deltoid ligament repair
C. Medializing heel slide with lateral column shortening through the anterior calcaneus
D. Medializing heel slide with a flexor digitorum longus transfer to the navicular

ANSWERS

35.1 **B.** The spring ligament connects the calcaneus and navicular, holding up the talar head and helping support the medial arch.

35.2 **D.** The posterior tibia tendon inserts on the navicular. Its primary action is to invert the hindfoot and can be assessed with the single heel raise test.

35.3 **C.** A flatfoot deformity that does not correct on exam is considered rigid and therefore classified as stage III. Arthritis is commonly present.

35.4 **C.** A medial heel post helps tilt the heel out of valgus. The arch support helps to maintain the medial arch. Metatarsal posts are generally used for pain under the metatarsals, and the carbon-graphite insert above is generally used for patients with arthritis in the great toe joint.

35.5 **D.** The heel must be cut and translated medially to bring the calcaneus out of valgus. The flexor digitorum transfer to the navicular helps restores inversion power to the foot.

CLINICAL PEARLS

- AAFD usually is caused by failure of the ligaments supporting the medial arch along with the posterior tibial tendon.
- Patients with AAFD present with hindfoot valgus and an inability to do a single heel raise.
- Standard weightbearing radiographs often diagnose flatfoot deformity due to decreased first tarsometatarsal angle on a lateral view, increased forefoot abduction through the talonavicular joint on an anteroposterior view, and a hindfoot alignment view showing increased heel valgus.
- MRI can also show the failure of the posterior tendon and medial arch ligaments.
- Conservative treatment generally consists of orthotics and bracing.
- Surgical reconstruction usually consists of an osteotomy of the calcaneus and a tendon transfer in the foot in patients with flexible deformity.

REFERENCES

Deland JT. Adult-acquired flatfoot deformity. *J Am Acad Orthop Surg*. 2008;16:399-406.

Deland JT, Page A, Sung IH, O'Malley MJ, Inda D, Choung S. Posterior tibial tendon insufficiency results at different stages. *HSS J*. 2006;2:157-160.

Haddad SL, Myerson MS, Younger A, Anderson RB, Davis WH, Manoli A 2nd. Symposium: adult acquired flatfoot deformity. *Foot Ankle Int*. 2011;32:95-111.

Johnson KA, Strom DE. Tibialis posterior tendon dysfunction. *Clin Orthop Relat Res*. 1989:196-206.

Myerson MS. Adult acquired flatfoot deformity: treatment of dysfunction of the posterior tibial tendon. *Instr Course Lect*. 1997;46:393-405.

Younger AS, Sawatzky B, Dryden P. Radiographic assessment of adult flatfoot. *Foot Ankle Int*. 2005;26:820-825.

CASE 36

A 37-year-old man arrives in the emergency department after a motorcycle accident in which he hit a tree traveling at approximately 50 mph. He was helmeted and denies any loss of consciousness. His blood pressure is 130/80 mmHg, his heart rate is 90 beats/minute, and his temperature is 99°F. He complains of significant pain localized to his right foot. On physical exam of the right foot, the skin is found to be intact. However, there is significant swelling over the dorsum of the foot as well as plantar ecchymosis. His foot is tender, predominantly over the midfoot and forefoot. The patient will not move his toes secondary to pain. His sensation is grossly intact. The posterior tibial pulse is palpable, whereas the dorsalis pedis pulse is only appreciated with a Doppler probe. Capillary refill of the toes is brisk and less than 2 seconds. His pain does not worsen with passive dorsiflexion of the toes.

- What initial radiographic studies are most appropriate?
- What is the most likely diagnosis?
- Given the mechanism of injury, what other considerations must be taken before initiating appropriate treatment for the patient's foot?
- How is this injury classified?
- What is the most appropriate treatment for this patient?

ANSWERS TO CASE 36:
Lisfranc Injury

Summary: A 37-year-old man complains of severe right foot pain after a motorcycle accident in which he hit a tree at approximately 50 mph. On physical exam of his foot, diffuse tenderness and dorsal swelling are noted, as is medial plantar ecchymosis.

- **Radiographs to order:** Anteroposterior (AP), lateral, and 30-degree oblique views of the right foot.
- **Most likely diagnosis:** Tarsometatarsal joint complex injury, commonly referred to as a Lisfranc injury.
- **Other considerations:** Given the high-energy mechanism of injury, this patient must be managed with strict adherence to advanced trauma life support protocol. A complete trauma workup and evaluation should be performed before orthopaedic intervention for the left foot.
- **Classification of Lisfranc injury:** Although multiple classifications exist, none have been proven to be useful for determining treatment or prognosis. One commonly used descriptive classification describes homolateral, isolated, and divergent patterns.
- **Treatment:** Open-reduction internal fixation when soft tissue swelling subsides.

ANALYSIS

Objectives

1. Be familiar with the general presentation of a Lisfranc injury.
2. Understand the workup and imaging studies required for diagnosis of a Lisfranc injury.
3. Know the treatment options for and complications associated with Lisfranc injuries.

Considerations

This patient's history and presentation are common for an injury to the tarsometatarsal (TMT) joint complex. The diffuse pain and swelling, specifically over the midfoot and forefoot, are consistent with a high-energy injury mechanism, such as a motorcycle accident, which is often associated with Lisfranc injuries. **Additionally, the medial plantar ecchymosis is often thought to be pathognomonic for this injury.** The absence of a palpable dorsalis pedis pulse is likely due to the soft tissue swelling over the dorsum of the foot, another common finding. Although the patient's clinical picture is consistent with a Lisfranc injury, **up to 20% of these initially go undiagnosed.** The swelling is concerning, as compartment syndrome of the foot can be seen in association with injuries to the TMT joint complex. The practitioner must carefully and serially examine the patient in this setting and even consider measuring compartment pressures if they believe an acute compartment syndrome is present. The orthopaedic workup of this patient should also include imaging of the right foot, including AP, lateral, and oblique views. A secondary survey should also be performed to rule out additional musculoskeletal injuries requiring care. In the emergency department, this patient's foot should be splinted, iced, and elevated to control swelling, as the timing of potential operative intervention is dependent on this. Soft tissue swelling can delay operative treatment of Lisfranc injuries by up to several weeks. **In addition to an orthopaedic surgery consultation, this patient requires an evaluation by the trauma team; intracranial, thoracic, abdominal, and spine injuries can be present concurrently.**

APPROACH TO: Lisfranc Injuries

DEFINITIONS

JACQUES LISFRANC: A field surgeon in Napoleon's army. He described an amputation involving the TMT joint due to a severe gangrene that developed when a soldier fell from a horse with his foot caught in a stirrup.

LISFRANC JOINT: This refers to the TMT joint complex, an osseous and capsule-ligamentous network that includes the 5 metatarsals (MTs), their articulations with the cuneiforms and cuboid, and the Lisfranc ligament, a strong interosseous attachment between the medial cuneiform and second MT.

LISFRANC INJURY: Refers to a spectrum of processes involving the TMT joint complex, including both fractures and dislocation. It does not delineate a specific injury.

HOMOLATERAL LISFRANC INJURY: All 5 metatarsals are displaced in the same direction.

ISOLATED LISFRANC INJURY: 1 or 2 metatarsals are displaced from the others.

DIVERGENT LISFRANC INJURY: The metatarsals are displaced in both the coronal and sagittal planes.

COMPARTMENT SYNDROME: A surgical emergency that occurs as a result of increased pressure within a muscle compartment, at times compromising blood flow and damaging nerves, muscle, and surrounding soft tissue structures. It is often encountered in the setting of trauma and extremity fractures. Although a clinical diagnosis, intracompartmental pressure measurements of greater than 30 mmHg or a less than 30-mmHg difference between the patient's intracompartmental pressure and diastolic blood pressure are consistent with the diagnosis of compartment syndrome (see Case 13).

CLINICAL APPROACH

Anatomy

The Lisfranc joint divides the midfoot and the forefoot, forming an oblique line running from the lateral aspect of the proximal forefoot to the medial aspect of the distal forefoot. Bony elements provide the primary structural support to this articulation, with ligamentous contributions adding additional stability. The 3 medial MTs articulate with the 3 cuneiforms; the fourth and fifth MTs articulate with the cuboid. The middle cuneiform–second MT articulation forms the **keystone** of the arch, preventing mediolateral MT motion at the Lisfranc joint. This transverse arch also prevents plantar displacement of the 3 medial MTs. The most significant and strongest ligamentous structure is the **oblique interosseous ligament,** referred to as Lisfranc ligament. Originating on the lateral surface of the medial cuneiform, it passes in front of the intercuneiform ligament and ultimately inserts on the medial aspect of the second MT base near the plantar surface.

Mechanism

Direct and indirect injury patterns can damage the Lisfranc joint. Direct mechanisms, **most commonly crush injuries,** are due to high-energy blunt trauma to the dorsum of the foot. These often result in worse clinical outcome as compared with indirect types, secondary to the associated soft tissue trauma. The indirect mechanism usually involves axial loading of a plantarflexed foot, external rotation on a pronated forefoot, or an abduction stress to the midfoot. Indirect mechanisms are stratified into high-energy and low-energy subtypes. Motor vehicle accidents are the most common cause of high-energy Lisfranc injury. **Low-energy injuries include those incurred during athletic competition.** The fracture pattern and direction of dislocation in direct injuries are dependent on the force vector applied. Indirect injuries are more predictable and most commonly involve failure of the weaker dorsal TMT ligaments in tension with subsequent dorsal or dorsolateral MT dislocation.

Workup and Diagnosis

The diagnosis of high-energy Lisfranc injuries is straightforward; physical exam will reveal swelling and many times obvious deformity, including widening or flattening of the forefoot. Additionally, it might be an open injury with disruption of the skin and subcutaneous tissue. TMT joint injury and intercuneiform disruption is suggested in the presence of a gap between the first and second toes, known as a **positive gap sign.** Although associated vascular injury is rare, it may be difficult to palpate a dorsalis pedis pulse secondary to swelling. The clinician must also consider a concurrent **compartment syndrome** with severe swelling and pain with passive dorsiflexion of the toes. If unsure, measurement of pressures is warranted.

In the setting of a low-energy injury, physical exam may only reveal a patient with an inability to bear weight and possibly midfoot and forefoot swelling. Paying attention to the reported mechanism and the clinical appearance of the foot is pivotal to making the correct diagnosis. An additional finding may be **plantar arch ecchymosis,** which is considered pathognomonic for Lisfranc injury. To increase the accuracy of diagnosis, various tests and stress maneuvers have been described to aid in the diagnosis of subtle injury. Of note, pain on passive abduction and pronation of the forefoot is suggestive of injury to the TMT complex.

Initial imaging to obtain include nonweightbearing anteroposterior (AP), lateral, and 30-degree oblique views of the foot (Figures 36–1A, 36–1B, and 36–1C).

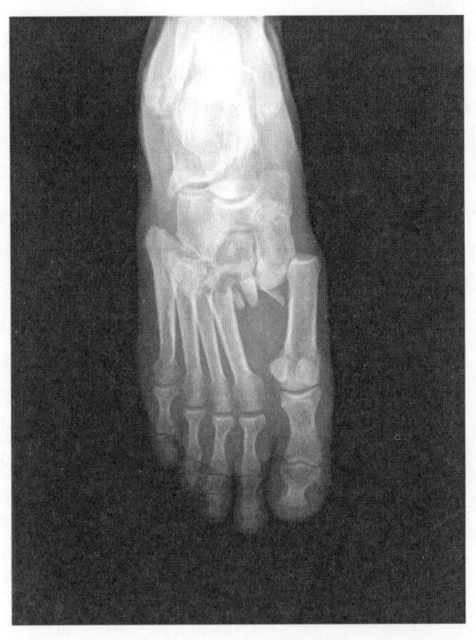

A

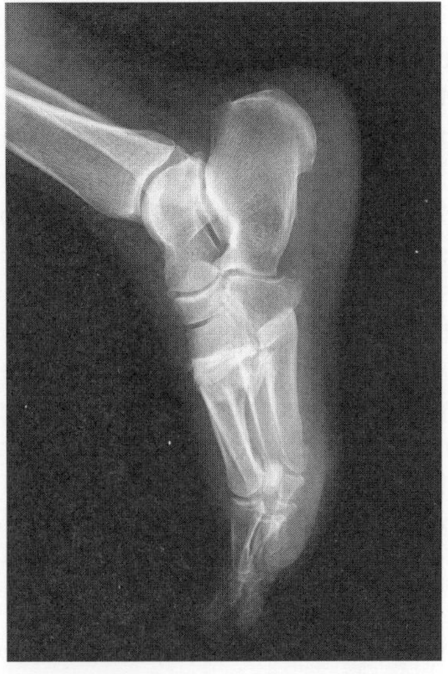

B

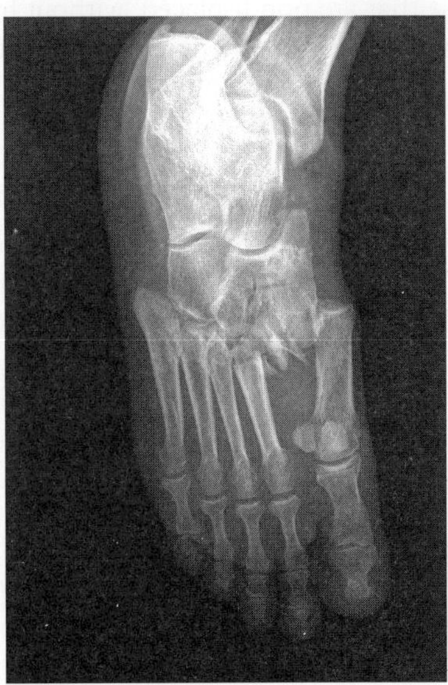

C

Figure 36–1. (**A**) AP, (**B**) lateral, and (**C**) oblique radiographs demonstrating a divergent Lisfranc injury of the right foot.

However, 50% of subtle Lisfranc injuries will have normal nonweightbearing imaging. Thus to diagnose these injuries, a **weightbearing film** with both feet on a single cassette or an **abduction-pronation stress view** should be obtained. Admittedly, these are rarely obtained secondary to pain, necessitating a bone scan or magnetic resonance imaging. Computed tomography may be beneficial as a diagnostic adjunct, as it is effective at delineating fractures.

On the AP radiograph, findings suggestive of a Lisfranc injury include incongruity at the first and second MT joints, misalignment of the medial border of the second MT and medial border of the middle cuneiform, and a diastasis of ≥2 mm between the first and second MTs as compared with the contralateral foot (Figure 36–1A). The oblique radiograph should show alignment of the medial border of the fourth MT and the medial border of the cuboid in a normal foot (Figure 36–1C). Misalignment may suggest a TMT joint complex injury. Potentially seen on this view as well as the AP is the **"fleck" sign,** as described by Myerson et al. It refers to the presence of a small bony fragment between the base of the second MT and the medial cuneiform and represents an avulsion of either the proximal or distal attachment of the Lisfranc ligament. The lateral radiograph will show flattening of the longitudinal arch and/or dorsal displacement at the second TMT joint (Figure 36–1B). The fifth MT is normally plantar in relation to the medial cuneiform. Flattening of the midfoot arch positions the medial cuneiform plantar to the fifth MT.

TREATMENT

Indications for both operative and nonoperative treatment exist, all with the goal of reestablishing a painless and stable foot. Any disruption of normal anatomy warrants surgical correction. Nonoperative treatment is limited to stable TMT joint complex injuries and include those that are nondisplaced, without fracture, and stable under radiographic stress examination. Treatment involves protected weightbearing in a Cam Walker® boot, with frequent follow-up radiographs to ensure no change in alignment. It takes approximately 4 months to recover from a nonsurgical Lisfranc injury.

In unstable Lisfranc injuries, open-reduction internal fixation is performed to restore anatomic alignment. Commonly, screw fixation is used to fix the first, second, and third TMT joints, whereas the fourth and fifth may be pinned with K-wires. Although this is one common approach to operative management, many forms of fixation are available and depend on both the nature of the injury and the surgeon's preference. Although controversial, TMT joint arthrodesis is recommended by some for purely ligamentous Lisfranc injuries. Traditionally, this procedure was considered a salvage operation for failed ORIF and in cases of posttraumatic arthritis. Postoperatively, protected weightbearing for 3 to 5 months and therapy emphasizing passive midfoot range of motion are allowed. Regardless of the modality, anatomic alignment is the standard to decrease the risk of posttraumatic arthritis, chronic instability, and pain.

COMPREHENSION QUESTIONS

36.1 A 40-year-old equestrian complains of right midfoot pain associated with difficulty ambulating for the last 2 days, when her foot got caught in a stirrup while riding. Radiographs show a 4-mm diastasis between the first and second metatarsals. What is the most appropriate treatment?

A. Open-reduction internal fixation
B. Nonweightbearing in a short leg cast
C. Weightbearing as tolerated in an aircast
D. Chevron osteotomy

36.2 A football player who is lying on the ground after being tackled attempts to stand up. While he is still prone on the ground, another player falls directly on his left heel. He immediately experiences midfoot pain and is unable to place any weight on his left foot. In this setting, what should the team physician be most concerned about?

A. High ankle sprain
B. Achilles tendon rupture
C. Lisfranc injury
D. Ankle fracture

36.3 A 54-year-old woman sustains a twisting injury to her foot. An AP radiograph of the foot reveals a 4-mm diastasis between the first and second metatarsals. Which structure connects the medial cuneiform to the base of the second metatarsal?

A. Chopart ligament
B. Deltoid ligament
C. Lisfranc ligament
D. Spring ligament

ANSWERS

36.1 **A.** The patient has sustained an injury to her TMT joint complex. The Lisfranc ligament, which connects the base of the second metatarsal to the medial cuneiform, has been disrupted. Anatomic reduction of the Lisfranc joint is necessary and in this case requires open reduction and internal fixation. Postoperatively, protected weightbearing for 3 to 5 months and therapy emphasizing passive midfoot range of motion are allowed. Posttraumatic arthritis, midfoot instability, and pain are the long-term outcomes of a nonreduced joint.

36.2 **C.** Lisfranc injuries are common in football players, with up to approximately 4% of American football players sustaining them each season. External rotation on a pronated forefoot is responsible for this and can lead to an unstable Lisfranc ligamentous injury. Other sports in which TMT joint complex injuries are encountered include equestrian events and windsurfing, in which the use of a stirrup can lead to one's forefoot being abducted around a fixed hindfoot. When this occurs, dislocation of the second metatarsal and lateral displacement of the other metatarsals occurs.

36.3 **C.** This woman sustained a TMT joint complex injury, as evidenced by the large diastasis between the first and second metatarsals. The most significant and strongest ligamentous structure of the TMT joint complex is the oblique interosseous ligament, more commonly referred to as the Lisfranc ligament. Originating on the lateral surface of the medial cuneiform, it passes in front of the intercuneiform ligament and ultimately inserts on the medial aspect of the second MT base near the plantar surface. A, B, and D are incorrect—the Chopart, or bifurcate, ligament provides stability to the calcaneocuboid joint; the Deltoid ligament stabilizes the medial side of the ankle; and the Spring ligament stabilizes the talonavicular joint.

CLINICAL PEARLS

- The Lisfranc joint refers to the TMT joint complex, an osseous and capsuloligamentous network that includes the 5 metatarsals, their articulations with the cuneiforms and cuboid, and the Lisfranc ligament.
- Radiographic findings indicative of a Lisfranc injury include diastasis of ≥2 mm between the first and second MTs as compared with the contralateral foot, the fleck sign, flattening of the longitudinal arch of the foot, and dorsal displacement at the second TMT joint.
- The goal of both operative and nonoperative management of Lisfranc injuries is restoration of the normal anatomy of the TMT joint complex.
- Open-reduction internal fixation is the predominant surgical intervention for unstable Lisfranc injuries.
- Posttraumatic arthritis, chronic instability, and pain are the long-term complications associated with inadequate and nonanatomic reduction of the Lisfranc joint and its structures.

REFERENCES

Davies MS, Saxby TS. Intercuneiform instability and the "gap" sign. *Foot Ankle Int*. 1999;20:606-609.

Myerson MS, Fisher RT, Burgess AR, Kenzora JE. Fracture dislocations of the tarsometatarsal joints: end results correlated with pathology and treatment. *Foot Ankle*. 1986;5:225-242.

Nunley JA, Vertullo CJ. Classification, investigation, and management of midfoot sprains: Lisfranc injuries in the athlete. *Am J Sports Med*. 2002;30:871-878.

Ross G, Cronin R, Hauzenblas J, Juliano P. Plantar ecchymosis sign: a clinical aid to diagnose occult Lisfranc tarsometatarsal injuries. *J Orthop Trauma*. 1996;10:119-122.

Thompson MC, Mormino MA. Injury to the tarsometatarsal joint complex. *J Am Acad Orthop Surg*. 2003;11:260-267.

Watson TS, Shurnas PS, Denker J. Treatment of Lisfranc joint injury: current concepts. *J Am Acad Orthop Surg*. 2010;18:718-728.

CASE 37

A 51-year-old man presents to the emergency department (ED) after falling 6 feet from a ladder onto his left foot while moving heavy boxes. The patient has no past medical history, works as a self-employed engineer, and is a nonsmoker. On initial presentation, he complains of isolated left foot and heel pain. He states he cannot bear any weight on his affected limb. Physical exam of the foot reveals no open wounds, marked soft tissue swelling, ecchymosis, and tenderness to palpation. Sensation to light touch is grossly preserved, but his ankle and foot range of motion is significantly limited by pain. Pedal pulses are palpable and symmetric to the contralateral side. Initial radiographic evaluation with anteroposterior (AP), lateral, and Harris views of the foot are shown in Figures 37–1, 37–2, and 37–3.

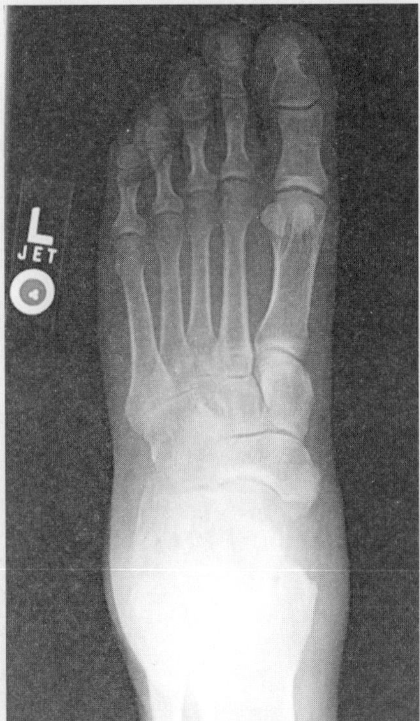

Figure 37–1. AP view of the foot.

- What is the most likely diagnosis?
- What additional studies should be obtained?
- What are the treatment options?
- What are the potential complications?

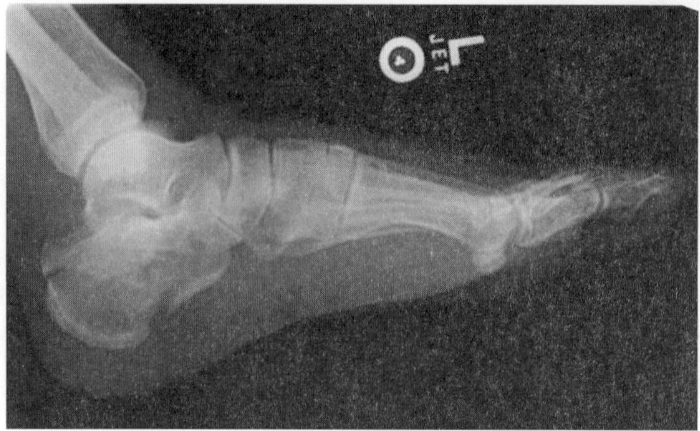

Figure 37–2. Lateral view of the foot.

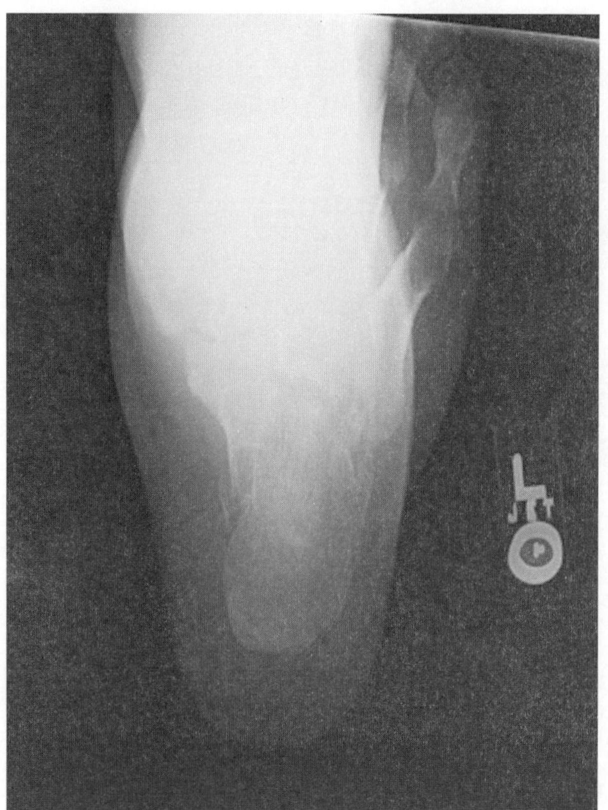

Figure 37–3. Harris view of the foot.

ANSWERS TO CASE 37: Calcaneus Fracture

Summary: A 51-year-old man presents with left foot pain, swelling, and ecchymosis after a 6-foot fall. He is unable to bear weight on his left foot. Radiographs are consistent with a left displaced intraarticular joint depression calcaneus fracture.

- **Most likely diagnosis:** Displaced intraarticular joint depression calcaneus fracture.
- **Additional studies:** To further define the calcaneus fracture pattern and plan for definitive management, an axial computed tomography (CT) scan of the left calcaneus should be obtained. Coronal and sagittal plane reconstructions are frequently useful as well. Physical exam of the spine with further imaging is indicated, as there is a 10% incidence of associated spine injuries with calcaneus fractures. Although this patient complains of isolated foot pain, other regions such as the ipsilateral hip and knee should also be examined for pain, and if pain is present, appropriate radiographs of the affected area should be obtained.
- **Treatment options:** Nonoperative with immobilization in a nonweightbearing short leg splint or cast; open-reduction internal fixation.
- **Potential complications:** Wound complications/infection, calcaneal malunion, peroneal tendon irritation, anterior ankle impingement, subtalar arthritis, calcaneocuboid arthritis.

ANALYSIS

Objectives

1. Identify the calcaneus fracture pattern using AP, lateral, and Harris radiographs.
2. Define and measure the Bohler angle and the critical angle of Gissane.
3. Recognize the fracture pattern on CT scan and apply the Sanders classification.
4. Understand the indications for open-reduction internal fixation.
5. Identify common complications of either nonoperative or operative treatment.

Considerations

On initial presentation of a fractured calcaneus, the patient's chief complaint will be pain about the hindfoot and an inability to bear weight on the affected limb. Observation of the skin and soft tissues may reveal soft tissue swelling, ecchymosis, and fracture blisters. The limb must be fully uncovered and circumferentially examined. A detailed motor and sensory examination should be performed. Because of the violent nature of the axial heel loading, there often exist fine disturbances to the plantar sensory nerves, which should be fully documented. A pulse exam must similarly be documented. Any lacerations, typically medially, reflect an open calcaneal fracture unless proven otherwise. Open fractures, especially those associated with contamination, should undergo emergent debridement and irrigation in the operative theatre.

Extensive soft tissue swelling may also predispose the patient to compartment syndrome of the foot. **There are 9 compartments within the foot, which are individually defined by an inflexible investing fascia.** As muscle swelling increases, the closed spaces within the foot do not permit an increase in volume, and the individual compartment becomes pressurized. This pressure head exceeds the venous outflow pressure, which results in ischemia to the nervous and muscular components in a time-dependent manner. The most common signs are increasing pain requirements and pain on passive stretch, specifically great toe abduction and adduction. Diagnosis requires a coherent patient, not under the influence of excessive sedating medications. If the patient is unable to interact appropriately, pressure measurements may be objectively obtained through needle manometry. If compartment syndrome is present, the compartments must be emergently released via surgical fasciotomies.

In addition to the calcaneus fracture, the patient may present with additional injuries. A thorough history and physical exam should be performed, with additional imaging obtained as indicated. **Approximately 10% of patients with calcaneus fractures have associated spine injuries, and upward of 26% of patients have other extremity injuries.** Missed injuries can be avoided by a careful clinical and radiographic evaluation of the coherent patient at the time of injury.

APPROACH TO:

Calcaneus Fracture

DEFINITIONS

INTRAARTICULAR: With respect to the calcaneus, a fracture that extends into the subtalar joint. More specifically, a fracture that exists within the posterior facet of the talocalcaneal articulation.

EXTRAARTICULAR: The fracture does not extend into the subtalar joint, particularly the posterior facet of the talocalcaneal articulation.

BOHLER ANGLE: An angle created from the intersection of 2 radiographic lines observed on a lateral calcaneus x-ray. The first line connects the most cephalad point of the calcaneal anterior process with the most cephalad point of the calcaneal posterior facet. The second line connects the most cephalad point of the calcaneal posterior facet with the most cephalad point of the calcaneal tuberosity. An uninjured calcaneus typically demonstrates an angle between 20 and 40 degrees.

CRITICAL ANGLE OF GISSANE: Another angle created from the intersection of 2 radiographic lines observed on the lateral calcaneus x-ray. The first line runs tangential along the superior aspect of the anterior process. The second line runs tangential to the superior border of the posterior facet. A typical value for the uninjured calcaneus measures between 95 and 105 degrees.

CLINICAL APPROACH

Etiology

Fractures of the calcaneus typically result from high-energy trauma such as falls from a height or motor vehicle collision and represent approximately 2% of all fractures.

DIAGNOSIS

Initial radiographic evaluation of a suspected calcaneus fracture should include an AP of the foot, lateral of the foot, and a Harris axial projection, along with AP, lateral, and mortise views of the ankle. These radiographs will help classify the fracture pattern, whether joint depression or tongue type. The diagnosis is most evident on the lateral projection, which will demonstrate the degree of calcaneal compression quantified by the **Bohler angle** (Figure 37–4). **The degree of height loss has prognostic implications, with a smaller Bohler angle correlating with poorer functional outcomes.** CT will help identify each fracture line and fracture fragment. Reformats in the coronal and sagittal planes parallel the findings in the Harris axial and lateral views, respectively. Additional information can be obtained from the CT, including an evaluation of lateral wall expulsion and peroneal tendon impingement or dislocation.

From the CT scan, the fracture can be classified according to **Sanders.** The posterior facet is divided into 3 fragments: lateral, central, and medial. With the addition of the sustentaculum, there are 4 defined fragments. The primary fracture line is identified and the number of fragments created by the fracture line is noted. A letter is assigned to where the fracture line crosses the posterior facet. The number and location of posterior facet fracture lines have been demonstrated to correlate with outcomes after surgical fixation, with poorer outcome measures associated with more comminuted patterns. The collective information obtained by careful evaluation of the radiographs and CT scan aid in definitive management and preoperative planning.

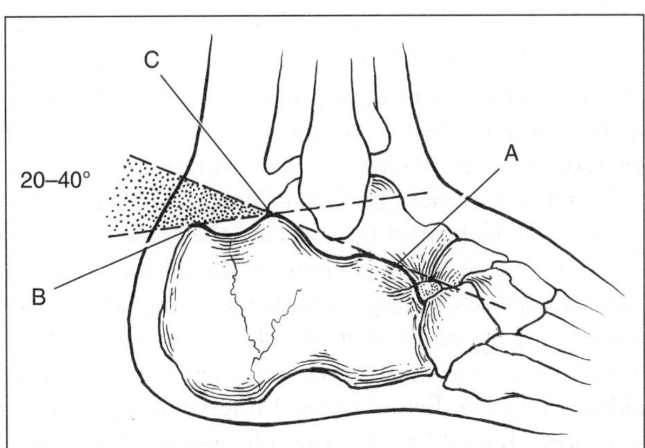

Figure 37–4. Calcaneus fracture: Bohler angle. The Bohler angle is formed by the intersection of lines drawn tangentially to the **(A)** anterior and **(B)** posterior elements of the **(C)** superior surface of the calcaneus. A normal angle is approximately 20 to 40 degrees. (Reproduced, with permission, from Knoop KJ, Stack LB, Storrow AB, et al. *Atlas of Emergency Medicine.* 3rd ed. New York, NY: McGraw-Hill; 2009:Fig. 11-83.)

TREATMENT

Nonoperative

Nonoperative treatment consists of early ankle and subtalar range-of-motion exercises and **nonweightbearing for approximately 3 months.** Initial management consists of splinting the foot and ankle in neutral dorsiflexion to prevent an equinus contracture, ice, elevation, and pain control. Once the swelling subsides, the splint is removed while ankle and subtalar range-of-motion exercises are performed. Clinical and radiographic follow-up is carried out at routine intervals to document healing. Specific indications for nonoperative treatment include a nondisplaced fracture, a patient too physiologically compromised to tolerate surgery, or a nonambulatory patient. In addition, patients unable or unwilling to comply with postoperative weightbearing restrictions are best managed nonoperatively. Factors that affect local wound healing, such as a history of smoking, severe peripheral vascular disease, or insulin-dependent diabetes, are relative contraindications to surgery.

Open-Reduction Internal Fixation

Historically, fractures of the calcaneus were treated nonoperatively by means of re-impacting the fracture by striking the lateral heel with a hammer. Surgeons would rather perform this procedure over open surgery because of fears over infection, malunion, nonunion, and need for amputation. With the development of aseptic techniques and the modern principles of reduction and fixation, calcaneal surgery could be performed with an improved complication profile. A prospective, randomized, controlled multicenter trial by **Buckley et al** warrants mention. In this study, 309 patients were prospectively randomized to either nonoperative or operative treatment and followed for a minimum of 2 years. Operative treatment demonstrated improved outcomes in women, patients not receiving worker's compensation, young men (<30 years of age), patients with a higher Bohler angle, patients with a lighter workload, and patients with a simple displaced intraarticular fracture pattern. Anatomic reductions also improved outcomes. Patients treated nonoperatively were more likely to require late arthrodesis. As our understanding of the outcomes of nonoperative and operative treatment improves, we can identify those patients best managed by open-reduction internal fixation.

Once the decision has been made to proceed with open-reduction internal fixation, timing and surgical treatment goals must be discussed. Timing of surgery is an important consideration. Calcaneal fractures are the result of high-energy trauma, and the associated soft tissue injury is often extensive. Incisions across a compromised soft tissue envelope risk postoperative wound complications and deep sepsis. Serous and hemorrhagic fracture blisters should be unroofed and treated with dry bandages until epithelialization occurs. Despite signs of healing, the blister beds should be avoided if possible. Before surgical intervention, the foot must achieve soft tissue quiescence. This readiness of the soft tissues is indicated by the appearance of fine skin wrinkles with passive foot dorsiflexion, known as a positive **"wrinkle test."** A waiting period of 10 to 14 days is common before proceeding to surgery. Although waiting for an appropriate surgical window is critical, treatment within the first 3 weeks is recommended to avoid a malunion. This is a situation in which the fracture heals in an undesirable position. The malunited calcaneus is frequently shortened and in varus.

The goal of surgical intervention is to anatomically restore the calcaneus. Critical components in this restoration include anatomic reduction of the posterior facet and reconstitution of calcaneal height, width, and length. Medial and lateral approaches to fixation have been described. An **extensile lateral approach** is most often used. The vertical limb of the incision is made anterior to the lateral border of the Achilles tendon and continued in a right angle fashion horizontally along the border of the foot where the glabrous and plantar skin meet. This approach allows for direct reduction of the anterior process, the posterior facet, and the tuberosity. Kirschner wires can be used to temporarily hold the reduction, which should be checked fluoroscopically and under direct visualization. Calcaneal height is checked on the lateral view. Width and varus heel positioning is imaged on the axial view. The reduction of the posterior facet is directly visualized and can be imaged through the use of the Broden view. Once the reduction is satisfactory, the Kirschner wires are replaced with screws or a combination of screws and plates for the final construct. Careful handling of the flap is crucial during wound closure to minimize the risk of skin necrosis and wound complications. A Hemovac drain is typically left in place and a splint applied in neutral dorsiflexion to prevent an equinus contracture. Postoperative radiographs and CT are performed to check the accuracy of the reduction. The patient is made nonweightbearing for approximately 3 months, at the discretion of the treating surgeon. During the healing period, range-of-motion exercises for the ankle and subtalar joint can be initiated as soon as the incision appears stable and healing. Postoperative follow-up is at routine intervals to document fracture healing. Good to excellent results can be achieved with an anatomic articular reduction.

Complications

Subtalar Arthritis: Posttraumatic arthritis of the subtalar joint can develop after both nonoperative and operative treatment. A nonanatomic articular reduction and cartilage damage from the injury itself are the primary contributing factors. Patients will primarily complain of pain. The pain is dependent on activity and worsens as the day progresses. As a result of subtalar stiffness, patients will complain that it is **difficult to navigate over uneven walking surfaces.** Radiographic evaluation with standard x-rays and CT may reveal joint space narrowing, osteophyte formation, and subchondral sclerosis. Injecting a local anesthetic into the subtalar joint and documenting relief of symptoms can confirm the diagnosis. Nonoperative measures include nonsteroidal anti-inflammatory medications, shoe wear modifications, or custom orthoses. These measures should be tried before operative intervention is considered. If nonoperative measures fail, operative treatment consists of a **subtalar fusion.**

Wound Complications/Infection: The most common complication after open-reduction internal fixation is related to the surgical wound. Wound complications including **dehiscence** and **infection** have been noted to occur in up to 20% of patients with closed fractures. The reported rates of deep infections and calcaneal osteomyelitis range from 0% to 20% in closed fractures and from 19% to 31% in open fractures. Cellulitis and superficial wound sloughs can be treated with dressing changes and the administration of antibiotics. Persistent drainage or purulence necessitates open debridement coupled with administration of antibiotics. In the case of superficial infection, the hardware can be retained. If a deep infection is noted or there is evidence of diffuse osteomyelitis at the time of open debridement, the hardware must be removed. Patient selection, meticulous surgical technique, and compliance with postoperative protocols can minimize the risks of wound complications.

Calcaneocuboid Arthritis: Arthritis can develop after both nonoperative and operative treatment secondary to an imperfect reduction of the anterolateral fragment. Similar to the diagnosis of subtalar arthritis detailed previously, physical exam, radiographs, and a trial injection can be performed to elucidate whether the calcaneocuboid joint is the source of the patient's pain. First-line treatment is nonoperative with nonsteroidal anti-inflammatory medications, shoe wear modifications, or custom orthoses. If nonoperative treatment fails, calcaneocuboid fusion may be considered and is typically performed in conjunction with a talonavicular and talocalcaneal fusion.

Peroneal Irritation: This occurs more commonly in patients managed nonoperatively. During the axial loading event, the lateral wall often becomes a separate fragment, which translates laterally. Both the peroneus longus and brevis tendons traverse the lateral calcaneus in this region and are subjected to compression and irritation. Dislocations or subluxations are common. Operative treatment addresses both the lateral wall displacement and the peroneal tendon instability. In operative cases, postoperative scarring or prominent hardware is more frequently the culprit. The initial treatment is nonoperative with nonsteroidal anti-inflammatory medications and shoe wear modifications or orthotics. Elective surgery includes removal of hardware, lateral wall reconstruction, or exostectomy, along with a peroneal tendon reconstruction. These procedures should be considered if the patient is experiencing pain refractory to nonoperative measures.

Anterior Ankle Impingement: Anterior ankle impingement can occur after nonoperative or operative treatment. The impingement is the result of loss of calcaneal height and a decreased lateral talocalcaneal angle. With nonoperative management or incomplete restoration of calcaneal height, the talus adopts a pathologic horizontal position. The result is direct contact with the dorsal talar neck and the anterior tibial plafond. On clinical evaluation, the patients present with pain and **restriction in ankle dorsiflexion.** Often the examiner can feel a firm block when the ankle is passively dorsiflexed. Surgical management can include exostectomy of the talar osteophytes, but **distraction subtalar bone block fusion is the preferred procedure.** The goal of this procedure is to restore the calcaneal height and thus create an improved lateral talocalcaneal angle.

Calcaneal Malunion: Malunion can occur in both nonoperative and operative management of calcaneal fractures. **Varus angulation of the hindfoot is the most common residual deformity.** This usually occurs from a varus malunion of the tuberosity. Treatment with subtalar fusion and a calcaneal osteotomy has been described, with variations, by several authors. To plan the malunion repair, Stephens and Sanders developed a CT classification for malunions. Type I involves a large lateral exostosis with or without arthrosis of the subtalar joint and is treated with peroneal tenolysis and a lateral exostectomy. Type II involves a lateral exostosis with arthrosis across the subtalar joint and is treated with peroneal tenolysis, a lateral exostectomy, and in situ subtalar fusion. Type III involves a lateral exostosis, severe subtalar arthrosis, and varus or valgus angulation of the calcaneal body and is treated with peroneal tenolysis, a lateral exostectomy, subtalar fusion, and a calcaneal osteotomy.

COMPREHENSION QUESTIONS

37.1 A 29-year-old man presents with significant right hindfoot swelling and pain after a 25-foot jump from a cliff. Imaging confirms a comminuted intraarticular calcaneus fracture involving the posterior facet. As the treating physician, you request that radiographs of the spine be obtained. What percentage of patients with fractures of the calcaneus have associated spine injuries?

A. 10%

B. 30%

C. 50%

D. 80%

37.2 Which of the following factors is associated with worse outcomes after operative treatment of fractures of the calcaneus?

A. Female sex

B. Age < 30 years

C. Worker's compensation

D. Bohler angle > 0 degrees

E. Simple articular fracture pattern

37.3 A 42-year-old man presents with a displaced comminuted intraarticular calcaneus fracture. On physical exam, there is extensive soft tissue swelling and hemorrhagic blisters. The patient is splinted and discharged home, as the soft tissues are not ready for open-reduction internal fixation. He returns to clinic 10 days later with clawing of his toes. What is the most likely explanation for this finding?

A. Tendon laceration from displaced fracture fragment

B. Nerve injury from displaced fracture fragment

C. Compartment syndrome

D. Weakness secondary to pain and prolonged immobilization

ANSWERS

37.1 **A.** Approximately 10% of patients who present with calcaneus fractures have associated spine injuries. A thorough history and physical exam, with additional imaging as indicated, is important to avoid missed injuries.

37.2 **C.** A prospective, randomized, controlled multicenter trial by Buckley et al followed 309 patients for a period of 2 to 8 years. Overall the outcomes for nonoperative and operative management were not found to be different. After closer examination of the patient population, operative treatment demonstrated improved outcomes in women, patients not receiving worker's compensation, young men (<30 years), patients with a higher Bohler angle, patients with a lighter workload, and patients with a simple displaced intraarticular fracture pattern. Anatomic reductions also improved outcomes. Patients treated nonoperatively were more likely to require late arthrodesis.

37.3 **C.** Foot compartment syndrome is a known complication of calcaneus fractures. There are 9 compartments within the foot, which are individually defined by an inflexible investing fascia. As muscle swelling increases, the closed spaces within the foot do not permit an increase in volume, and the individual compartment becomes pressurized. This pressure head exceeds the venous outflow pressure, which results in ischemia to the nervous and muscular components in a time-dependent manner. If this is unrecognized, nerve and muscle death occur. This can result in contractures of the muscles in the affected compartments, which is evident on clinical evaluation.

CLINICAL PEARLS

- Fractures of the calcaneus represent high-energy trauma with a significant incidence of associated spine and extremity injuries. A thorough history and physical exam are crucial at the time of presentation.
- AP, lateral, and Harris radiographs should be ordered along with a CT scan in the axial plane with sagittal and coronal reconstructions to evaluate the fracture pattern and plan for treatment.
- Open-reduction internal fixation should be delayed until soft tissue swelling is reduced and blisters have epithelialized.
- Wound complications including dehiscence and infection are the most common problems associated with operative management.
- Outcomes after operative treatment are best in women, non–worker's compensation cases, young (age <30 years) men, higher Bohler angle (>0 degrees), patients with a lighter workload, and those with simple articular fracture patterns.

REFERENCES

Benirschke SK, Kramer PA. Wound healing complications in closed and open calcaneal fractures. *J Orthop Trauma*. 2004;18:1-6.

Buckley R, Tough S, McCormack R, Pate G, Leighton R, Petrie D, Galpin R. Operative compared with nonoperative treatment of displaced intra-articular calcaneal fractures: a prospective, randomized, controlled multicenter trial. *J Bone Joint Surg Am*. 2002;84-A:1733-1744.

Howard JL, Buckley R, McCormack R, Pate G, Leighton R, Petrie D, Galpin R. Complications following management of displaced intra-articular calcaneal fractures: a prospective randomized trial comparing open reduction internal fixation with nonoperative management. *J Orthop Trauma*. 2003;17:241-249.

Sanders R. Current concepts review: displaced intra-articular fractures of the calcaneus. *J Bone Joint Surg Am*. 2000;82-A:225-250.

Sanders R, Fortin P, DiPasquale T, Walling A. Operative treatment in 120 displaced intraarticular calcaneal fractures. Results using a prognostic computed tomography scan classification. *Clin Orthop*. 1993;290:87-95.

Sanders R, Gregory P. Operative treatment of intra-articular fractures of the calcaneus. *Orthop Clin North Am*. 1995;26:203-214.

CASE 38

A 19-year-old woman presents to the office complaining of dull right thigh pain for the past 2 months. She denies any trauma or inciting events over that time. The pain was initially present only while walking and after other physical activities but has progressed and is present at rest. It now disrupts her sleep at night. She is otherwise healthy and denies any fevers, chills, weight loss, or night sweats. On physical exam, her right lower extremity is neurovascularly intact. Her knee has full range of motion, and there is no warmth or erythema. However, you do note mild swelling of her distal thigh and on palpation appreciate a mass in that region. An anteroposterior (AP) radiograph of the distal femur is shown in Figure 38–1.

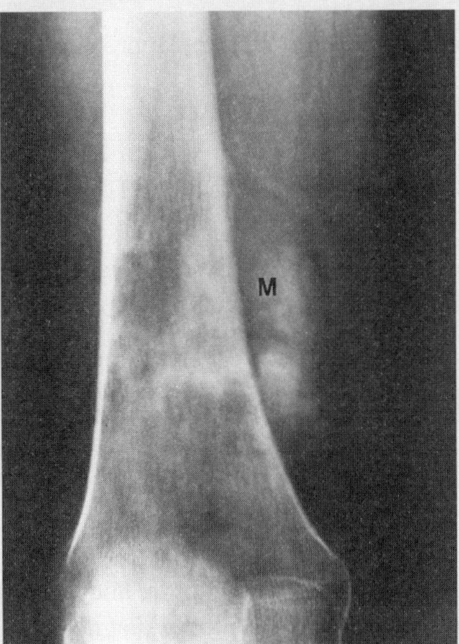

Figure 38–1. AP view of the distal femur. Many of the radiographic features of this osteosarcoma mark it as a malignant tumor. The abnormal area of mottled lucent and sclerotic tumor in the metaphysis fades gradually into the shadows of surrounding normal bone. It is difficult to see where the tumor begins and ends; there is a large soft-tissue mass adjacent to the bone (M). The periosteum has been unable to maintain a shell of mineralized new bone around this mass. The sclerotic areas within the bone and the mineralized portions of the soft-tissue mass both have a relatively amorphous, smudged appearance that is seen with calcified osteoid matrix. (Reproduced, with permission, from Chen MYM, Pope TL, Ott DJ. *Basic Radiology.* 2nd ed. New York, NY: McGraw-Hill; 2011:Fig. 6-24.)

- What is the most likely diagnosis?
- What are the next steps in the workup?
- What is the treatment approach?

ANSWERS TO CASE 38: Osteosarcoma

Summary: This is a 19-year-old otherwise healthy woman who presents with a 2-month history of dull right thigh pain that was initially activity dependent but has progressed and is now most severe at rest, especially at night. She denies any fevers, chills, night sweats, or recent weight loss. A mass in her distal thigh is palpated on examination. An AP plain radiograph illustrates a soft-tissue mass adjacent to a mottled lucent and sclerotic lesion in the metaphysis of her right femur.

- **Most likely diagnosis:** Pathologic bone tumor, specifically osteosarcoma.
- **Next steps in workup:** Magnetic resonance imaging (MRI) of the right lower extremity, tissue biopsy, computed tomography (CT) scan of the chest, and a bone scan.
- **Treatment approach:** Multidisciplinary approach ultimately dependent on tumor grade and type of osteosarcoma.

ANALYSIS

Objectives

1. Understand the important history, physical exam, and radiographic findings consistent with a diagnosis of osteosarcoma.
2. Know the essential components of the workup for a musculoskeletal lesion, specifically an osteosarcoma.
3. Appreciate the need for a multidisciplinary approach to treatment and how the Musculoskeletal Tumor Society Staging System (MSTS, Enneking) influences it.

Considerations

There are many important clinical, radiographic, and pathologic findings that will aid the orthopaedist in establishing the proper diagnosis in the setting of a likely musculoskeletal tumor, as in this case. Diagnosis begins with the history and physical exam. Concerning findings in this patient include her progression of pain symptoms, to the point where it awakens her from sleep, and the presence of a palpable mass. Age is another important consideration, especially for establishing an appropriate differential diagnosis. Furthermore, some tumors have a sex predilection; osteosarcoma is more common in males. Laboratory tests are not typically diagnostic for bone tumors, but may be helpful once a diagnosis is made. Imaging must begin with at least 2 plain radiographic views of the lesion. An MRI is typically obtained after and has become the imaging modality of choice for most musculoskeletal tumors. Nuclear imaging and CT are also performed for evaluation of metastases, staging, and surveillance. Biopsy of the lesion allows for histologic analysis, which determines tumor grade and significantly impacts treatment options and ultimate prognosis. After this workup, a multidisciplinary treatment plan can be developed in conjunction with both the oncologist and orthopaedic surgeon.

APPROACH TO:
Osteosarcoma

DEFINITIONS

CODMAN TRIANGLE: A radiographic finding of new subperiosteal bone created when a lesion elevates the periosteum away from bone. Although it can appear triangular, it is often a pseudotriangle on plain radiographs with a 2-sided appearance owing to tumor growing at a faster rate than the periosteum can expand.

MSTS (ENNEKING) STAGING SYSTEM: Most recognized staging system for malignant bone tumors. It is based on tumor grade (low, high), extent (intracompartmental, extracompartmental), and the presence or absence of metastases. In general, low-grade, localized tumors are stage I; high-grade, localized tumors are stage II; and metastatic tumors (regardless of grade) are stage III. Each stage is further categorized into type a and b subsets, representative of intra- versus extracompartmental disease, respectively.

LIMB-SALVAGE SURGERY: A constellation of surgical procedures designed to achieve removal of a malignant tumor and reconstruction of a limb with an acceptable oncologic, functional, and cosmetic result.

CLINICAL APPROACH

Osteosarcoma is the most common bone sarcoma, affecting approximately 560 children and adolescents annually in the United States. Its incidence peaks in the second decade of life and is most commonly seen at sites of rapid bone turnover, such as the distal femur, proximal tibia, proximal humerus, and proximal femur. Although most cases of osteosarcoma are sporadic, those that carry the **retinoblastoma tumor suppressor gene (*RB1*)** or who have **Li-Fraumeni syndrome (*p53* gene)** are predisposed.

There are multiple subtypes of osteosarcoma, including low-grade, high-grade, and telangiectatic intramedullary variants, as well as parosteal, periosteal, and high-grade surface types. This discussion pertains to the classic, most common subtype, which accounts for approximately 80% of all osteosarcomas, the high-grade intramedullary osteosarcoma.

The history and physical exam are crucial in the initial diagnosis of osteosarcoma. A common presenting complaint is new-onset pain over several months duration; it may occur at rest, disrupt sleep, or only occur after physical activity. This complaint must be investigated with due diligence by the clinician. Pain associated with weightbearing or activity is typically due to an inflammatory process. However, pain at rest or at night is biologic pain possibly secondary to the growth of a lesion in bone. A patient with an osteosarcoma may also present with a palpable mass in the extremity that is painful. Symptoms such as fevers, chills, weight loss, and fatigue are late signs of disease.

After a physical exam, plain radiographs of the region in question must be obtained. An osteosarcoma classically arises from the metaphyseal region of a bone and appears as a **mixed sclerotic and lytic lesion** that can infiltrate bone and

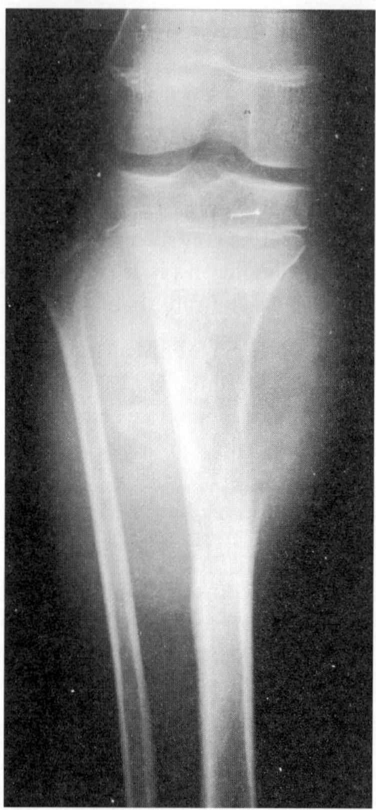

Figure 38–2. Osteosarcoma with Codman triangle, a new area of subperiosteal bone formed when a tumor raises the periosteum away from the bone. (Reproduced, with permission, from Doherty GM. *Current Diagnosis & Treatment: Surgery.* 13th ed. New York, NY: McGraw-Hill; 2010:Fig. 40-38.)

surrounding cortex, causing a periosteal reaction and soft tissue mass. A **Codman triangle** may be seen on radiographs (Figure 38–2). Plain radiographs concerning for a malignant bone lesion require advanced imaging, such as an MRI, to evaluate for surrounding soft tissue, neurovascular, and bone marrow involvement, as well as skip lesions, which represent discontinuous metastases.

A biopsy of the lesion is required when the imaging, examination, and history are consistent with a pathologic process; it is the only definitive means of determining whether a tumor is benign or malignant. An orthopaedic oncologist must perform the biopsy, which, if improperly obtained, can compromise the ability to perform limb salvage procedures. Definitive osteosarcoma resection must include the biopsy tract, as it too can be contaminated with tumor cells. In the setting of osteosarcoma, histologic analysis often shows **diffuse cellular atypia with nuclear pleomorphism and "lacey" osteoid matrix production.**

Laboratory testing is not diagnostic for osteosarcoma, but does play a role in its workup and management. Before initiation of chemotherapy, laboratory values (ie, complete blood count with differential, basic metabolic profile, renal and liver function values) must be obtained to provide a baseline assessment of organ function.

Additionally, elevated alkaline phosphatase (up to 2-3 times the normal value) and lactate dehydrogenase levels are considered poor prognostic factors.

Chest CT and bone scan evaluate for metastatic disease, which is the most important prognostic and staging factor in osteosarcoma. In approximately 10% of patients, pulmonary or lymph node metastases are detected at presentation. It is not uncommon for osteosarcoma to have early hematogenous metastases. Micrometastases, which are undetectable with conventional imaging, are likely present in the lungs in most patients on initial presentation and without appropriate treatment will become evident on imaging within 1 to 2 years. A bone scan will be "hot" in osteosarcoma, specifically in areas of tumor. Those areas of the body showing increased metabolic activity must be further evaluated with imaging.

The majority of patients with osteosarcoma present as having Enneking stage IIB disease at diagnosis. For most types, treatment is multimodal. Two to three cycles of neoadjuvant chemotherapy are commonly given before wide-margin surgical resection is performed, which involves achieving the largest possible margin without unnecessary functional sacrifice. **Fortunately, approximately 90% of patients with osteosarcoma are able to undergo limb salvage procedures and do not require amputation.** The excised segment of bone may be replaced with a prosthesis and/or allograft. Postoperative chemotherapy is also typically used. Radiation is not used in the treatment of osteosarcoma.

The overall 5-year survival rates of patients with osteosarcoma are 60% to 80%. With the initiation of neoadjuvant chemotherapy protocols, 5-year survival rates are almost 80% in patients with nonmetastatic disease and 10% to 20% in patients with metastatic disease. **In addition to elevated alkaline phosphatase and lactate dehydrogenase, poor prognostic factors include metastatic disease at diagnosis, a poor response to chemotherapy (defined as <90% necrosis of resected tumor), and pathologic fracture.**

COMPREHENSION QUESTIONS

38.1 Which of the following most accurately lists the most common location of osteosarcoma in increasing frequency?

A. Proximal tibia < axial skeleton < proximal humerus < proximal femur

B. Axial skeleton < proximal humerus < proximal femur < proximal tibia

C. Axial skeleton < proximal humerus < proximal tibia < proximal femur

D. Proximal humerus < axial skeleton < proximal tibia < proximal femur

38.2 In addition to metastases, which of the following is also a poor prognostic indicator in the setting of osteosarcoma?

A. High alkaline phosphatase

B. Pain

C. Low lactate dehydrogenase

D. A and B

38.3 A 14-year-old male presents with an 8-month history of increasing right knee pain and swelling. He is otherwise healthy, but is a known carrier of the retinoblastoma gene. A mass is found on the posterior aspect of his knee, and a biopsy is taken. If found to be an osteosarcoma, what would histologic analysis of the specimen likely show?

A. Densely packed uniform small blue-stained cells in sheets

B. Numerous multinucleated giant cells

C. Diffuse cellular atypia with nuclear pleomorphism and "lacey" osteoid matrix production

D. Cystic spaces filled with blood

ANSWERS

38.1 **C.** The distal femur is the most common location of osteosarcoma. This is followed by the proximal tibia, proximal humerus, and then the axial skeleton (ie, spine and sacrum).

38.2 **A.** Poor prognostic factors include elevated alkaline phosphatase and lactate dehydrogenase, metastatic disease at diagnosis, a poor response to chemotherapy (defined as $<90\%$ necrosis of resected tumor), and pathologic fracture.

38.3 **C.** Histologic analysis of osteosarcoma often reveals diffuse cellular atypia with nuclear pleomorphism and "lacey" osteoid matrix production. Other malignant characteristics include stromal cells with atypia, a high nuclear to cytoplasmic ratio, and abnormal mitotic figures. A describes a Ewing sarcoma, B a giant cell tumor, and D an aneurysmal bone cyst.

CLINICAL PEARLS

- The history and physical exam are crucial in the initial diagnosis of osteosarcoma.
- MRI is effective at evaluating an osteosarcoma because it can clearly identify surrounding soft tissue, neurovascular and bone marrow involvement, and skip lesions, which represent discontinuous metastases.
- Chest CT and bone scan are used to evaluate for metastatic disease.
- The majority of patients with osteosarcoma present with **Enneking** stage IIB disease at diagnosis.
- Treatment commonly involves neoadjuvant chemotherapy, limb-salvage surgery, and postoperative chemotherapy.
- The overall 5-year survival rates of patients with osteosarcoma are 60% to 80%.

REFERENCES

Leet, Arabella I. Chapter 64: Pediatric tumors and hematologic diseases. In: Aiona MD. *OKU 10: Orthopaedic Knowledge Update*. Rosemont, IL: American Academy of Orthopaedic Surgeons; 2011:827.

Messerschmitt PJ, Garcia RM, Abdul-Karim FW, Greenfield EM, Getty PJ. Osteosarcoma. *J Am Acad Orthop Surg*. 2009;17:515-527.

CASE 39

A 73-year-old man is seen in the outpatient clinic with complaints of right knee pain, 6 months in duration. He denies recent trauma and is otherwise without significant medical problems. He states that over the past several years, he has had a progressive "dull ache" in his knee. The near constant pain wakes him at least 3 times per week. Last month, he started using a golf cart instead of walking between holes and now borrows a friend's cane when walking long distances. He states that his right leg feels "unstable." He denies fevers, weight loss, and recent illnesses, and he takes only acetaminophen as needed for pain relief. Family history is unremarkable. On physical exam of his right knee, there is no obvious effusion, erythema, or drainage. He has joint line tenderness, most prominent on the lateral aspect of his knee, and he exhibits a slight genu valgum. There is crepitus with range of motion. A 5-degree flexion contracture is noted when he is fully extended, and he can only flex the knee to 100 degrees. He is neurovascularly and ligamentously intact. He has brought an x-ray of his right knee, taken last month at his primary care doctor's office (Figure 39–1).

- What is the most likely diagnosis?
- What are the next steps in the workup for this condition?
- What are the next steps in the management of this condition?

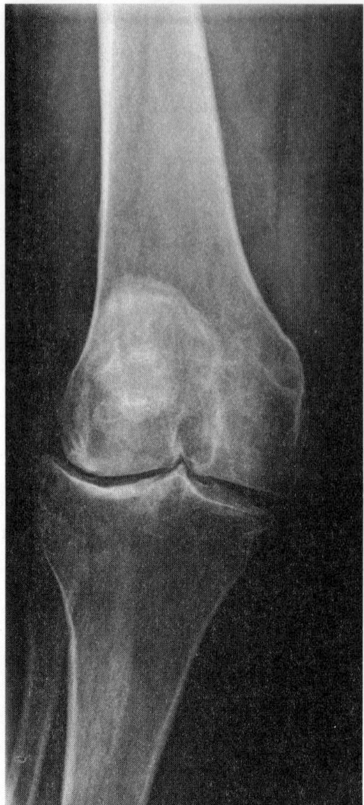

Figure 39–1. AP radiograph of the right knee.

ANSWERS TO CASE 39:

Total Knee Arthroplasty

Summary: A relatively healthy 73-year-old man presents with progressive right knee pain. His pain is severe enough that it has caused him to change his daily activities, has caused him to start using a cane, and wakes him at night. Exam reveals crepitus, lateral joint line tenderness, and a limited range of motion. He denies a history of traumatic injury and exhibits neither signs nor symptoms of infection.

- **Most likely diagnosis:** Osteoarthritis (degenerative joint disease) of the right knee.
- **Next diagnostic test:** Obtain plain radiographs of bilateral knees, including weightbearing posteroanterior and lateral views in approximately 45 degrees of flexion, a tunnel or notch view, and Merchant (sunrise) views of the patellofemoral joint.

- **Next step in therapy:** Conservative therapy including nonsteroidal anti-inflammatory drugs (NSAIDs; ibuprofen, naproxen, diclofenac, or selective COX-2 inhibitors); physical therapy is sometimes recommended to help strengthen the muscles around the knee, including the hamstrings, gastrocsoleus complex, and quadriceps. Assistive devices such as canes, crutches, and walkers can be used as well to offset some of the joint reactive forces stressing the knee.

ANALYSIS

Objectives

1. Recognize the presentation of DJD of the knee and understand the salient aspects of patient history necessary to guide treatment.
2. Develop a standard treatment algorithm for DJD of the knee.
3. Understand the surgical options available for the treatment of knee arthritis.
4. Understand common potential complications after total knee arthroplasty.

Considerations

There are several differential diagnoses that must be considered in any patient with nonacute traumatic joint pain. Common etiologies include osteoarthritis, also referred to as degenerative joint disease (DJD), inflammatory arthritis, osteonecrosis, and posttraumatic arthritis. Given this patient's atraumatic history and his lack of fevers, joint erythema, or other systemic inflammatory symptomatology, osteoarthritis is the most likely diagnosis. Specifics for workup of these alternate diagnoses are considered later in this chapter. This 73-year-old male presents with signs, symptoms, and radiographic findings consistent with right knee osteoarthritis, specifically the lateral compartment. In a patient who has had no previous intervention to address his symptoms, **the first priority is pain relief.** There are many options for pain relief, including acetaminophen, NSAIDs, corticosteroid injections, and narcotics. Ideally, narcotics are reserved for short-term relief in individuals with intractable pain, refractory to all other modalities. Following analgesia recommendations, attempts should be made to address pathologic changes in the mechanics of knee. The available treatment options are bracing, physical therapy, and assistive devices for ambulation. Other conservative modalities include intraarticular viscosupplementation with hyaluronic acid analogues or derivatives (Synvisc®) and corticosteroid injections.

APPROACH TO:
Osteoarthritis of the Knee

DEFINITIONS

ARTHROPLASTY: The surgical replacement and reconstruction of a functional joint.

OSTEONECROSIS: The death of bone tissue secondary to impaired or disrupted blood supply, often as the result of trauma or disease. Osteonecrosis is marked by severe, localized pain and by structurally weakened bone that may flatten and collapse. This process is also known as aseptic or avascular necrosis (AVN).

POLYMETHYLMETHACRYLATE (PMMA): A synthetic polymer used commonly as cement for the implantation of knee and hip prostheses

CLINICAL APPROACH

Differential Diagnosis

As discussed, there are several causes of knee pain that must be considered before the diagnosis of osteoarthritis is made. Like DJD, **inflammatory arthropathies such as gout, chronic septic arthritis, and rheumatologic processes may present with insidious, atraumatic knee pain.** Several conditions in this wide spectrum of inflammatory diseases are discussed in greater depth elsewhere in this text. As a general rule, however, if there is suspicion for underlying infectious, rheumatologic, or crystalline process, further workup should be performed and includes obtaining blood and synovial fluid samples. Although the specific laboratory tests to be ordered are chosen on a case-by-case basis, general studies typically always obtained include a complete blood count (CBC), erythrocyte sedimentation rate (ESR), C-reactive protein (CRP), and synovial fluid gram stain, crystal analysis, cell count and aerobic and anaerobic cultures.

Avascular necrosis of the knee can also be a cause of this gentleman's pain. There are several etiologies of this condition. First, spontaneous osteonecrosis of the knee, an idiopathic condition that commonly affects women older than 55 years, is typically unilateral and affects only 1 condyle. The other causes include excessive alcohol use, sickle cell anemia, trauma, or corticosteroid use and usually affect patients younger than 45 years. Both conditions may present with slow-onset knee pain, sometimes worst at night, and typically affect the medial compartment. As with DJD, these conditions may respond to arthroplasty when conservative treatments fail.

Finally, **posttraumatic arthritis** is an accelerated degenerative process of the knee that results from previous damage to the knee's articular surfaces. It is managed in much the same way as DJD, with conservative measures first and arthroplasty for end-stage disease.

TREATMENT OF OSTEOARTHRITIS

Nonoperative (Conservative) Treatment

Despite the surgical focus of this text, it must be stressed that **the initial management of DJD is almost always nonoperative.** The conservative interventions described previously are usually successful in attenuating patients' DJD symptoms, at least in the short term. **How long, exactly, DJD can be managed nonoperatively varies greatly between individuals.** Several studies show significant short-term pain relief and functional improvement using corticosteroid injections and viscosupplementation, but results, again, are unpredictable.

It is important to recognize that none of these aforementioned treatments are a cure for DJD. Therefore, when discussing the natural history of osteoarthritis with patients, it is important to explain that it will progress as long as they partake in weightbearing activities. Because **the lifespan of a prosthetic joint is finite**—and most prone to wear in younger, active individuals—arthroplasty interventions are generally delayed until the patient can no longer tolerate conservative measures.

Operative Treatment

Once a patient has failed all conservative therapy, surgery may be indicated. There are several surgical options available and include total knee arthroplasty, osteotomies, arthroscopic interventions, and unicompartmental arthroplasty.

Arthroscopy and Osteotomies

Arthroscopic interventions are reserved for young patients with mild, localized disease in the setting of mechanical symptoms (ie, joint clicking, locking, or instability). Arthroscopic treatments are guided at debridement, chondroplasty, and removal of chondral loose bodies commonly found in osteoarthritic disease. Arthroscopy also plays a diagnostic role in determining the severity of arthritic disease, as some patients with advanced, debilitating arthritis may have deceptively benign-appearing x-rays.

Another surgical option that does not involve prostheses are osteotomies, or wedge-shaped bone cuts, that alter the alignment of the knee joint. When patients present with disproportionately worn compartments, the alignment of the knee can be altered to divert weightbearing pressures from the affected side. Ideal patients for this procedure are younger than 50 years, with isolated unicompartmental disease and a normal range of motion. They should also have competent ligaments, active flexion beyond 90 degrees, and minimal evidence of a flexion contracture. A varus or valgus osteotomy can be used to offload the lateral or medial compartments, respectively. In general, varus-producing osteotomies are performed on the femur, and valgus-producing osteotomies are performed on the tibia.

Arthroplasty

Before discussing total joint arthroplasty, it is worthy to mention the increasing popularity of unicompartmental knee arthroplasty (UKA). This procedure is restricted to patients with unicompartmental noninflammatory osteoarthritis, deformities of less than 10 degrees (varus or valgus), and an intact anterior cruciate ligament. Medial compartment replacement is by far the most commonly performed UKA, as the prevalence of medial-sided arthritis far exceeds that of isolated lateral disease.

In the correct patient population, advantages of UKA over total joint replacement include faster recovery, less rehabilitation, and smaller incisions.

The most commonly performed procedure for knee arthritis in the United States is total knee arthroplasty (TKA). Typically, patients are older than 50 years, have disease in all 3 compartments, and have experienced changes in their activity levels secondary to pain. TKA involves a resurfacing procedure of the distal femur and proximal tibia and typically the undersurface of the patella. **The goals are to reconstruct a stable knee with a functional range of motion, to restore knee alignment and smooth patella tracking, and to relieve pain.** There are a great variety of TKA prosthetic designs whose nuances extend beyond the scope of this discussion. Most modern TKA systems, however, share these same goals, and indeed there is no definitive evidence that supports the superiority of one modern TKA system over another.

Complications

The common complications that are associated with TKA include infection, deep vein thrombosis, aseptic loosening, osteolysis, periprosthetic fracture, failure of the extensor mechanism, and postoperative stiffness or arthrofibrosis.

Infections in an artificial joint, although rare (< 1%), are one of the most devastating complications of TKA. Periprosthetic joint infections (PJIs) can present in a multitude of ways. While some patients present with acute pain, swelling, and redness, others have a more insidious onset of symptoms. In general, any patient with a TKA and new-onset pain should be evaluated for infection, amongst other causes of pain. Diagnosis can be challenging and relies on physical exam findings, laboratory studies (ESR, CRP), and synovial fluid analysis. Although a positive gram stain and/or cultures make the diagnosis easy, many times these tests are negative. When this occurs, many believe that a synovial fluid white blood cell count of greater than 1100 cells/mL and a polymorphonuclear level of greater than 64% is consistent with a PJI, regardless of gram stain and culture findings. The management of PJI is challenging. In general, acute infections (defined as those of less than 3 weeks duration) are treated with a surgical irrigation and debridement and polyethylene exchange. Unfortunately, a PJI of greater than 3 weeks duration requires a complete explantation of the total knee system, placement of an antibiotic-eluting spacer where the total knee was, and 4 to 6 weeks of intravenous antibiotics. After this, a replantation of the total knee may be performed.

Finally, patients undergoing total joint replacements are notoriously at risk for deep vein thrombosis (DVT). DVTs occur in up to 5% to 15% of patients undergoing arthroplasty and are considered the most common complication of TKA. Most surgeons and hospitals go to considerable lengths to reduce DVT rates, including frequent mobilization postoperatively, placement of sequential compression stockings and compression stockings, and the use of anticoagulation medications such as postoperative heparin, low-molecular-weight heparin, warfarin, aspirin, and several other drugs. Unfortunately, despite significant efforts, the rates of DVT in arthroplasty patients remain relatively high.

COMPREHENSION QUESTIONS

39.1 A 55-year-old construction worker presents to your office with complaints of right knee pain, several years in duration. Examination of the right knee is notable for a slight flexion contraction, painful range of motion (ROM), and palpable crepitus during ROM. The left knee by comparison has a greater, albeit limited ROM that is not painful. Standing radiographs show significant medial and lateral compartmental joint space narrowing with sclerotic and osteophytic changes in bilateral knees. He has not yet been treated for his condition. What is the best next step in the management of this patient?

A. Right total knee arthroplasty

B. Right knee medial unicompartmental arthroplasty

C. Right knee lateral unicompartmental arthroplasty

D. NSAIDs and acetaminophen, recommend physical therapy

E. Bilateral knee total arthroplasties

39.2 A 52-year-old woman with a history of rheumatoid arthritis is referred to your clinic with right knee pain. For the past 3 years, her rheumatoid arthritis has been well controlled with a disease-modifying anti-rheumatic drug (DMARD) regimen; however, she continues to have persistent knee pain. On exam you note a comparatively varus right knee with a painful and limited ROM. She is ligamentously intact and is tender to palpation only on the anteromedial aspect of her knee. Radiographs show significant narrowing of the right knee medial compartment, with relative sparing of the patellofemoral and lateral compartments. There are sclerotic and cystic changes on the medial aspect of her knee only. Having failed nonoperative interventions, which of the following is the most appropriate surgical intervention for this patient?

A. Right total knee arthroplasty

B. Right knee lateral unicompartmental arthroplasty

C. Right knee medial unicompartmental arthroplasty

D. Right knee corrective osteotomy

39.3 A 73-year-old woman is on postoperative day 3 for a total knee replacement. The procedure was without complication, but as a result of postoperative pain, she has been slow to mobilize. You are called to evaluate the patient for increasing tachycardia (heart rate 115 beats/minute) and sudden-onset tachypnea (respiratory rate 30 breaths/min). Blood pressure and temperature are within normal limits. She has received a dose of intravenous morphine 30 minutes before your evaluation and currently states her pain is "only a 3/10." Electrocardiogram, cardiac enzymes, and chest x-ray are obtained and demonstrate no acute changes or abnormalities. She is a smoker and has a history of breast cancer. Which of the following is the most likely diagnosis?

A. Acute myocardial infarction

B. Pneumonia

C. Pulmonary embolism

D. Fat embolism

E. Blood loss anemia with secondary hypovolemia

ANSWERS

39.1 **D.** Nonoperative measures are almost always trialed before arthroplasty is performed for patients with DJD. Although this patient has radiographic degenerative changes, he is asymptomatic on the left, and thus bilateral TKA would be contraindicated. The presence of bilateral compartment disease is a contraindication to unicompartmental arthroplasty should the patient fail conservative treatment.

39.2 **A.** Although this patient's arthritis is confined to the medial space, the presence of rheumatoid arthritis is a contraindication to unicompartmental replacement. Corrective osteotomies may correct the patient's varus alignment but do nothing to address the underlying joint pathology.

39.3 **C.** Pulmonary emboli (PE) are an unfortunate and not too uncommon complication of knee or hip arthroplasty. Most occur second to embolized DVTs, which result from immobilizations, surgical trauma, insufficient postoperative thrombus prophylaxis, and underlying risk factors, such as this patient's history of tobacco use and malignancy. The next step should be a CT angiogram of the chest (the diagnostic gold standard) or a ventilation perfusion scan. Although pneumonia and acute myocardial infarction may account for her symptoms, they are less likely given the normal chest x-ray and cardiac enzymes/electrocardiogram changes, respectively. Blood loss anemia with subsequent hypovolemic shock is also common; however, it is less likely given her normal blood pressure. Fat embolism may occur in the setting of joint replacement procedures, but more often occurs intraoperatively or immediately postoperatively with placement of intramedullary components. Remember that PEs rarely cause electrocardiogram changes and are not typically diagnosable on regular chest x-rays.

CLINICAL PEARLS

- Standard radiographic imaging of patient with DJD of the knee includes standing AP radiographs of bilateral knees, extension- and flexion-lateral radiographs of the affected knee, and a Merchant-view radiograph.
- First-line therapies for DJD of the knee are almost always nonoperative in nature. They include interventions such as physical therapy, nonsteroidal anti-inflammatories, and intraarticular corticosteroid injections.
- Total knee arthroplasty is the treatment of choice for end-stage osteoarthritis in patients who have failed conservative measures.
- A synovial fluid white blood cell count of greater than 1100 cells/mL and a polymorphonuclear level of greater than 64% is concerning for a PJI.

REFERENCES

Flynn JM, ed. Knee reconstruction and replacement. In: *Orthopaedic Knowledge Update: Ten*. Rosemont, IL: American Academy of Orthopaedic Surgeons; 2011:469-478.

Miller MD, ed. Adult reconstruction. In: *Review of Orthopaedics*. 5th ed. Philadelphia: Saunders Elsevier; 2008: 306-358.

CASE 40

A 65-year-old woman presents to her primary care physician with complaints of right "groin" pain that radiates to the buttock. She has noticed some mild pain in her right hip for the past 2 years, but has had severe pain over the last 4 months. She describes the pain as being "4/10" but at times can be an "8/10." The quality of the pain is a dull ache, and she denies any weakness, numbness, or tingling in her leg below the knee; however, the pain recently has kept her from getting sleep at night. She is currently using a cane for ambulation around her community and has to rest every 4 to 5 blocks because of pain. She also notes difficulty putting on her shoes and socks and getting in and out of the car. Her symptoms are refractory to ibuprofen and acetaminophen. She denies any recent trauma, infections, or dental work. Vital signs are within normal limits. When she ambulates, she leans her body to the right side during stance phase while maintaining a level pelvis. When she is lying flat on her back, she is able to flex her right hip to 90 degrees but has severe pain past this point. She has limited abduction of her right hip compared with the left. She has 0 degrees of right hip internal rotation and 20 degrees of external rotation. When holding her left knee to her chest and extending the right hip, the right posterior thigh does not fully lie on the exam table. She has a negative straight leg raise bilaterally and is neurovascularly intact in both lower extremities.

- ▸ What is the most likely diagnosis?
- ▸ What is your next diagnostic step?
- ▸ What are the nonoperative treatment options?
- ▸ What are the surgical treatment options?

ANSWERS TO CASE 40:

Hip Osteoarthritis

Summary: A 65-year-old woman presents with a chief complaint of right "groin" pain that radiates to the buttock. She is having difficulty performing activities of daily living and sleeping, and her pain is not relieved by anti-inflammatory medications. She has not had a traumatic event or recent infections. On physical exam, she has painful and limited range of motion of her hip, with a flexion contracture.

- **Most likely diagnosis:** Right hip osteoarthritis.
- **Next diagnostic step:** Anteroposterior (AP) pelvis radiograph and AP and lateral radiographs of the right hip (Figures 40–1 and 40–2).
- **Nonoperative treatment options:** Nonsteroidal anti-inflammatory drugs (NSAIDs), physical therapy (eg, stretching and range-of-motion exercises, modalities, pool therapy), and corticosteroid injections.
- **Surgical treatment option(s):** Total hip replacement.

ANALYSIS

Objectives

1. Understand the etiologies of arthritis.
2. Be familiar with the treatment options for hip arthritis.
3. Understand the indications for total hip arthroplasty.

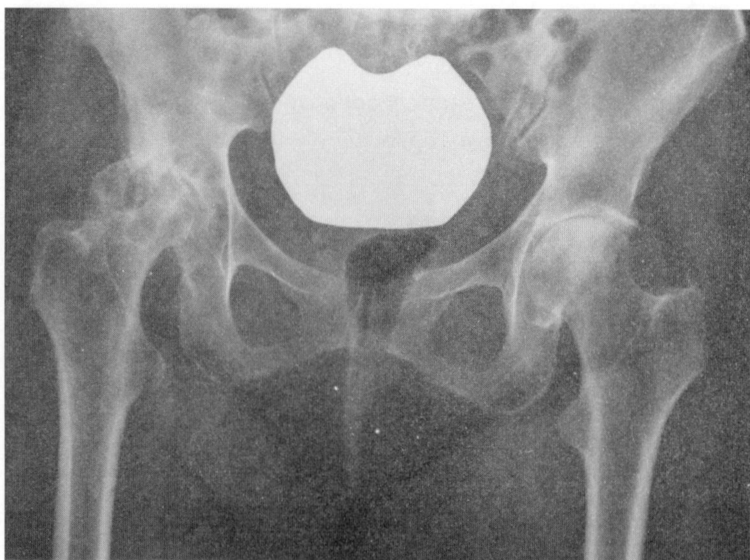

Figure 40–1. AP pelvis radiograph demonstrating osteoarthritis in the right hip.

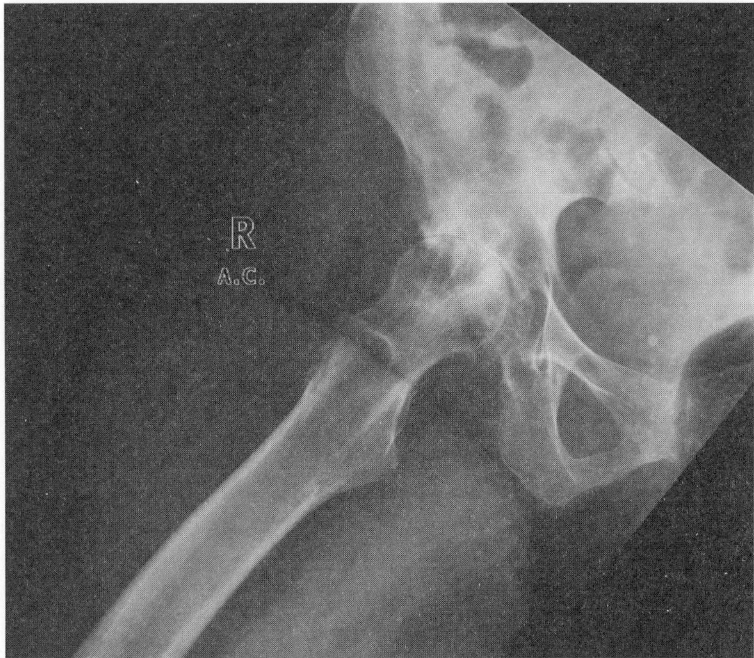

Figure 40–2. Frog-leg lateral radiograph of the right hip demonstrating osteoarthritic changes.

Considerations

This 65-year-old patient presents with **"groin" pain,** which is the typical location of pain that is coming from the hip joint. Patients often complain additionally of **radiating pain to the buttock, lateral thigh, or knee.** Sometimes patients who have hip arthritis will actually present with "knee pain." This is called referred pain and is thought to be caused by irritation of the obturator nerve or, less commonly, the femoral nerve. "Hip pain" can also be due to problems in the spine and pelvis. On physical exam, **pain with resisted straight leg raise and resisted hip flexion and groin pain with hip flexion and internal rotation** are more commonly seen in hip disease and less commonly with low back disease. This patient also had **limitations in hip range of motion,** which is common with end-stage osteoarthritis. Although pain in the **hip can radiate** *down to* **the knee, lumbar spine disease (eg, sciatica) will often radiate** *below* **the knee and into the foot.** If the diagnosis is unclear or if the patient has both hip and lumbar spine pathology, a **diagnostic injection of anesthetic and corticosteroids** into the hip joint can be performed to determine whether the pain is coming primarily from the hip. If the pain is alleviated with the injection, the pain is likely coming from the hip. It is important to obtain a quality **AP pelvis radiograph as well as AP and lateral radiographs** of the affected hip when there is concern for arthritis (Figures 40–1 and 40–2). If the patient complains of radiating pain, AP and lateral radiographs of the lumbar spine and/or weightbearing AP/lateral/Merchant x-rays of the knee may be required.

APPROACH TO: Hip Osteoarthritis

DEFINITIONS

OSTEOARTHRITIS: Progressive, degenerative disorder of the joints caused by a gradual loss of cartilage and bone resulting in pain, stiffness, and bony overgrowth

REFERRED PAIN: Pain perceived in a body location other than the location of pathology

CLINICAL APPROACH

Etiologies

Osteoarthritis is the most common form of end-stage arthritis in the community; other types of arthritis include **juvenile rheumatoid arthritis, rheumatoid arthritis, posttraumatic arthritis, inflammatory arthritis (eg, systemic lupus erythematosus), secondary arthritis from avascular necrosis, and septic arthritis.** It is important to determine the etiology of the underlying arthritis, as this may affect surgical decision making and postoperative management. Radiographs are often helpful in determining the etiology of arthritis. **Osteoarthritis** will show evidence of **asymmetric joint space narrowing, osteophyte formation, subchondral sclerosis, and subchondral cysts,** whereas **rheumatoid arthritis** will demonstrate **symmetric joint space narrowing, bony erosions, and osteopenia.** Osteoarthritis of the hip may also occur secondary to previous traumatic injuries, developmental dysplasia of the hip, osteonecrosis of the hip, and femoroacetabular impingement.

Clinical Presentation

The majority of patients who present with hip pain will not require surgery. As with any painful condition, when taking a patient's history, it is important to ask (1) location of the pain, (2) whether or not the pain radiates to another location, (3) alleviating or aggravating factors, (4) what the patient has tried to alleviate the pain, (5) quality of the pain, (6) quantity of the pain, (7) duration of the pain, (8) when the pain occurs, and (9) associated symptoms, including numbness, weakness, fevers, weight loss, involvement of other joints, and so forth.

As discussed, patients with arthritis (particularly osteoarthritis) present with groin pain that can radiate to the buttock, lateral proximal femur, thigh, or knee. Patients often describe the pain as a **constant, dull ache** that **worsens with physical activity** and is relieved, at least partially, with rest. Patients often tolerate the pain, taking anti-inflammatories or acetaminophen for many years. Often, what compels patients to finally seek treatment is restricted motion that **prevents them from performing activities of daily living,** including dressing and driving, or **pain that interferes with their ability to sleep.**

On physical exam, they often have relatively normal vital signs (unless they have an underlying medical condition) and ambulate with a **coxalgic gait.** A coxalgic gait is when the patient **lurches his or her torso to the affected side but keeps the pelvis level.** This is different from a Trendelenburg gait (a sign of hip abductor weakness), in which the patient leans his or her torso to the affected side but the pelvis is *not* level and is different from the antalgic gait seen with knee pathology, in which the patient limits the amount of time he or she weight bears on the affected knee during stance phase. As a result of loss of cartilage or bone, patients may have a **limb length discrepancy,** which may also cause an abnormal gait. With the patient supine, patients often have **painful, restricted range of motion.** A **Thomas test,** in which the patient holds his or her unaffected knee to the chest and attempts to extend the affected hip, can help the clinician to determine whether the patient also has a **hip flexion contracture.** Patients with hip pathology also have **pain with resisted hip flexion and resisted straight leg raise.** Radiographic evaluation of a painful hip includes a quality **AP pelvis** radiograph (Figure 40–1) and an **AP and lateral radiograph** (Figure 40–2) of the affected hip. Magnetic resonance imaging (MRI) is rarely required to make the diagnosis of arthritis, but may be beneficial in eliminating other causes of hip pain or to diagnose early cartilage loss.

TREATMENT

Total hip arthroplasty is one of the most successful procedures in medicine. Indications for total hip replacement in general terms are **debilitating, end-stage arthritis of the hip that limits activities of daily living.** Orthopaedic surgeons generally evaluate pain, success (or lack of success) of nonoperative interventions, baseline function, mobility, and radiographic evidence of joint space damage in their decision to recommend surgery. In addition, patients must have **failed nonoperative treatment interventions,** including physical therapy (eg, stretching and range-of-motion exercises, modalities, pool therapy), nonsteroidal anti-inflammatories, and intraarticular corticosteroid injections.

A variety of implants and bearing surfaces are currently available. The most common current bearing options include metal on metal, metal on polyethylene, ceramic on ceramic, ceramic on-polyethylene, and Oxinium on polyethylene. With each of the previously mentioned types of bearings, the femoral head is former and the acetabular liner is latter. There are advantages and disadvantages to each type of bearing surface. In older adults, the most commonly used bearing surface is metal on polyethylene. In addition, both the acetabular and femoral components can be cementless or cemented, depending on the patient's age and bone quality and surgeon preference.

COMPREHENSION QUESTIONS

40.1 A 58-year-old golfer presents to your office with complaints of progressive right groin pain, 2 years in duration. Lately he has been having difficulty walking between holes on the golf course. On examination, he is overweight, exhibits an antalgic gait, and has markedly limited range of hip motion. Which of the following choices will provide the most information to the orthopaedic surgeon regarding the presence of degenerative joint disease?

A. AP pelvis plain x-ray
B. CT scan of the pelvis
C. AP pelvis, AP, and lateral plain radiographs of the affected hip
D. AP and lateral comparison plain x-rays of the unaffected hip
E. MRI of the pelvis

40.2 A 68-year-old male active tennis player presents to your practice with a 4-year history of left groin pain. His pain has been worsening over the last year, and he is now unable to participate in the local singles league. He has moderate relief with NSAIDs and acetaminophen in the past, but states these are no longer fully effective. An orthopaedic spine surgeon has evaluated him in the recent past for degenerative disc disease but only treated him with NSAIDs and prednisone for what he recalls as a "slipped disc." On exam, the patient has a limited range of hip motion and pain with internal rotation. Straight leg raise above 70 degrees causes pain to radiate down his leg. X-rays show mild degenerative changes in his bilateral hips. What is the next best step in management of this patient?

A. Left total hip arthroplasty
B. Left hip hemiarthroplasty
C. Immediate referral back to his spine surgeon for further workup
D. Intraarticular corticosteroid injection
E. Continue NSAIDs and acetaminophen, recommend physical therapy, and add a low-dose narcotic for daily pains

40.3 A 63-year-old obese woman is referred to your office for evaluation for arthritis, diagnosed on x-rays ordered by her primary care physician. The patient complains that she gets left hip pain when power-walking with her dog. She states she has an aunt who had relief of chronic pain from a hip replacement last year and wants you to perform the same "miracle operation." A careful history, physical exam, and appropriate imaging confirm the diagnosis of left hip osteoarthritis. Which of the following is *not* an appropriate first-line treatment?

A. Activity modification
B. Weight loss
C. Physical therapy for quadriceps strengthening
D. Intraarticular steroid injection
E. Total hip arthroplasty

ANSWERS

40.1 **C.** AP pelvis, AP hip, and frog-leg lateral radiographs are the standard films to obtain of the hip when evaluating a patient for degenerative joint disease. CT scans and MRI are typically unnecessary in the setting of osteoarthritis.

40.2 **D.** It is unclear by this question whether his symptoms are from osteoarthritis or spinal pathology. In these situations, intraarticular corticosteroid injections may play a diagnostic role in addition to being therapeutic. The simultaneous injection of lidocaine or similar local anesthetics should provide near-immediate relief of symptoms if his pain is arthritic in nature. Although referral and/or consultation with a spine surgeon is appropriate, this patient may well have symptomatic osteoarthritis of the hip and should not be simply sent to see someone else. Although NSAIDs, acetaminophen, and physical therapy play an important role in his therapy, they do not necessarily provide the diagnostic evidence needed to determine the source of his pain; secondary, chronic narcotics should almost never be used in the treatment of degenerative joint disease. Of course, total hip arthroplasty or hemiarthroplasty should not be performed until the surgeon is certain of the underlying diagnosis and has exhausted nonoperative treatments when effective.

40.3 **E.** Activity modification, physical therapy (especially that directed at quadriceps strengthening), weight loss, and intraarticular steroids are all first-line nonoperative treatments for osteoarthritis. Total hip arthroplasty is reserved for patients who have failed conservative measures and whose arthritis is adversely affecting their ability to accomplish activities of daily living.

CLINICAL PEARLS

- The most common cause of end-stage hip arthritis in the United States is osteoarthritis.
- Most patients with intraarticular hip pathology present with groin pain that may or may not radiate to other locations around the hip joint or the knee.
- If it is unclear whether or not a patient is having hip, back, or pelvis pain, a diagnostic intraarticular injection of anesthetic and corticosteroids may help elicit the source of the underlying pain.
- Standard radiographic imaging of patient with hip arthritis includes an AP pelvis radiograph and an AP and lateral radiograph of the affected hip.
- First-line therapies for degenerative disease of the hip are almost always nonoperative in nature. They include interventions such as physical therapy (eg, stretching and range-of-motion exercises, modalities, pool therapy), nonsteroidal anti-inflammatories, and intraarticular corticosteroid injections.

REFERENCES

Hochberg MC, et al. Guidelines for the medical management of osteoarthritis. Part I. Osteoarthritis of the hip. American College of Rheumatology. *Arthritis Rheum*. 1995;38:1535-1540.

Huo MH, et al. What's new in total hip arthroplasty. *J Bone Joint Surg Am*. 2011;92:2959-2972.

Pluot E, et al. Hip arthroplasty. Part 1: prosthesis terminology and classification. *Clin Radiol*. 2009;64: 954-960.

CASE 41

A 63-year-old left-hand dominant man presents to your office with complaints of progressive left shoulder pain. He reports a remote history of blunt trauma to the shoulder, sustained after a fall from a ladder. After that fall, the patient returned to his job at the post office despite mild residual discomfort with activity. Recently the pain has been more persistent, and he is having difficulty handling parcels at work. He reports loss of sleep due to night pain and has had no relief with steroid injection provided by his primary care physician. On examination, the patient is overweight, with symmetrical appearance of the shoulder musculature. He can raise his left arm to the level of his shoulder in forward elevation and can abduct 60 degrees. He has external rotation of the shoulder to approximately 10 degrees and can internally rotate to reach his low lumbar region. His left arm strength at the extremes of motion is only mildly diminished relative to his right, but his left arm range of motion is markedly restricted. There is palpable crepitus overlying the shoulder. He is neurovascularly intact. X-rays are obtained of the left shoulder demonstrating significant glenohumeral joint space narrowing with mild flattening of the humeral head. Osteophytes are present on the glenoid rim and on the inferior articular surface of the humerus. The anteroposterior view shows the humeral head to be concentrically aligned with the glenoid without evidence of proximal migration.

- ▶ What is the most likely diagnosis?
- ▶ What are the treatment options for his condition?

ANSWERS TO CASE 41: Shoulder Arthroplasty

Summary: A 63-year-old left-hand dominant man presents with posttraumatic degenerative changes of the left shoulder and significant disability. Examination demonstrates intact rotator cuff function. X-rays of the left shoulder demonstrate significant glenohumeral joint space narrowing with mild flattening of the humeral head. Osteophytes are present on the glenoid rim and on the inferior articular surface of the humerus. The anteroposterior view shows the humeral head to be concentrically aligned within the glenoid without evidence of proximal migration.

- **Most likely diagnosis:** Posttraumatic arthritis of the glenohumeral joint.
- **Interventions:** Nonoperative interventions include steroid injections, physical therapy, and pharmacologic agents (anti-inflammatories, analgesics). Operative interventions include hemiarthroplasty, total shoulder arthroplasty, or reverse total shoulder arthroplasty.

ANALYSIS

Objectives

1. Understand the relevant anatomy of the shoulder musculature, bony anatomy, and related biomechanics.
2. Identify the key features of radiographic evaluation of the shoulder anatomy.
3. Understand the surgical options for treating advanced degenerative joint disease of the shoulder and the clinical considerations that guide treatment decisions.

Considerations

This is a 63-year-old left-hand dominant man who presents with degenerative changes of the left shoulder. Clinical findings must be considered in the context of the patient's overall functional demands on the shoulder, his overall health status, and his degree of symptoms. On exam, irreparable or chronic rotator cuff deficiency necessitates reverse-total shoulder arthroplasty to enable elevation or abduction of the arm. For low-demand patients lacking rotator cuff function, hemiarthroplasty (replacement of the humeral head) may relieve pain but is unlikely to increase functional range of motion. With rotator cuff function intact, as it is in this patient, either standard total or hemiarthroplasty is possible, depending on the degree of glenoid arthritis. Significant glenoid involvement necessitates additional resurfacing, and total shoulder arthroplasty may be performed provided that there is sufficient glenoid bone remaining to support the implant.

APPROACH TO: Shoulder Arthroplasty

DEFINITIONS

SHOULDER HEMIARTHROPLASTY: Prosthetic replacement of the humeral head.

TOTAL SHOULDER ARTHROPLASTY: Prosthetic replacement of the humeral head in combination with prosthetic resurfacing of the glenoid.

REVERSE TOTAL SHOULDER ARTHROPLASTY: Prosthetic resurfacing of both the glenoid and humeral articular surfaces with reversed placement of the ball and socket components. The hemispherical ball component is fixed to the glenoid, and the humeral head is replaced with a cup prosthesis.

CLINICAL APPROACH

Shoulder Anatomy and Normal Glenohumeral Biomechanics

The shoulder joint is comprised of the glenohumeral articulation and the surrounding soft-tissue envelope including the joint capsule, associated ligamentous structures, and the rotator cuff musculature. The glenohumeral joint functions as a **ball-and-socket joint** and enables significant mobility but is inherently unstable due to the relatively small size of the glenoid and minimal congruence afforded by its shallow concavity (Figure 41–1). Muscles acting across the joint to move the extremity create force vectors that tend to displace the glenohumeral articulation. To prevent dislocation, the joint is stabilized by both static and dynamic forces that counteract the displacing forces to permit coordinated motion of the joint.

Static stabilizers include the glenoid labrum, the joint capsule, the glenohumeral ligaments, negative intraarticular pressure or adhesive fluid properties, and the glenoid concavity and joint version. Degenerative process and traumatic injury to these structures can result in significant and disabling functional pain, joint laxity, or gross instability. The glenoid labrum is a fibrocartilaginous ring around the periphery of the glenoid that doubles the depth of the concavity. Similarly, integrity of the joint capsule and its associated ligamentous structures provide additional constraints to joint displacement at varying positions of the arm. Adhesive fluid properties and **negative intracapsular pressure** resist joint dislocation or distension. Alterations in synovial fluid production or quality can affect the physiology of articular tissues and is related to several pathologic processes. Degenerative wear or trauma to the bony anatomy of the glenohumeral joint surfaces can result in chronic pain and joint instability due to an insufficient or distorted glenoid surface or distorted and asymmetric humeral head.

Dynamic stabilizers of the shoulder include periscapular muscles, the biceps tendon, and the rotator cuff musculature. Periscapular muscles function to reposition the glenohumeral joint in a mechanically advantageous orientation by coordinating scapulothoracic and glenohumeral motion. Thus, normal kinematics of the shoulder requires normal neuromuscular function in addition to unimpaired motion at

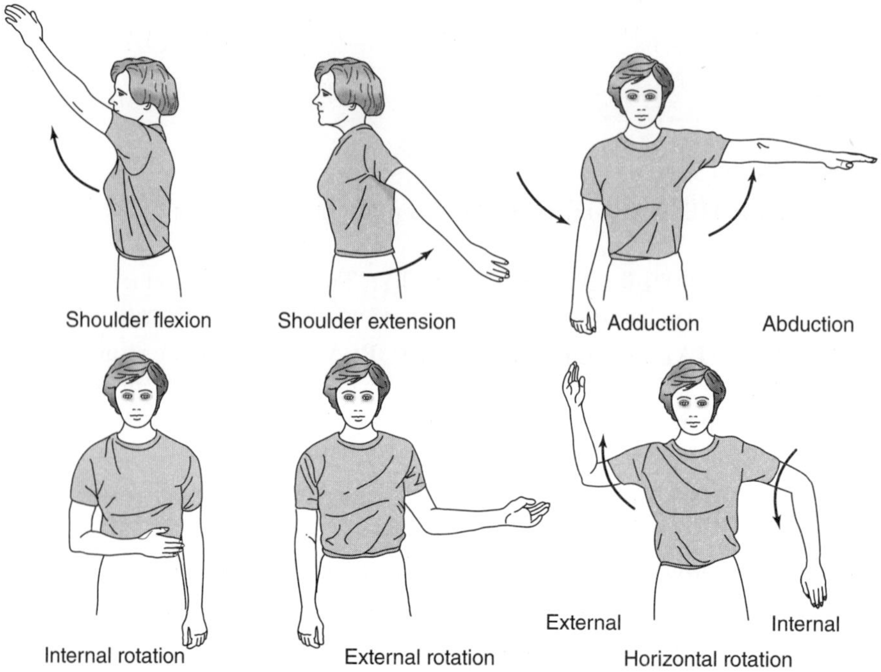

Figure 41–1. Basic shoulder motions. (Reproduced, with permission, from Skinner HB. *Current Diagnosis & Treatment in Orthopedics.* 4th ed. New York, NY: McGraw-Hill; 2006:Fig. 4-23.)

the scapulothoracic, glenohumeral, acromioclavicular, and sternoclavicular joints. Dysfunction of these structures impairs coordinated motion, results in compromised biomechanical function at the glenohumeral joint, and predisposes to traumatic injury and accelerated degenerative wear. The function of the long head of the biceps tendon in shoulder stabilization is controversial. Although some studies have shown increased joint laxity in the absence of an intact biceps tendon, functional evaluations have not demonstrated significant clinical differences. In contrast, the muscles of the rotator cuff are the primary stabilizers of the glenohumeral articulation during arm motion. The principal function of the rotator cuff is to compress the humeral head against the glenoid and resist shear forces generated by the pull of muscles acting across the joint (eg, the deltoid, pectoralis major, latissimus dorsi, teres major, and biceps brachii). In particular, deltoid contraction during arm elevation tends to pull the humeral head proximally, and the rotator cuff is required to depress the head and permit the glenohumeral articulation to act as a fulcrum for arm elevation during deltoid contraction (Figure 41–2).

Rotator Cuff Muscle Function and Testing

The rotator cuff muscles all originate from the scapula and insert along the margin of the humeral head articular surface on the greater and lesser tuberosities. The **subscapularis** muscle originates from the entire anterior surface of the scapular body, and its tendon passes anterior to the humeral head to insert on the lesser tuberosity.

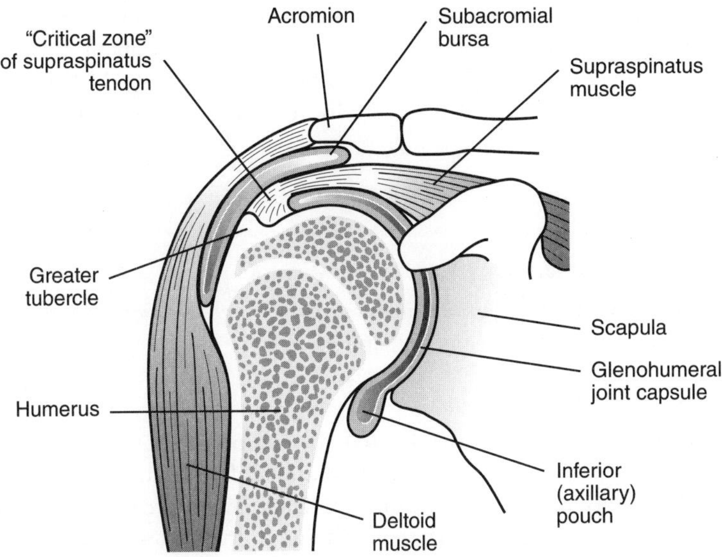

Figure 41–2. Coronal section of the shoulder illustrating the relationships of the glenohumeral joint, the joint capsule, the subacromial bursa, and the rotator cuff (supraspinatus tendon).

The subscapularis contributes to joint stability by helping to prevent anterior dislocation of the shoulder joint, and contraction results in internal rotation of the arm. The **supraspinatus** and **infraspinatus** originate from the posterior scapular body above and below the scapular spine, respectively. Their tendons become confluent at their insertion on the superolateral aspect of the humeral head. They prevent proximal humeral head migration during deltoid-mediated arm elevation and are essential for any arm flexion or abduction. The **teres minor** muscle originates from the lateral border of the scapular body and passes posterior to the humeral head to insert on the posterior aspect of the greater tuberosity. The teres minor creates an external rotation force on the arm. Rotator cuff testing is achieved by assessing the isolated functional integrity of the four rotator cuff muscles on physical exam. Deficiencies noted on exam suggestive of surgically correctable tears are generally confirmed with magnetic resonance imaging (MRI). For patients requiring shoulder arthroplasty for painful arthritis or irreparable fracture of the humeral head, the integrity of the rotator cuff and the patient's functional status determine the appropriate procedure.

Radiographic Evaluation

Radiographic imaging should proceed stepwise. Initial imaging for painful shoulder conditions should be initiated with plain radiographs. Anteroposterior (AP) imaging will demonstrate joint space, articular surface degeneration, any proximal head migration suggestive of a large tear or significant attenuation of the superior rotator cuff, and superior or inferior osteophytes. Lateral (scapular Y) images permit careful inspection of the anatomy of the acromion. This is useful when rotator cuff impingement is a concern based on history or exam. An axillary view will show glenoid version (orientation), glenoid bone loss, and anterior or posterior osteophytes. Computed tomography (CT) scans provide the most detail about bony anatomy and can be invaluable in preoperative planning for arthroplasty. MRI is used when the integrity of the rotator cuff is uncertain or additional soft-tissue pathology is being investigated.

TREATMENT

Nonoperative Treatment

Nonoperative therapy for glenohumeral arthritis includes activity modification, physical therapy, steroid injection, and analgesics.

Total Shoulder Arthroplasty

Total shoulder arthroplasty is indicated for symptomatic degenerative shoulder conditions in patients with an **intact rotator cuff.** Because the glenohumeral articulation is relatively unconstrained, significant sheer forces are created at the joint when muscles acting across the joint are used. In the absence of the dynamic and coordinated counterforce generated by rotator cuff function, these shear forces would result in malposition of the humeral head during arm motion, eccentric forces across the prosthetic articulation, and eventual glenoid component loosening. For this reason, **total shoulder arthroplasty (TSA) is contraindicated in the setting of irreparable rotator cuff deficiency.** TSA is also contraindicated in the setting of significant glenoid erosion or irreparable glenoid bone loss from trauma or arthritis because of the technical requirements involved in glenoid prosthetic resurfacing and implant fixation. The benefits of TSA also require that the patient have intact brachial plexus and deltoid muscle function.

Shoulder Hemiarthroplasty

Shoulder hemiarthroplasty is appropriate when there is symptomatic shoulder arthritis without significant glenoid involvement. This can occur after traumatic injury to the humeral head (eg, with dislocation), avascular necrosis (eg, with sickle cell disease or steroid use), or primary osteoarthritis. Similarly, hemiarthroplasty can be used as the initial procedure to address comminuted multipart fractures of the proximal humerus that are unlikely to have a good outcome with primary fracture repair. With mild degenerative changes of the glenoid, gentle recontouring of the articular surface can sometimes permit arthroplasty without requiring glenoid prosthetic resurfacing. Hemiarthroplasty is also appropriate for select patients with chronic rotator cuff deficiency who have very low functional demands and painful shoulder arthritis. In these patients, humeral head replacement and excision of osteophytes can provide significant symptom improvement, although objective shoulder function may be adversely impacted due to the muscular deficiencies.

Reverse Total Shoulder Arthroplasty

Low-demand patients with painful arthritis who lack rotator cuff function can benefit from reverse total shoulder arthroplasty. The absence of rotator cuff function results in pseudoparalysis of the arm. When attempting to raise the arm, the deltoid contraction causes the entire humerus to slide proximally because the rotator cuff cannot maintain the humeral head position in the glenoid. The result is that the arm slides up and down the body, but remains at the side. **Reversing the ball and socket configuration of the implants so the cup is on the humerus and the ball is on the scapula changes (ie, medializes) the center of rotation of the shoulder joint and provides a fulcrum for the arm to pivot on.** This allows the deltoid to raise the arm despite the absence of rotator cuff function.

Reverse shoulder arthroplasty can restore function but has significant limitations and is considered a salvage procedure for patients older than 70 years with intact deltoid function but irreparable rotator cuff tears and limited preexisting shoulder function. The complication rate is increased relative to standard shoulder arthroplasty.

Technical Considerations

An AP radiograph will generally reveal degenerative arthritis (including osteophytes or joint space narrowing from cartilage thinning) and can demonstrate proximal humeral head migration, indicating rotator cuff deficiency. **An axillary view will demonstrate any posterior glenoid erosion, which is the most common bony glenoid deficiency with osteoarthritis of the shoulder.** CT scans provide excellent anatomic detail and can allow precise determination of bony erosion and glenoid version (or mechanical orientation). MRI is helpful in determining rotator cuff anatomy, acuity of injury, and degree of muscular atrophy.

The **deltopectoral approach** for shoulder arthroplasty takes advantage of an internervous plane between the axillary nerve (supplying the deltoid muscle) and the medial and lateral pectoral nerves (supplying the pectoral muscles). The subscapularis tendon is the only musculotendinous structure that has to be cut before opening the joint capsule anteriorly, and it must be carefully repaired at the end of the case to allow for internal rotation and to keep the humeral head from dislocating anteriorly.

Component size and position must be carefully evaluated to ensure effective muscle function at the shoulder, maintain biomechanical joint stability, and avoid painful motion. Component version (ie, axial rotational orientation) must be determined with consideration given to preoperative anatomy and assessed intraoperatively in relation to the distal extremity.

Rehabilitation

Early postoperative rehabilitation is **limited by the subscapularis tendon repair** and healing. Patients are initially maintained in a shoulder immobilizer to support the arm and maintain a position of internal rotation. External rotation is avoided to prevent damage to the subscapularis tendon repair. Therapy is initiated with passive range of motion exercises (eg, shoulder pendulums) that progress to active assisted and active stretching before starting a strengthening regimen.

Complications

Complications include component loosening, failure of the subscapularis tendon repair, component malposition, postoperative stiffness, dysfunction or instability due to improper soft-tissue balancing, periprosthetic fracture, heterotopic ossification, or infection.

COMPREHENSION QUESTIONS

41.1 An 80-year-old woman who lives independently falls at home and sustains an irreparable fracture of the proximal humerus. She reports a history of painful shoulder arthritis and a long-standing inability to raise her arm over her head. She is otherwise healthy. Which of the following is the best therapy?

A. Perform rotator cuff repair before performing a total shoulder arthroplasty
B. Surgical intervention is contraindicated by her age
C. Total shoulder arthroplasty
D. Reverse total shoulder arthroplasty

41.2 Two weeks after undergoing shoulder hemiarthroplasty for advanced arthritis, a 66-year-old man slips at home and reinjures his shoulder. The patient presents complaining of anterior shoulder pain that is worse with attempted motion. X-rays show no evidence of fracture or component loosening, but the humeral head is anteriorly dislocated. What is the most likely mechanism of his injury?

A. Supraspinatus tear
B. Subscapularis tear
C. Labral injury
D. Biceps tendinitis
E. Occult fracture

41.3 A 65-year-old retired laborer presents to your office with complaints of generalized right shoulder pain with motion. He has had subtle aching in this shoulder for the past 2 years. Initially his pain was in the evening after a long day's work, but he now complains that the ache is constant and wakes him from sleep. His symptoms are refractory to 2 steroid injections. On exam, he is able to forward flex the arm to 120 degrees and has good strength with internal and external rotation. X-rays of the right shoulder show degenerative changes of the humeral head and glenoid with sclerotic changes and joint space narrowing. There are osteophytes surrounding the glenoid. The humeral head is appropriately located within the glenoid. Which of the following would be most appropriate for this patient?

A. Rotator cuff repair alone
B. Shoulder hemiarthroplasty
C. Total shoulder arthroplasty
D. Reverse total shoulder arthroplasty
E. Staged rotator cuff repair, followed by delayed shoulder hemiarthroplasty

ANSWERS

41.1 **D.** The patient is elderly but lives independently and would likely suffer significant disability and decreased quality of life without intervention. No mention is made of medical comorbidities that would contraindicate surgical consideration. She has a long-standing history of rotator cuff deficiency that would be irreparable because of its chronicity and consequent muscular atrophy and tendon retraction. The lack of a functional rotator cuff is a contraindication to total shoulder arthroplasty. The patient could benefit from a reverse total shoulder arthroplasty to address both the irreparable proximal humerus fracture and the rotator cuff deficiency. A shoulder hemiarthroplasty would also be appropriate, as it would address her fracture and permit an approximate return to baseline function, but it would not improve her ability to elevate her arm like a reverse arthroplasty would.

41.2 **B.** The deltopectoral approach to the shoulder requires that the subscapularis be divided near its tendinous insertion onto the proximal humerus to expose the anterior joint capsule before arthrotomy and to enable wide exposure for arthroplasty. At the end of the procedure, the subscapularis must be repaired to permit active internal rotation and to prevent anterior dislocation of the humeral head. Postoperatively, patients are immobilized with their arm internally rotated to prevent tension from being applied to the subscapularis repair by active or passive forces. Postoperative anterior shoulder dislocations can occur in conjunction with rupture of the subscapularis repair from trauma or failure of the repair.

41.3 **C.** This patient has degenerative joint disease of the shoulder with osteoarthritic changes involving both the humeral head and the glenoid. There is no evidence of rotator cup arthropathy, given his good active range of motion and the reduced humeral head on x-ray. Therefore, the surgical choices come down to hemi- versus total arthroplasty. Because there are long-standing degenerative changes to the glenoid in addition to the humeral head, this patient would more likely benefit from a total shoulder arthroplasty.

CLINICAL PEARLS

- Understand the function of the rotator cuff in normal glenohumeral biomechanics as a dynamic counter to shear forces that act to destabilize the joint, and recognize the particular importance it plays in depressing the humeral head to permit deltoid-mediated overhead motion.
- Reverse total shoulders are only appropriate in low-demand patients with disability resulting from glenohumeral arthritis in the setting of rotator cuff deficiency.
- Hemiarthroplasty is appropriate for symptomatic humeral head arthritis or irreparable proximal humeral head fractures, but will not address rotator cuff insufficiency.
- Total shoulder arthroplasty is only appropriate in patients requiring resurfacing of both the humeral and glenoid surfaces who have a functioning rotator cuff.

REFERENCES

Galatz LM. *Orthopaedic Knowledge Update: Shoulder and Elbow 3*. Rosemont, IL: American Academy of Orthopaedic Surgeons; 2008.

Miller MD, ed. Adult reconstruction. In: Miller MD, ed, *Review of Orthopaedics*. 5th ed. Philadelphia: Saunders Elsevier; 2008:340-342.

CASE 42

A 55-year-old man with a history of hypertension, hyperlipidemia, and obesity presents complaining of a painful right elbow, which awoke him from sleep the morning of his presentation. He denies any recent trauma. The pain is localized to the right elbow, which he notes is warm and extremely tender to even the lightest touch. The pain is much worse when he moves his arm at the elbow. He had no relief with acetaminophen. He has not had fevers, and he does not have pain in any other joints. He reports that he has had similar episodes of joint pain in the past affecting his left first toe and right ankle; he hasn't had an episode in more than a year, however. He recently started taking a daily baby aspirin and routinely takes hydrochlorothiazide and atorvastatin. The patient is obese and claims to be a social drinker, typically consuming 5 to 7 glasses of red wine per week. On exam, he is afebrile, with vital signs within normal limits except for some mild hypertension. His right elbow is swollen, erythematous, warm, and exquisitely tender to palpation, with a decreased range of motion secondary to pain. An effusion is appreciable in the elbow. The remainder of the joint exam is unremarkable, and there is no erythema extending beyond the elbow. No tophi are identified. Arthrocentesis of the right elbow is performed, and 5 mL of cloudy-yellow aspirate is obtained. The sample is positive for negatively birefringent monosodium urate crystals. No organisms are identified on a Gram stain, and the fluid is sent for culture. The patient's serum uric acid level is 8 mg/dL, and his renal function is normal.

- ▶ What is the most likely diagnosis?
- ▶ What diagnosis must be excluded?
- ▶ What are the acute management options in this patient?
- ▶ What is the best long-term management plan for this patient?

ANSWERS TO CASE 42: Gout

Summary: A 55-year-old man with a history notable for hypertension, hyperlipidemia, obesity, and likely acute intermittent gout presents with acute monoarticular arthritis of the right elbow. He takes a daily baby aspirin and is on hydrochlorothiazide. The exam is remarkable for an afebrile obese male with a tender, warm, and swollen right elbow with decreased range of motion and no tophi. His labs are remarkable for monosodium urate crystals (MSU) seen on microscopy and an elevated serum uric acid level. His normal renal function will be important when considering treatment options.

- **Most likely diagnosis:** Acute gout flare.
- **Diagnosis to exclude:** Septic arthritis.
- **Acute treatment:** Several treatment options are available and include nonsteroidal anti-inflammatory drugs (NSAIDs) and/or oral prednisone. Colchicine is an alternative agent. Intraarticular steroid injections are also an option.
- **Long-term management:** Allopurinol, a type of xanthine-oxidase inhibitor, is helpful in the prophylaxis of future gout flares.

ANALYSIS

Objectives

1. Know the basic differential diagnosis of an acute monoarticular inflammatory arthritis.
2. Know the workup of acute monoarticular inflammatory arthritis.
3. Understand the natural history of gout.
4. Be familiar with medications used in the acute management of gout flares.
5. Be familiar with the chronic management of gout.

Considerations

Gout is the most common inflammatory arthritis in men older than 40 years. Like most individuals who suffer from gout, this patient is a middle-aged man (age and sex being nonmodifiable risk factors) with comorbidities that included obesity, hypertension, and hyperlipidemia (all modifiable risk factors). He presented with the acute onset of a monoarticular arthritis. He was found to have an elevated uric acid level, which is the strongest risk factor for gout, but it is not always present in the setting of an acute flare. Normal levels may vary by age and laboratory, but levels greater than 6.8 mg/dL are associated with decreased systemic solubility of uric acid and thus increased risk of gout. Medications such as thiazide diuretics, including hydrochlorothiazide, and low-dose aspirin (eg, baby aspirin) have also been associated with gout. The patient described prior episodes of arthritis that were most likely gout flares, including a classic presentation with podagra, or gout of the first metatarsophalangeal (MTP) joint.

APPROACH TO: Gout

DEFINITIONS

PODAGRA: Gout affecting the first MTP joint.

MONOSODIUM URATE CRYSTALS: Seen in synovial fluid of joints affected by gout.

CALCIUM PYROPHOSPHATE DEHYDRATE CRYSTALS: Found in synovial fluid of joints affected by pseudogout.

CLINICAL APPROACH

Differential Diagnosis

Crystal-induced arthritis can be due to MSU crystals, as in gout, or calcium pyrophosphate dehydrate crystals, as in pseudogout. The 2 are distinguished using polarized microscopy, which reveals ***negatively*** **birefringent needle-shaped crystals in gout and** ***positively*** **birefringent crystals in pseudogout.** The crystals in pseudogout may be a number of different shapes. Septic arthritis may also present as acute monoarticular arthritis and must be excluded with Gram stain and culture of the synovial fluid. Other causes of acute monoarticular arthritis include inflammatory conditions (eg, psoriatic arthritis, reactive arthritis), infections (eg, Lyme disease), osteoarthritis, sickle cell disease, and traumatic injury.

Risk Factors

There are a number of risk factors for gout other than hyperuricemia; they include purine-rich diets or those incorporating large quantities of alcohol (especially wine and beer), physical inactivity, being postmenopausal, renal impairment, treatment with diuretics (eg, hydrochlorothiazide), obesity, and family history (particularly in young men or premenopausal women). Hospitalization itself is a risk factor for gout flares. Notably, gout and cardiovascular disease (CVD) share many risk factors, and hyperuricemia has been shown to be an independent risk factor for CVD either via direct effect of uric acid or indirectly through associated systemic inflammation.

Workup of Crystal-Induced Arthropathy

Although the history and physical exam can be helpful, the gold standard for diagnosis of crystal-induced arthropathy is arthrocentesis with crystal analysis. Clinical practice varies, however, and some physicians are comfortable enough with a typical story (eg, podagra, an elevated uric acid level, and response to treatment) to confidently treat gout without crystal analysis. The absence of crystals on synovial fluid analysis rules out crystal-induced arthropathy; as a corollary, the presence of crystals makes the diagnosis of crystal-induced arthropathy likely but does not rule out other conditions, specifically septic arthritis. Notably, in-between episodes of gout flares, arthrocentesis of previously affected joints in individuals not on uric acid-lowering medications will demonstrate crystals and a mild inflammatory aspirate. A Gram stain and culture of synovial fluid are necessary to rule out septic arthritis; be aware that a negative Gram stain does not rule out a septic joint per se, so one is often left to rely on clinical suspicion. **Synovial fluid cell counts in crystal-induced arthropathy are typically between 30,000 and 50,000 cells/μL but may be greater.** In pseudogout, plain films of the affected joint may demonstrate chondrocalcinosis, or mineralization of the articular cartilage, visible on plain x-rays. In severe gout, plain films may show "punched out" lesions, or lytic lucencies near the articular surfaces, as well as overgrowth of the adjacent periosteal membranes.

Natural History of Gout

Humans suffer from gout because we lack the enzyme uricase and either overproduce or under-excrete uric acid (90% of patients with gout). The progression of gout is stratified into 3 phases. The first involves asymptomatic hyperuricemia. Of note, not all patients with hyperuricemia will develop gout. The second phase encompasses the acute, intermittent gout flare. It is characterized by involvement of a single joint, which may be different with subsequent flares. Symptoms typically last for 7 to 10 days. The third stage is chronic tophaceous gout, in which patients have persistent symptoms worsened by acute episodes of often polyarticular arthritis, as well as crystal deposition (tophi) in joints and soft tissue (eg, the ear lobes). A discussion of secondary gout is beyond the scope of this chapter but may be seen in conditions such as myeloproliferative disease, in which high cell turnover leads to hyperuricemia.

Acute and Chronic Medical Management of Gout

Basic dietary strategies (ie, avoiding beer and meats) can reduce uric acid levels, but not enough to prevent recurrent gout attacks. Thus, patients typically require medical therapy once the acute episode has resolved, which will lower serum uric acid levels. The patient, such as the one described here, likely has acute intermittent gout and is currently suffering from an acute gout flare. Now is not the appropriate time to initiate uric acid–lowering medications, as this can worsen precipitation of gout crystals. There are many options for treatment of gout flares, and the choice of one over the other is often dictated by the patient's comorbidities (ie, renal failure), especially in the hospitalized patient. **The goal of treatment in the acute setting is to control pain and reduce disability.** The sooner that treatment is initiated, the faster the resolution of symptoms occurs.

A randomized clinical trial performed in the outpatient setting demonstrated the equivalence of oral corticosteroid and the NSAID naproxen for the treatment of an acute gout flare in terms of pain management. No NSAID has been demonstrated to be more effective than any other; their use is limited by gastrointestinal and renal toxicity and should be avoided in patients with a history of myocardial infarction, heart failure, or renal disease. Oral prednisone (or other oral corticosteroids) may be administered with a starting dose of 40 to 60 mg/day for several days followed by a 10- to 14-day taper or, alternatively, several days of 40 to 60 mg/day without a taper. Oral corticosteroids may lead to or worsen preexisting hyperglycemia and may affect mood and appetite; chronic steroid therapy has more severe side effects. Intraarticular corticosteroid injection of a large joint affected by gout is also reasonable if there is no suggestion of a septic joint. Adrenocorticotropic hormone may be administered parenterally and is also effective, although it is less commonly used than other treatment options. Colchicine is typically used when prednisone and/or NSAIDs cannot be administered. Colchicine possesses a narrow therapeutic window, and side effects include nausea, vomiting, and diarrhea. When used appropriately, it can be very effective, although it often has a slower onset to action than NSAIDs or steroids. Debate exists over the optimal dosing regimen for colchicine in the treatment of acute flares. **Colchicine should be avoided in patients with renal or hepatic disease.** The use of intravenous colchicine is rare. For patients in whom none of these medicines can be administered safely, immobilization and pain management with opioids and ice are often the only options until the flare resolves on its own (typically approximately 7 days).

Several weeks after the patient's acute episode has resolved, it is reasonable to initiate a uric acid–lowering agent (goal uric acid <6 mg/dL), as is typically done in patients with a history of gout flares or tophi (clinically or radiographically) and hyperuricemia. Using uric acid–lowering agents will help prevent the transition in this patient from acute intermittent gout to chronic tophaceous gout and reduce the incidence of flares. **Allopurinol** is a xanthine oxidase inhibitor used to reduce uric acid levels. It must be dose-adjusted in renal impairment and has been associated with potentially fatal hypersensitivity reactions. For those who fail allopurinol or experience a hypersensitivity reaction, febuxostat is available; it is also a xanthine oxidase inhibitor. **Probenecid** is a uricosuric agent that inhibits renal tubular reabsorption of uric acid; it is also used as a uric acid–lowering agent. Pegloticase is an expensive recombinant form of uricase administered via infusion and carries a risk of infusion reaction. It is important to use either colchicine or NSAIDs as prophylaxis against acute gout flares during the first 6 months of uric acid–lowering therapy. If uric acid–lowering agents cannot be used, daily colchicine may be used for indefinite prophylaxis.

COMPREHENSION QUESTIONS

42.1 A 55-year-old man has had 2 gout attacks in the last year, most recently about 6 weeks ago. His serum uric acid level at today's visit is 9.3 mg/dL. He has been on daily colchicine prophylaxis since his last gout attack. He drinks socially, enjoying a "gin and tonic" once or twice a week. His body mass index is 24 kg/m^2, and he has no currently painful joints on examination. Which of the following is the next best step in the management of this patient?

A. Advise him to reduce the amount of alcohol he drinks.

B. Advise him to lose weight.

C. Advise him to discontinue colchicine and begin allopurinol.

D. Advise him to continue colchicine and begin allopurinol.

E. Advise him to discontinue colchicine altogether.

42.2 You are asked to see a 70-year-old woman with a swollen right knee that is warm and tender. You perform an arthrocentesis and observe positively birefringent rhomboid-shaped crystals on polarized microscopy. The Gram stain shows no organisms, and the synovial fluid culture grows no organisms. Which of the following is the most likely diagnosis?

A. Gout

B. Pseudogout

C. Rheumatoid arthritis

D. Systemic lupus erythematosus

42.3 Which of the following is a **false statement** regarding the causes of hyperuricemia?

A. The most common cause of hyperuricemia is under excretion.

B. Myeloproliferative disorders are a secondary cause of uric acid overproduction.

C. Primary under excretion of uric acid is related to hereditary excretion defects.

D. Ethanol increases urate production and increases urate excretion.

ANSWERS

42.1 **D.** Allopurinol should be started as prophylaxis and should be initiated while taking colchicine or an NSAID to prevent a gout flare. Urate-lowering treatments, such as allopurinol, should not be administered during an acute attack. Although weight loss and decreasing alcohol consumption are generally helpful in the management of gout, this patient is not overweight and does not admit to consuming an excessive amount of alcohol. Stopping colchicine without a prophylactic agent raises his risk of future flares.

42.2 **B.** Pseudogout is caused by calcium pyrophosphate dehydrate crystals, which are weakly birefringent positive on polarized microscopy. Pseudogout most commonly affects the knee and, unlike gout, is more common in women than men. Polyarticular gout and pseudogout may mimic rheumatoid arthritis. The lack of symmetry, prolonged morning stiffness, positive serologies, and systemic symptoms may help differentiate polyarticular crystal arthropathy from rheumatoid arthritis.

42.3 **D.** Ethanol increases urate production but *decreases* urate excretion. Ninety percent of hyperuricemia is due to under excretion of uric acid. It is now known that primary underexcretion of gout is related to hereditary defects that involve the transport of uric acid in renal tubules. Renal insufficiency as well as drugs and toxins are secondary causes of uric acid under excretion.

CLINICAL PEARLS

- An elevated serum uric acid level is the strongest risk factor for gout but may not be present during an acute flare.
- The gold standard for the diagnosis of crystal-induced arthropathy is arthrocentesis with crystal analysis.
- Septic arthritis must be considered when assessing the patient with acute monoarticular arthritis.
- Hyperuricemia is an independent risk factor for cardiovascular disease.
- Uric acid–lowering agents must not be initiated during an acute flare and should be coadministered initially with colchicine or NSAID prophylaxis.

REFERENCES

Dalbeth N, So A. Hyperuricemia and gout: state of the art and future prospective. *Ann Rheum Dis*. 2010;69:1738-1743.

Janssens HJ, Jannsen M, van de Lisdonk EH, et al. Use of oral prednisolone or naproxen for the treatment of gout arthritis: a double-blind, randomised equivalence trial. *Lancet*. 2008;371:1854-1860.

Klippel J, Stone J, Crofford L, White P, eds. *Primer on the Rheumatic Diseases*. 13th ed. New York: Springer; 2008.

CASE 43

An otherwise healthy 45-year-old woman presents to your clinic complaining of bilateral wrist pain. Over the last 4 weeks she has noticed that her wrists have been swollen and warm, and she has had difficulty completing tasks (eg, cleaning, turning door knobs) as a result of pain. The pain is particularly bad in the morning, when she also notices that both wrists are extraordinarily stiff; it typically takes at least 60 minutes for the stiffness to improve, and running them under warm water often helps. She has also felt quite fatigued. She recalls no recent viral-like illness, rashes, or sick contacts. She has been using ibuprofen every day for the pain with some relief of her symptoms, but she has developed an upset stomach as a result. On your exam, you find that both wrists are swollen, warm, and generally boggy. When you rotate her hand at the wrist she complains of exquisite pain that limits the range of motion. When you evaluate the small joints of her hands, you note multiple swollen, tender, and warm proximal interphalangeal (PIP) and metacarpophalangeal (MCP) joints that have a restricted range of motion because of pain. The remainder of her exam is unremarkable. She has a 20 pack-year smoking history. She does not recall a family history of arthritis or other connective tissue disease.

- ▶ What is the most likely diagnosis?
- ▶ What laboratory tests would you order to confirm your diagnosis?
- ▶ What would you expect to find on the radiographs of this patient's hands?
- ▶ What are some extraarticular manifestations of this disease?
- ▶ What medication would you begin for long-term treatment of her disease?

ANSWERS TO CASE 43:

Rheumatoid Arthritis

Summary: A premenopausal woman presents to you with a several-week history of a debilitating symmetrical polyarthritis that is associated with prolonged morning stiffness and fatigue. Her exam demonstrates active synovitis, without findings to suggest extraarticular manifestations of rheumatoid arthritis. She has had no recent viral illness, reports no significant family history, and has a significant smoking history. Her exam has no findings that would suggest an alternative diagnosis.

- **Most likely diagnosis:** Rheumatoid arthritis (RA).
- **Laboratory testing:** Standard laboratory tests include erythrocyte sedimentation rate (ESR), C-reactive protein (CRP), rheumatoid factor titer, and anticyclic citrullinated peptide (CCP) titer. Of these, anti-CCP is the most specific for rheumatoid arthritis.
- **Hand x-rays:** In RA patients with aggressive, advanced, or insufficiently treated disease, x-rays of the hands (and feet) often reveal juxtaarticular erosions (Figure 43–1B) and joint space narrowing (Figure 43–1C), which are both progressive and irreversible. X-rays early in the disease course may be normal (Figure 43–1A) or may show evidence of osteopenia.
- **Extraarticular manifestations of RA:** Rheumatoid nodules, ocular symptoms (eg, keratoconjunctivitis, scleritis), vasculitis, cardiac disease (eg, pericarditis, valvular heart disease, conduction abnormalities), neurologic disease (eg, nerve entrapment, mononeuritis multiplex), pulmonary disease, anemia, and cutaneous findings

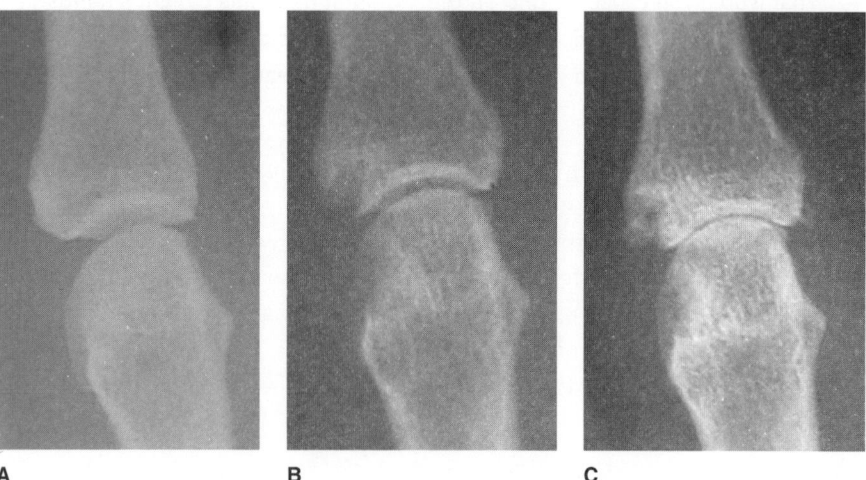

Figure 43–1. Plan posteroanterior radiographs of a metacarpophalangeal joint in patients with rheumatoid arthritis. (Reproduced, with permission, from Imboden J, Hellmann DB, Stone JH. *Current Rheumatology Diagnosis & Treatment.* 2nd ed. New York, NY: McGraw-Hill; 2007:Fig. 15-3.)

- **Medication to begin:** Methotrexate for long-term management of RA, with close reassessment of effectiveness, recognizing the potential need to switch or add medications

ANALYSIS

Objectives

1. Be familiar with the general presentation and diagnosis of rheumatoid arthritis.
2. Be familiar with the use of rheumatoid factor, anti-CCP, and radiology in the diagnosis of RA.
3. Understand the basic approach to treating rheumatoid arthritis.
4. Understand the prognosis of patients with RA.

Considerations

Rheumatoid arthritis is a heterogeneous group of systemic diseases characterized by a symmetric inflammatory polyarthritis that, if untreated, leads to joint erosions, disability, and a shortened life expectancy. It is more common in women than men, people of northern European and North American ancestry, and people older than 65 years of age. The annual incidence of RA is estimated to be 0.5 per 1000 persons. This patient has a fairly characteristic presentation of RA, with indolent symmetrical polyarthritis primarily affecting smaller joints and a history of prolonged morning stiffness. Notably, our patient had no recent viral-like illness to suggest a related polyarthritis, which may be difficult to distinguish from RA. She has a history of smoking, which in population studies has been identified as a risk factor for RA.

APPROACH TO: Rheumatoid Arthritis

DEFINITIONS

DISEASE-MODIFYING ANTI-RHEUMATIC DRUGS (DMARDs): A diverse group of medications unified by their shared ability to reduce inflammation and prevent disease progression. Methotrexate is the most commonly used DMARD.

BIOLOGIC DMARDs: DMARDs that are developed and produced in live cell systems. Examples include tumor necrosis factor inhibitors such as infliximab and etanercept.

TUMOR NECROSIS FACTOR: A cytokine in the inflammatory cascade that is overexpressed and overproduced in rheumatoid arthritis.

CLINICAL APPROACH

Differential Diagnosis

When evaluating a patient with inflammatory polyarthritis, **differential diagnoses** include connective tissue disorders such as **rheumatoid arthritis, mixed connective tissue disease, vasculitis, and systemic lupus erythematosus (SLE); crystal-induced arthropathy; viral-induced arthritis** such as those caused by hepatitis C and parvovirus B-19; and **seronegative spondyloarthropathies** such as psoriatic arthritis. The history and physical exam can often help guide your assessment. Laboratories such as RF and anti-CCP, as described later, may suggest RA but can also be positive in other connective tissue disorders. A high antinuclear antibody (ANA) titer may suggest an alternative or overlap syndrome that includes SLE. People who regularly interact with children, such as schoolteachers, may be at risk for parvovirus B-19, whereas intravenous drug users are at increased risk for hepatitis C; antibody assays are available for both conditions. **Primary osteoarthritis is a non-inflammatory arthritis,** although secondary osteoarthritis may occur secondary to inflammatory joint diseases.

Diagnosis

Obtaining a detailed history of the disease process is paramount in accurately diagnosing rheumatoid arthritis. Early in the disease, smaller joints (eg, PIPs, MCPs, metatarsophalangeals [MTPs], wrists) are affected; with time, larger joints including the knees, ankles, and elbows may be affected. **The distal interphalangeal (DIP) joints are almost always spared in RA.** Often, there **is symmetric joint involvement** (both within a single joint and when comparing both sides of the body), and **patients describe prolonged morning stiffness** (>60 minutes). Early disease is characterized by joint inflammation, whereas untreated, late disease is notable for joint deformity. A number of different sets of criteria have been developed to diagnose patients with rheumatoid arthritis. One set of guidelines relies on a point system based on joint involvement, serology, acute phase reactants, and the duration of symptoms.

Role of Serologies and Radiology in RA

RF is an antibody (typically immunoglobulin M) targeted against the Fc portion of immunoglobulin G, which is positive in most patients at some point in their disease course. The sensitivity and specificity of RF are estimated to be 66% and 82%, respectively; bacterial endocarditis, older age, and other conditions have been associated with a weakly positive RF. Anti-CCP antibodies are also found in patients with RA, with a sensitivity and specificity of 70% and 95%, respectively. Typically, **anti-CCP positive patients suffer from more severe disease and are less likely to achieve remission,** as are those with high RF titers. Approximately 50% to 85% of patients with RA are positive for RF, anti-CCP, or both during their disease course; some patients never test positive for RF or anti-CCP, and others test positive before experiencing any symptoms. Radiographs early in the disease may show **periarticular osteopenia** but the more common finding is **juxtaarticular bone erosion and symmetrical joint space narrowing** (as compared with asymmetric narrowing in osteoarthritis). The role of magnetic resonance imaging and ultrasound in the assessment of RA is still being defined.

Extraarticular Manifestations of RA

Because 50% of patients are affected by extraarticular manifestations of RA at some point, patients should periodically be assessed for such involvement. Sjogren syndrome, which is characterized by dry eyes and mouth, is the most common extraarticular manifestation. Rheumatoid nodules are found on pressure points (eg, elbows) in patients with RA, typically those positive for rheumatoid factor; they are firm, nontender, and adherent to the periosteum. Complaints of dyspnea or difficulty breathing should raise concern for associated interstitial lung disease. As with other chronic inflammatory conditions, RA patients are at increased risk for cardiovascular disease.

TREATMENT

The primary goal of treatment is remission with no evidence of active disease. Based on studies of historical cohort data, 5% to 15% of patients achieve drug-free remission, but many patients will relapse. At a minimum, treatment should limit the severity of disease and disability, leading to an improvement in the patient's quality of life. Frequent (every 2-3 months) reassessment of disease activity is necessary to determine treatment effectiveness. The key to treating rheumatoid arthritis is the early initiation of DMARDs, particularly methotrexate. **Thus, nearly all patients with RA are started on methotrexate at diagnosis unless contraindicated, in which case sulfasalazine or leflunomide may be substituted.** Alternatively, for more severe disease, multiple DMARDs (eg, methotrexate and leflunomide) may be initiated simultaneously to gain control of disease activity, or biologic DMARDs may be introduced.

The addition of biologic DMARDs (eg, tumor necrosis factor [TNF] inhibitors, anti-CD20 therapy, anti-interleukin 1 therapy, T-cell costimulator modulators, and anti-interleukin 6 therapy) to the rheumatologist's armamentarium represents a milestone in RA treatment because of their effectiveness, but the precise role of biologics, especially in early disease, is controversial, and the aim of numerous active clinical trials. Of the biologics, TNF inhibitors are typically reached for first and combined with a classic DMARD (eg, methotrexate). The biologics, as a class, are not benign and carry increased risk of infection (eg, usual infections as well as reactivation of tuberculosis and viral hepatitis).

Factors to consider when initiating treatment include the severity of the illness, medication cost, and the risk of side effects. **Management of flares may be undertaken with short courses of high-dose steroids to bridge to DMARDs, with an emphasis on a short course to limit side effects (eg, osteoporosis, diabetes, glaucoma).** Nonsteroidal anti-inflammatory medications (NSAIDs) limit pain as well as inflammation in flares but are limited by gastrointestinal intolerance and an increased risk of cardiac disease. Analgesics may be useful for the management of severe pain, but their use should also be minimized.

PROGNOSIS OF RHEUMATOID ARTHRITIS PATIENTS

Advances in our knowledge of the natural history of RA and the development of more sophisticated treatment modalities have led to significantly improved outcomes in RA. Without treatment, RA is typically a progressive disease that will leave patients disabled with chronic pain and at increased risk for other conditions, such as cardiovascular disease, the most common cause of death in RA patients. Evidence suggests that the severity of RA may be lessening; it is not clear whether this is because more patients with mild disease are being identified, because of new drug development, or because of more aggressive treatment strategies. A number of conditions have been associated with RA, including infection, osteoporosis, lymphoproliferative disorders, and cardiovascular disease. Reducing risk factors for these comorbidities, particularly cardiovascular disease, is important to improving life expectancy in patients with RA.

COMPREHENSION QUESTIONS

43.1 A 38-year-old woman is referred to your office with bilateral wrist, MCP, and PIP pain. Her pains are worst in the morning and become tolerable after taking ibuprofen. She complains of mild subjective fevers but has no other constitutional symptoms and no remarkable family history. Anti-CCP and RF titers are positive. A diagnosis of rheumatoid arthritis is made, and she is started on a DMARD regimen. How do you counsel her regarding her life expectancy?

A. She has no different life expectancy than age-matched controls.

B. She has a longer life expectancy than age-matched controls.

C. She has a shorter life expectancy than age-matched controls because of increased risk of infection.

D. She has a shorter life expectancy than age-matched controls because of premature atherosclerosis in the setting of systemic inflammation.

43.2 You are working in a hand clinic and see a large population of patients with preexisting diagnoses of rheumatoid arthritis. Which of the following patients do you expect to have a more aggressive form of rheumatoid arthritis?

A. A 45-year-old woman who is positive for RF and anti-CCP.

B. A 65-year-old woman who is positive for RF and negative for anti-CCP.

C. A 60-year-old man who has a low positive ANA titer, a negative RF, and a negative anti-CCP.

D. A 60-year-old woman with a negative RF and a negative anti-CCP.

43.3 A 50-year-old woman presents to your office with complaints of morning pains in her PIPs, MCPs, and wrists. After positive serologic testing, the diagnosis of rheumatic arthritis is made. Which of these treatment regimens is most appropriate?

A. Ibuprofen 800 mg orally every 8 hours until symptoms improve

B. Methotrexate 15 mg orally once weekly and prednisone 40 mg orally daily, with a short taper of prednisone

C. Etanercept 50 mg subcutaneously every week

D. Prednisone 40 mg orally once daily until symptoms improve

43.4 A 62-year-old woman with a 15-year history of rheumatoid arthritis is seen in your office for follow-up. Her symptoms are predominantly located in her bilateral MCPs and PIPs and have been moderately controlled on a DMARD regimen. Follow-up x-rays of her hands are obtained. Which of the following radiographic descriptions is most commonly associated with rheumatoid arthritis?

A. Asymmetric joint space narrowing
B. Symmetric joint space narrowing and juxtaarticular bone erosions
C. Multiple fractures of different stages of healing
D. Bone erosion with an overhanging edge
E. Radio-opaque depositions throughout the joint space and mild joint effusion

ANSWERS

43.1 **D.** Patients with RA have a shorter life expectancy, thought to be related to systemic inflammation, which causes premature atherosclerosis. Life expectancy in RA patients, however, is likely improving as our management of RA becomes more aggressive and new treatment options are introduced. RA patients are at increased risk of infection, especially with some treatments, so it is important to administer the flu vaccine annually, as well as the pneumococcal vaccination.

43.2 **A.** The presence of RF and anti-CCP antibodies are both associated with more severe disease. A low titer ANA in most patients without additional symptoms to suggest an alternative diagnosis is likely of no immediate significance.

43.3 **B.** Steroids should not be used for extended periods of time but are useful to gain quick control of disease activity as a bridge to a DMARD, such as methotrexate, which is appropriate chronic therapy. Generally, TNF inhibitors, such as etanercept, and other biologic DMARDs are not used as first-line therapy except in severe disease. High-dose NSAIDs, such as ibuprofen, are not suitable monotherapy for RA, as they do not slow the progression of disease and carry potentially severe side effects.

43.4 **B.** Symmetric joint space narrowing and juxtaarticular bone erosions may be seen in rheumatoid arthritis. Very early in the disease course, periarticular osteopenia may be noted, or the joint may appear normal. In gout, x-rays may show bone erosions with an overhanging edge, suggestive of both atrophy and hypertrophy. Similarly, osteoarthritis may cause osteophyte growth with an overhanging edge–like appearance. Asymmetric joint space narrowing is seen in joints affected by osteoarthritis. Radio-opaque depositions throughout the joint space is descriptive of chondrocalcinosis, a radiographic finding most often associated with pseudogout. In pseudogout, radio-opaque calcium-pyrophosphate crystals are deposited in the joint and cause inflammatory states that may lead to joint effusions.

CLINICAL PEARLS

- RA is a chronic, progressive, symmetric inflammatory polyarthritis that causes bony erosions and joint deformity if untreated.
- At some point in the disease's course, most patients are positive for RF, anti-CCP, or both. Some patients are seronegative (negative for RF and anti-CCP).
- Sjogren syndrome is the most common extraarticular manifestation of RA. Anemia is also very common.
- Early treatment with DMARDs is key to limiting disease progression and subsequent disability.
- Continuous reassessment is necessary to measure disease activity and adjust the treatment regimen.

REFERENCES

Goekoop-Ruiterman YPM, de Vries-Bouwstra JK, Allart CF, et al. Clinical and radiographic outcomes of four different treatment strategies in patients with early rheumatoid arthritis (the BeSt study). *Arthritis Rheum*. 2005;52:3381-3390.

Klippel J, Stone J, Crofford L, White P, ed. *Primer on the Rheumatic Diseases*. 13th ed. New York: Springer; 2008.

Scott D, Wolfe F, Huizinga TW. Rheumatoid arthritis. *Lancet*. 2010;376:1094-1108.

Turgwell P, et al. Biologicals for rheumatoid arthritis. *BMJ*. 2011;343:d4027.

CASE 44

A 5-year-old African American boy is referred to your office for management of a nondisplaced right middle-third clavicle fracture after a witnessed fall from standing. He complains of mild pain over the clavicle, but has no other complaints. He has no history of previous fractures nor any other significant past medical history. His mother states that she strongly believes in "natural" medicine and is relieved when you explain her son will not need surgery on his clavicle. On further discussion, you learn that the entire family abides by a strict vegan diet and that his family has recently moved to the area from Minnesota. On physical exam, the patient is below the 10th percentile for both height and weight. He is appropriately tender over the right middle clavicle. There is no skin tenting or neurovascular dysfunction in the right upper extremity. Additional findings include bilateral outwardly bowed knees and a mild spinal kyphosis. His sclerae are white. The child's right arm is placed in a sling, and a prescription for low-dose acetaminophen with codeine is written.

- What is the most likely diagnosis?
- What is the pathophysiology for his condition?
- What is the next step in the workup?

ANSWERS TO CASE 44:
Rickets

Summary: This is a 5-year-old child with a nondisplaced clavicle fracture. He is well below height and weight averages for his age and has evidence of malnutrition and poor bone quality, including bilateral genu varum and kyphosis.

- **Most likely diagnosis:** Nutritional rickets.
- **Risk factors for nutritional rickets:** Decreased vitamin D intake from diet (vegan diet), dark skin tone, and decreased exposure to direct sunlight (previously living at northern latitudes).
- **Next appropriate diagnostic studies:** The next appropriate step is to obtain serum calcium, phosphorus, alkaline phosphatase, 25-hydroxyvitamin D, and 1,25-dihydroxyvitamin D levels. Radiographic survey should include images of the bilateral upper and lower extremities, skull, abdomen/pelvis, and chest.

ANALYSIS

Objectives

1. Understand the basic pathophysiology, clinical manifestations, and radiographic signs of rickets.
2. Understand the differences between nutritional and nonnutritional rickets.
3. Be familiar with the basic management of rickets and recognize when referral to subspecialists is necessary.

Considerations

The presence of a clavicle fracture in infants and young children grossly below norms of height, weight, and/or head circumference should alert examiners to the possibility of an underlying diagnosis of rickets or metabolic bone disorders. Further historical elements that are concerning for a diagnosis of rickets include poor diet, limited exposure to sunlight, and dark skin tone. Examiners should be sure to ask about previous history of fractures, familial history of metabolic bone diseases, and, as always, **carefully evaluate pediatric patients with fractures for the possibility of physical abuse.** Although this child presented with a clavicle fracture, a complete and thorough physical examination of all 4 extremities, spine, and skull should be performed. Careful examination of this patient revealed bilateral genu varum and kyphosis—significant findings that may have been missed if the examiner had only examined the symptomatic right upper extremity.

APPROACH TO:
Rickets

DEFINITIONS

OSTEOPENIA: Diffusely decreased bone mineral density (BMD) that can be diagnosed on plain x-ray. Defined formally by the World Health Organization as exhibiting a T-score between –1.0 and –2.5 on dual-emission x-ray absorptiometry (DXA) scanning.

OSTEOMALACIA: Defective mineralization of osteoid (the organic component of bone) affecting both children and adults. Osteomalacia is referred to as rickets when found in patients with open skeletal growth plates.

GENU VARUM: Outward (lateral) bowing about the knee. Considered a normal physiologic finding in patients with mild bowing up to 3 to 4 years of age, but is considered pathologic in older children.

GENU VALGUM: Inward bowing about the knee; sometimes referred to as "knock-knees."

CLINICAL APPROACH

Rickets is a nonspecific term that refers to a variety of pediatric disorders in which there is defective mineralization of bone. This leads to bone deformities such as bowing and growth retardation. **Osteomalacia** is a similarly generalized term describing the defective mineralization process of osteoid; when present in pediatric populations (or patients with open physes), it is referred to as rickets.

Etiologies and Pathophysiology

Rickets is caused by a **deficiency in vitamin D**—whether secondary to inadequate dietary intake, inadequate production from insufficient exposure to sunlight, defects in metabolic pathways, or genetic defects leading to an aberrant biochemical response to vitamin D.

Regardless of etiology, insufficient vitamin D in rickets leads **to insufficient circulating concentrations of calcium and/or phosphorous,** 2 minerals that comprise the inorganic components of healthy bone. Osteoid, or the organic collagenous scaffold of bone, becomes incompletely mineralized. As a result, bones are therefore "soft" and prone to bowing (chronic bending deformities typically in the long bones of the lower extremities), compression (commonly seen in vertebral bodies, leading to kyphosis), and fracture.

Nutritional Rickets

Rickets may be divided into nutritional and nonnutritional types. Nutritional rickets, perhaps more appropriately labeled vitamin D-deficient rickets, results from inadequate intake or inadequate production of vitamin D, secondary to insufficient exposure to sunlight. Vegan diets are notoriously implicated in rickets, as strict followers avoid almost all natural dietary sources of vitamin D, including fish, eggs, meats, and dairy. Patients who have been exclusively breast-fed without vitamin D supplementation are also at risk, because human breast milk alone is not a sufficient source of vitamin D. Similarly at risk are children living in northern regions (latitudes northward of New York City) and dark-skinned children whose abundance of melanin can shield the catalytic effects of ultraviolet light in the dermal production of previtamin D_3 from its cholesterol derivatives. Previtamin D_3 is a precursor to the active metabolite of vitamin D, 1,25-dihydroxyvitamin D_3. This hydroxylation process—the pathway by which vitamin D becomes biochemically active—occurs next in the liver, and finally in the kidneys. Renal and/or hepatic failure, therefore, can also lead to rickets. Figure 44–1 depicts the metabolic pathways by which vitamin D is synthesized and activated.

Nonnutritional Rickets

Nonnutritional rickets refers to a group of several genetic disorders affecting enzymes responsible for vitamin D metabolism. Although many mutations have been described, the most common form of nonnutritional rickets is familial hypophosphatemic rickets, caused by an X-linked mutation resulting in defective phosphate transport in the renal tubules. As a general rule, management should be referred to pediatric endocrinology specialists, as these diseases often have complex workups and disease-specific therapies.

Clinical Findings

Greenstick fractures after minimal trauma may be a heralding sign of rickets. Ambulatory toddlers often present with vague bone pain, waddling gate, and/or angular bowing of the lower extremity long bones with "genu varum," or outwardly bowed knees. Older children may instead exhibit genu valgum, or "knocked knees." Additional findings include pectus deformities and exaggerated curvatures of the spine marked by increased thoracic kyphosis and lumbar lordosis. Patients with severe forms of the disease may even exhibit generalized muscular weakness, tetany, or "floppiness" in infants, secondary to decreased concentrations of circulating calcium.

Laboratory and Radiographic Findings

All patients with histories or physical exams suspicious for rickets should receive laboratory testing for serum 25-hydroxyvitamin D, 1,25-dihydroxyvitamin D, calcium, phosphorus, and alkaline phosphatase levels. Patients with nutritional rickets will typically have findings of normal-to-low levels of serum calcium, low phosphate, low vitamin D, and increased levels of alkaline phosphatase and parathyroid hormone.

Radiographs of long bones typically show bowed diaphyses with widening of metaphyses. Metaphyses may also appear "cupped," with a central area of depression and are frayed at the periphery. Generalized osteopenia may be evident. Finally, chest x-ray may reveal rachitic rosary, or a beaded-like appearance of the ribs, secondary to heterogenous enlargement of the costal cartilage.

Management

Patients with nutritional rickets respond largely to dietary vitamin D supplementation. Breast-fed infants are recommended to receive oral supplementation with 400 international units (IU) of vitamin D daily and/or increased sunlight or ultraviolet light exposure. For infants, exposure to a half-hour of sunlight per week in the summer while wearing only a diaper, or 2 hours per week while clothed, is considered sufficient.

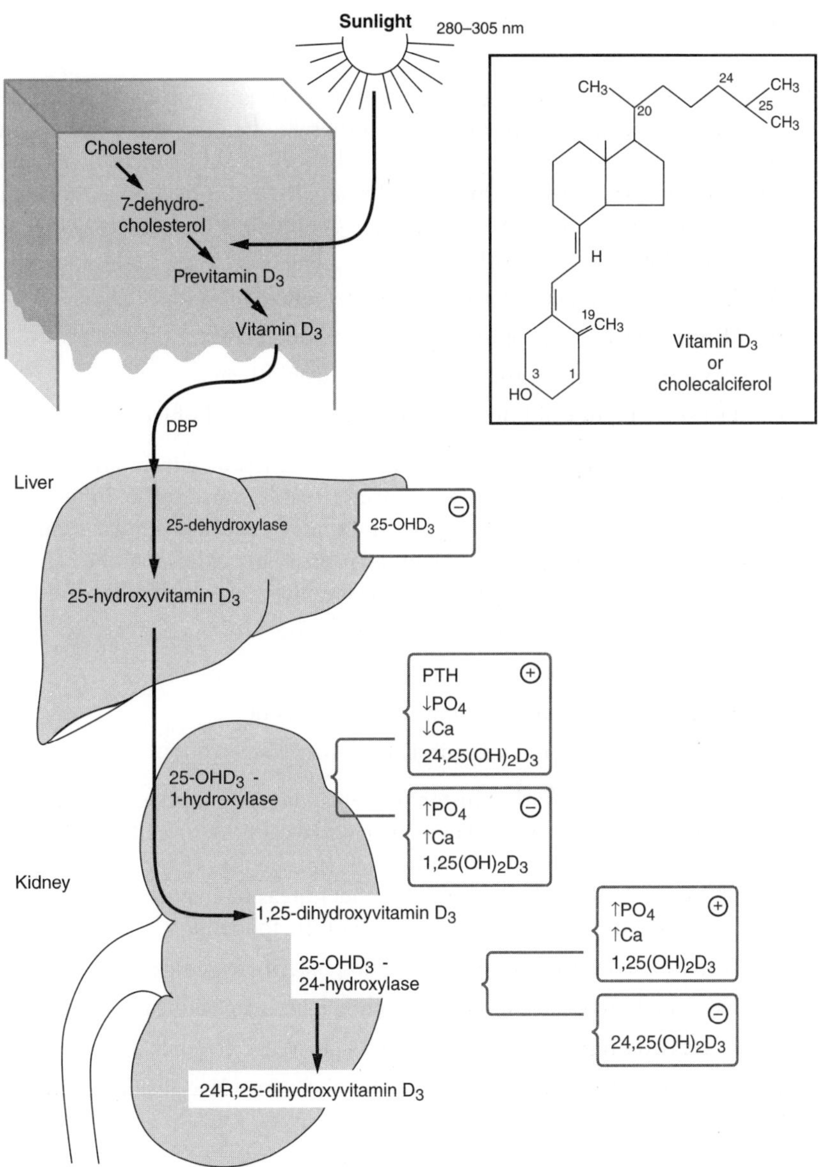

Figure 44–1. Metabolic pathways of vitamin D synthesis and activation. (Reproduced, with permission, from Toy EC, Yetman RJ, Girardet RB, et al. *Case Files: Pediatrics.* 3rd ed. New York, NY: McGraw-Hill; 2010:Fig. 7-1.)

The American Academy of Pediatrics recommends that all infants may benefit from vitamin D supplementation until they are able to drink 500 mL of vitamin D–fortified milk or formula daily. As stated, patients with nonnutritional rickets should generally be referred to a pediatric endocrinologist for further workup and management. In patients undergoing workup for surgical correction for long bone deformities, it is essential that the disease is metabolically stable.

COMPREHENSION QUESTIONS

44.1 A 6-year-old girl is seen in your office with complaints of insidious bilateral leg pain, 3 months in duration. She is otherwise healthy and is fair-skinned and freckled. Because of a strong family history of skin cancer, her parents rarely let her play outside. On physical exam, she exhibits mild genu valgum, or "knocked-knees." Plain radiographs are obtained. Which of the following is a radiographic feature likely to be seen?

A. Diffuse ground-glass opacities in the femoral diaphyses

B. "Rugger jersey" appearance of spine on lateral chest x-ray

C. Physeal widening of the proximal and distal tibiae

D. Dense metaphyseal lines of the proximal and distal tibiae

44.2 A mother and her 2 young sons are referred to your clinic. Although the mother appears normal, both boys are noticeably short and exhibit marked genu varum. The mother states that their father exhibits similar symptoms. Following workup, a diagnosis of familial primary hypophosphatemia (FPH) is made. This cause of nonnutritional rickets results from which of the following?

A. X-linked dominant mutation in PHEX gene

B. Autosomal dominant mutation in PHEX gene

C. Recessive mutation in vitamin D receptor gene

D. X-linked mutation in vitamin D receptor gene

44.3 A 13-year-old female with a history of celiac disease is referred to your clinic with complaints of generalized bone pain and weakness, as well as recent complaints of occasional muscle spasms. On exam, she is noted to have poor dentition, bowed long bones, and mildly tender areas of costochondral swelling. Laboratory testing will likely show which of the following?

A. Increased serum calcium, decreased phosphate, increased alkaline phosphatase

B. Decreased serum calcium, decreased phosphate, increased alkaline phosphatase

C. Decreased serum calcium, decreased phosphate, decreased alkaline phosphatase

D. Increased serum calcium, increased phosphate, increased alkaline phosphatase

ANSWERS

44.1 **C.** Nutritional rickets, which includes rickets secondary to inadequate sunlight exposure, may produce radiographic findings of physeal cupping and widening, generalized osteopenia, and genu varum or valgum. Physeal widening is caused by abnormal mineralization at the growth plate or chondroid calcification. This leads to a build-up of chondroid at the physis, which gives the appearance of widened physis on radiographs. A "rugger jersey" spine is seen in patients with secondary hyperparathyroidism of chronic renal failure or osteopetrosis. Dense metaphyseal banding may be indicative of lead poisoning or heavy metal deposition. Ground glass opacities are a relatively nonspecific finding, sometimes seen in fibrous dysplasia.

44.2 **A.** FPH is the most common form of nonnutritional vitamin D–independent rickets. It is caused by an X-linked dominant mutation in the phosphate-regulating neutral endopeptidase, or PHEX, gene. This mutation causes an excessive excretion of phosphate in the renal tubules.

44.3 **B.** Many patients suffering from gastrointestinal disorders have an elevated risk for developing nutritional rickets, due to malabsorption of vitamin D, a fat-soluble vitamin. Decreased absorption of vitamin D leads to a subsequent decrease in serum calcium and phosphorus concentrations. Decreased serum calcium and phosphorous will cause the increase in alkaline phosphatase.

CLINICAL PEARLS

- In developed countries, nutritional rickets is uncommon.
- Clavicle fractures in infants grossly below weight, height, and/or head circumference norms should alert the examiner to the possibility of an underlying diagnosis of rickets.
- Common radiographic findings of rickets include bowed long bone diaphyses with "cupped," "frayed," or widened metaphyses. Chest x-ray may reveal rachitic rosary, or a beaded-like appearance of the ribs.

REFERENCES

Brooks WC, Gross RH. Genu varum in children: diagnosis and treatment. *J Am Acad Orthop Surg.* 1995;3:326-335.

Flynn JM, ed. Bone metabolism and metabolic bone disease. *Orthopaedic Knowledge Update: Ten.* Rosemont, IL: American Academy of Orthopaedic Surgeons; 2011:189-192.

Tortolani PJ, McCarthy EF, Sponseller PD. Bone mineral density deficiency in children. *J Am Acad Orthop Surg.* 2002;10:57-66.

Toy EC, Yetman RJ, Girardet R, et al. *Case Files: Pediatrics.* 3rd ed. New York: McGraw-Hill Medical; 2003:65-73.

CASE 45

A 60-year-old white woman presents for a 6-week postoperative follow-up after intramedullary fixation of her intertrochanteric femoral neck fracture. She sustained the fracture after she tripped in her kitchen. In clinic, she gives a history of a low-energy distal radius fracture 5 years ago. She also believes that she recently has become shorter. Her family history is significant for multiple fractures in her mother and sister. She had an early menopause at the age of 40 and did not receive hormone replacement therapy. She has no other significant past medical history and is otherwise in good health. Physical exam reveals a 52-inch tall frail elderly woman with a body mass index (BMI) of 19 kg/m^2. Her height has decreased by 2.5 inches over the past several years. She has a significant kyphosis of her thoracic spine and an unsteady gait. Her surgical wound is healing well.

- ▶ What is the most likely diagnosis?
- ▶ What is the next diagnostic step?
- ▶ What is the best initial treatment?

ANSWERS TO CASE 45: Osteoporosis

Summary: A 60-year-old postmenopausal woman presents after sustaining multiple fragility fractures. She has a family history of fractures in first-degree relatives. She recently lost height and has significant kyphosis of the thoracic spine.

- **Most likely diagnosis:** Osteoporosis.
- **Investigations:** Dual-energy x-ray absorptiometry (DXA), complete metabolic panel, vitamin D, parathyroid hormone (PTH), and urine collagen N-telopeptide crosslinks (NTX).
- **Initial treatment:** Physical therapy, calcium and vitamin D supplementation, and bisphosphonates.

ANALYSIS

Objectives

1. Understand the pathogenesis of osteoporosis and underlying conditions leading to fragility fractures.
2. Develop a comprehensive approach to patients with osteoporosis including history, physical exam, appropriate laboratory investigations, and DXA.
3. Be aware of potential nonpharmacologic and pharmacologic treatments to prevent future fragility fractures.

Considerations

This case presents a postmenopausal woman who has suffered a low-energy hip fracture: a devastating sequelae of osteoporosis. **According to the most recent statistics, 50% of patients who sustain a hip fracture will never attain their previous functional status, and 25% will die within the first year after the fracture.** The annual cost of all osteoporotic fractures is as high as $18 billion; yet, as is the case with this patient, 80% of patients who have had a previous fragility fracture do not receive treatment for osteoporosis. The patient in this case has several risk factors that warrant an osteoporosis workup and treatment: female sex, white race, personal history of a previous fragility fracture, history of fracture in a first-degree relative, low BMI, and early menopause. Menopause leads to an increased risk of osteoporosis as a result of the loss of estrogen's suppressive effects on osteoclast-mediated bone resorption. Activation of osteoclasts results in rapid loss of bone mineral density (BMD), increasing the patient's risk of fracture. Furthermore, because estrogen is synthesized in peripheral adipose tissue, the patient's low BMI results in even lower estrogen levels. Being frail could indicate poor nutrition and potentially inadequate calcium and vitamin D intake, further increasing her risk of fracture. Her kyphosis and loss of height are also common complications of osteoporosis owing to compression fractures of the spinal vertebrae.

To prevent future fractures in this patient, a baseline DXA and lab investigations should be obtained to confirm the diagnosis of primary osteoporosis and rule out secondary causes. **Serum calcium and vitamin D must be corrected with daily supplementation.** Fall prevention needs to be addressed to decrease this patient's risk of future fracture. Pharmacologic treatment is indicated, and bisphosphonates are first-line agents. Bone markers are then used to monitor bisphosphonate treatment.

APPROACH TO: Osteoporosis

DEFINITIONS

FRAGILITY FRACTURES: Fractures after low-energy trauma such as a fall from standing height or less.

DUAL-ENERGY X-RAY ABSORPTIOMETRY (DXA): The standard tool to measure BMD for the diagnosis of osteoporosis. Bone mass is reported as a real density, which is then compared with both age-matched adults (Z-score) and young healthy adults (T-score). Z and T scores represent standard deviations from the mean established by the comparison group. Bone density is characterized by the lowest value at the spine, femoral neck, trochanter, or total femur. T-score values of 0 to –1 are considered normal; –1 to –2.5 indicates osteopenia; lower than –2.5 indicates osteoporosis.

PRIMARY OSTEOPOROSIS: A skeletal disorder characterized by compromised bone strength predisposing to an increased risk of fracture that occurs in individuals as they age or after menopause

SECONDARY OSTEOPOROSIS: Osteoporosis due to an underlying cause of bone loss and structural deterioration that can be treated, such as an endocrine abnormality, medication, or neoplastic condition. Table 45–1 outlines the causes of secondary osteoporosis.

FRAX: A fracture risk assessment tool developed by the World Health Organization, which merges BMD and clinical risk factors to establish a 10-year fracture risk.

CLINICAL APPROACH

Pathophysiology of osteoporosis

Bone strength is determined by 2 factors: bone quantity and quality. Bone quantity is assessed by DXA, which measures BMD. Bone quality, on the other hand, is a function of the microarchitecture and mineral and collagen composition of the extracellular matrix. In general, bone undergoes a dynamic process of renewal that involves coupling of both bone resorption and formation, known as bone remodeling. Bone remodeling, or turnover, is the principal factor that controls both the quality and quantity of bone in the adult skeleton.

Osteoporosis is characterized by low bone mass and the structural deterioration of bone tissue, which leads to bone fragility and an increased susceptibility to fractures.

Table 45–1 • UNDERLYING CAUSES OF SECONDARY OSTEOPOROSIS

Category	Disease
Disorders of bone mineral homeostasis	Rickets and osteomalacia
Endocrine abnormalities	Hyperparathyroidism Hyperthyroidism Hypogonadism Cushing syndrome
Medications	Alcohol Glucocorticoids Chemotherapy (methotrexate, cyclophosphamide) Radiotherapy Anticonvulsants (phenytoin, carbamazepine) Excess thyroid hormone replacement
Neoplasms	Multiple myeloma

Source: Courtesy of Joseph M. Lane, MD.

In osteoporosis, there is an imbalance between osteoclast-mediated bone resorption and osteoblast-mediated bone formation. **High-turnover osteoporosis** is characterized by an increased activity of osteoclasts, leading to bone loss and an abnormal bone microarchitecture. This is the most common form of osteoporosis and occurs in postmenopausal women or in patients with hyperparathyroidism. In **low-turnover osteoporosis,** a reduction in osteoblastic activity leads to reduced bone formation. This type of osteoporosis is seen in the elderly or after interventions that inhibit the activity of osteoblasts, including chemotherapy, radiotherapy, or corticosteroids. Any other underlying condition that disturbs the balance of bone remodeling can potentially lead to osteoporosis (Table 45–1).

Patient Evaluation

Osteoporosis is frequently recognized when a patient seeks medical attention for back pain, fragility fracture, or loss of height or spinal deformity due to vertebral compression fractures. Once osteoporosis is suspected, the patient should be evaluated with a comprehensive medical history and physical examination. The primary aim of the patient history is to identify modifiable and nonmodifiable risk factors (Table 45–2).

Findings on physical exam may include spinal deformities such as exaggerated thoracic kyphosis, loss of height from osteoporotic compression fractures (often >2 inches), and clinical signs of potential collagen disorders such as joint laxity, skin hyperextensibility, blue sclera, translucent teeth, and other skeletal abnormalities. Also, gait and balance should be examined to assess for increased risk of falls.

DXA is currently the reference standard for BMD measurement. Determining BMD at the spine and hip is needed to confirm the diagnosis of osteoporosis, assess the rate of BMD loss, and predict future fracture risk. **The National Osteoporosis Foundation (NOF) recommends DXA screening for all women over 65 years of age and men over 70 years regardless of risk factors, or younger postmenopausal women with one or more risk factors.**

Table 45–2 • RISK FACTORS FOR OSTEOPOROSIS
Nonmodifiable
Personal history of fracture
History of fracture in a first-degree relative
Female sex
Advanced age
White or Asian descent
Modifiable
Current cigarette smoking
Low body weight (<127 lb) or low body mass index (<20)
Low calcium and vitamin D intake
Excessive alcohol intake
Use of certain medications such as corticosteroids and anticonvulsants
Recurrent falls
Estrogen deficiency and early menopause

Source: Courtesy of Joseph M. Lane, MD.

Laboratory testing is performed to rule out secondary causes of osteoporosis, assess the severity of the disease, and establish baseline data to measure the response to therapeutic interventions. Serum calcium, 25-hydroxyvitamin D [25(OH)D], and parathyroid hormone (PTH) are measured to rule out osteomalacia, vitamin D deficiency, and hyperparathyroidism. Other tests include thyroid and renal function tests and a 24-hour urine calcium. Bone turnover can be assessed by measuring biochemical bone markers, categorized as markers of bone formation or bone resorption (Table 45–3). Bone markers are also used to measure response to treatment.

TREATMENT

Nonpharmacologic Treatment

The goal of treatment in patients with either osteoporosis or a fragility fracture is to prevent future fractures. Nonpharmacologic treatment to ensure proper bone health is crucial for every orthopaedic patient (see Figure 45–1). Calcium supplementation has been shown to decrease fracture rates and is recommended for all osteoporotic patients. Vitamin D has been shown to be important in maintaining calcium homeostasis, preventing falls and even improving muscle function. Serum monitoring of 25(OH)D and PTH levels is done to ensure that 25(OH)D levels are maintained

Table 45–3 • BIOCHEMICAL MARKERS OF BONE TURNOVER

Bone Formation Markers	Bone Resorption Markers
Enzymes secreted by osteoblasts Bone-specific alkaline phosphatase (BSAP)	**Enzymes secreted by osteoclasts** Tartrate-resistant acid phosphatase (TRAP) **Collagen degradation byproducts** Urine N-telopeptide crosslinks (NTX) Serum C-telopeptide crosslinks (CTX)

Source: Courtesy of Joseph M. Lane, MD.

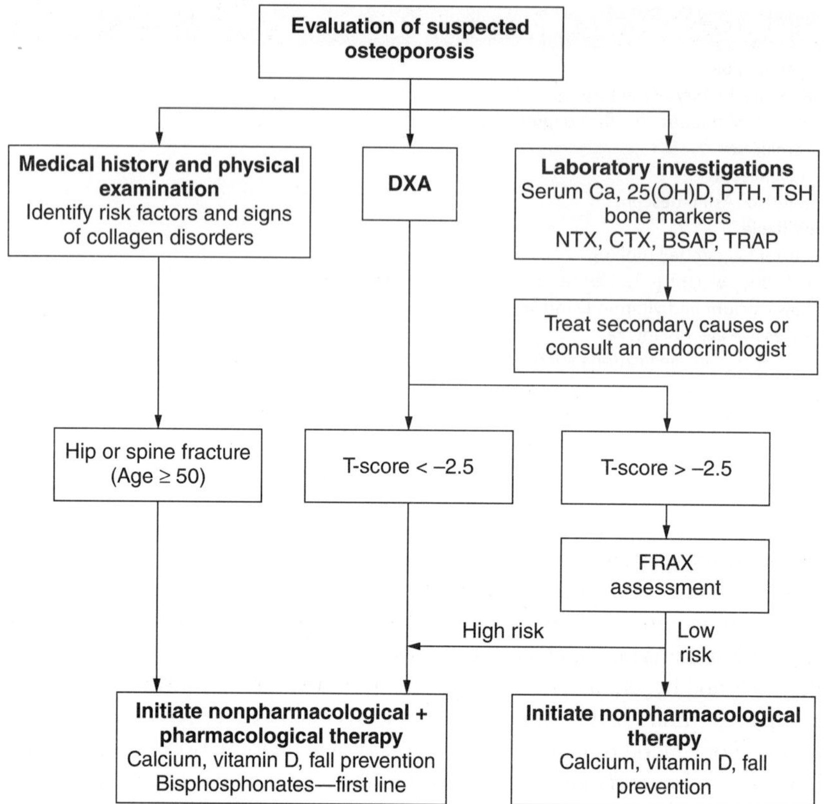

Figure 45–1. A flow chart showing a comprehensive management of fragility fractures in an osteoporotic patient. Ca, calcium; 25(OH)D, vitamin D; PTH, parathyroid hormone; NTX, N-telopeptide collagen crosslinks; CTX, C-telopeptide collagen crosslinks; BSAP, bone-specific alkaline phosphatase; TRAP, tartrate-resistant acid phosphatase. (Courtesy of Joseph M. Lane, MD)

in the normal range and to prevent elevations in serum PTH. In addition to optimizing calcium and vitamin D levels, physicians should focus on eliminating modifiable risk factors such as smoking, heavy alcohol consumption, and recurrent falls. **Fall prevention requires a multifactorial approach** that addresses vision deficits, balance and gait abnormalities, cognitive impairments, and dizziness. It is also important to eliminate medications that can affect alertness and balance.

Pharmacologic treatment

According to the National Osteoporosis Foundation (NOF), indications for pharmacologic treatment include men and postmenopausal women age 50 and older presenting with a hip or vertebral fracture, a T-score of –2.5 or below, or low bone mass (T-score between –1.0 and –2.5) accompanied by a high probability of future fracture as determined by the FRAX. Pharmacologic treatment for osteoporosis can currently be divided into 2 categories: antiresorptive and anabolic agents.

Antiresorptive agents such as bisphosphonates diminish rapid osteoclast-mediated resorption, whereas anabolic agents such as teriparatide build bone by stimulating osteoblast activity. Although both antiresorptive and anabolic agents have demonstrated antifracture efficacy, **bisphosphonates are considered the first-line treatment for patients with osteoporosis.**

Bisphosphonates have been proven to be effective in reducing fractures, improving BMD, and normalizing elevated serum bone markers. In patients with a fragility fracture, it is considered ideal to begin bisphosphonate treatment between 2 and 12 weeks after the fracture to ensure increased callus size and strength in healing. Bisphosphonates can be given orally, but can cause gastrointestinal complications, which may require intravenous delivery in some patients. **It is important to normalize serum calcium and vitamin D before initiating bisphosphonate treatment, as a common electrolyte abnormality attributed to bisphosphonates is hypocalcemia.**

Teriparatide is a recombinant human parathyroid hormone and is the only approved anabolic agent for the treatment of postmenopausal osteoporosis. Teriparatide can lead to an increase in BMD at the lumbar spine and reduce the risk of vertebral and nonvertebral fractures. **Although no consensus exists on when to treat osteoporosis with teriparatide, it should be considered in patients with continued bone loss or fragility fractures despite antiresorptive therapy, or patients with low turnover osteoporosis.** Teriparatide is contraindicated in patients with active metastatic skeletal disease, or patients with high risk for developing osteosarcoma, including patients with active Paget disease or a history of skeletal radiation. Currently, treatment is recommended for up to 24 months, followed by bisphosphonate therapy to maintain the improvement in BMD.

Raloxifene is a selective estrogen receptor modulator approved for the treatment of postmenopausal osteoporosis. Because of its side-effect profile, raloxifene is likely best used in postmenopausal women with osteoporosis who are unable to tolerate bisphosphonates, have no vasomotor symptoms or history of venous thromboembolism, and have a high breast cancer risk score. Other therapies for the treatment of osteoporosis include hormone therapy and calcitonin, which are not as effective as the first-line medications.

COMPREHENSION QUESTIONS

45.1 A 65-year-old white woman presents to your clinic after her first DXA. Her spine T-score is –2.2, and her right femoral neck T-score is –2.9. What is the best next step to reduce her risk of future fractures?

A. Calcium and vitamin D supplementation

B. Raloxifene

C. Calcium, vitamin D, and bisphosphonates

D. Calcium, vitamin D, and teriparatide

E. Bisphosphonates

45.2 A 70-year-old woman was prescribed alendronate for treatment of her osteoporosis. She presents to the clinic with a chief complaint of severe nausea, acidity, and heartburn after taking her medication. She had a history of gastrointestinal reflux disease and an "irritable stomach." Her NTX:Cr (N-telopeptide:creatinine) ratio was 45 (therapeutic range, 20-30). What is the most appropriate treatment option for this patient?

A. Risedronate
B. Ibandronate
C. Zoledronate
D. Teriparatide (PTH)
E. Raloxifene

45.3 A 58-year-old osteoporotic woman presents with persistent hypocalcemia after 3 months of adequate treatment with calcium and vitamin D. Today her corrected calcium is 8.7 (normal range: 8.8-10.2 mg/dL), vitamin D of 35 (normal range: 30-100 ng/mL), and PTH of 100 (normal range: 10-65 pg/mL). A 24-hour urinary calcium test is ordered. Additionally, which of the following tests should be part of her metabolic workup?

A. Thyroid-stimulating hormone (TSH)
B. Fasting blood glucose and hemoglobin A1C
C. 24-hour urinary creatinine
D. Anti-tissue transglutaminase antibodies (tTGA) or anti-endomysium antibodies
E. None of the above

43.4 A 78-year-old woman with known history of osteoporosis sustained a low-energy rib fracture. Despite the fact that she has been on alendronate for 4 years, her DXA T-score continues to decline. She is currently being treated conservatively with pain management. What is the appropriate next step in managing her osteoporosis?

A. Stop alendronate.
B. Lower the dose of alendronate.
C. Switch to risedronate.
D. Stop alendronate and start teriparatide.

ANSWERS

45.1 **C.** Because bone density is characterized by the lowest T-score at any site, the patient's femoral neck T-score places her in the osteoporotic range. The NOF recommends pharmacologic therapy for patients with T-scores below –2.5. Bisphosphonates are the first line of treatment and therefore should be initiated in this patient. Because bisphosphonate therapy can cause hypocalcemia, calcium and vitamin D should be corrected and monitored. Raloxifene (choice B) remains inferior to bisphosphonates, as it has not shown to reduce risk of hip fractures. Teriparatide (choice D) is currently reserved as a "rescue" drug for patients who fail bisphosphonate therapy.

45.2 **C.** Oral bisphosphonates include alendronate, risedronate, and ibandronate. In patients who have no underlying gastrointestinal sensitivity, side effects from oral bisphosphonates are uncommon. However, in subjects with a moderate history of gastrointestinal intolerance, side effects are much more common and may approach 20%. These adverse effects include irritation of the esophagus, acid eructation, nausea, and heartburn. Therefore, all patients are advised to take oral bisphosphonates on an empty stomach and wait at least 30 minutes in an upright position (sitting or standing) before eating or drinking. Because this patient is experiencing severe gastrointestinal (GI) symptoms while on alendronate, she should be treated with an intravenous bisphosphonate to bypass the GI tract. From the choices given, only zoledronate (choice C) is given intravenously. The NTX is relatively high, indicating inadequate suppression of bone turnover due to poor compliance. Intravenous zoledronate can correct the NTX within a few days.

45.3 **D.** Calcium is one of the major constituents of bone and, coupled with vitamin D has been shown to reduce the risk of fractures. The Institute of Medicine recommends 1000 to 1500 mg/day of daily calcium intake. The calcium management in this case, however, poses a challenge. The patient continues to have low serum calcium levels despite receiving adequate calcium and vitamin D. In such cases, further laboratory investigation is needed to rule out conditions or disorders that may increase urinary excretion or impair calcium absorption from the gut. Testing should include 24-hour urine calcium excretion and serologic studies to investigate for malabsorption disorders such as gluten-sensitive enteropathy (choice D). TSH (choice A) is not directly involved in maintaining calcium homeostasis. Testing for diabetes is not indicated in this scenario, as diabetes is unlikely to account for these malabsorption-related findings.

45.4 **D.** This case is an example of a patient who sustained a fragility fracture while on bisphosphonate therapy. Moreover, her DXA T-score continued to decline despite bisphosphonate therapy. In such cases, stopping the bisphosphonate and starting teriparatide to stimulate bone remodeling is recommended. Also, teriparatide stimulates callus formation, thus enhancing fracture healing and potentially reducing the rate of delayed union or nonunion.

CLINICAL PEARLS

- Careful evaluation of all patients with a fragility fracture will enable the orthopaedic surgeon to identify the cause of fracture and implement a treatment plan that can prevent subsequent fractures in this vulnerable population.
- DXA is the standard tool to measure BMD for the diagnosis of osteoporosis. A T-score between –1.0 and –2.5 indicates osteopenia, and below –2.5 indicates osteoporosis.
- Calcium and vitamin D supplementation is important for maintaining bone strength, enhancing muscle strength, preventing falls, and reducing the risk of fractures.
- Bisphosphonates are the standard treatment for osteoporosis, whereas teriparatide is reserved for patients at high risk of fracture with declining BMD despite bisphosphonate therapy.

REFERENCES

American Association of Clinical Endocrinologists medical guidelines for clinical practice for the diagnosis and treatment of postmenopausal osteoporosis. *Endocr Pract*. 2010;16(Suppl 3):1-37.

National Osteoporosis Foundation. Clinician's Guide to Prevention and Treatment of Osteoporosis. Washington, DC: National Osteoporosis Foundation; 2010.

Rebolledo BJ, Unnanuntana A, Lane JM. A comprehensive approach to fragility fractures. *J Orthop Trauma*. 2011;25:566-573.

Sweet MG, Sweet JM, Jeremiah MP, Galazka SS. Diagnosis and treatment of osteoporosis. *Am Fam Physician*. 2009;79:193-200.

Unnanuntana A, Gladnick BP, Donnelly E, Lane JM. The assessment of fracture risk. *J Bone Joint Surg Am*. 2010;92:743-753.

SECTION III

Listing of Cases

Listing by Case Number

Listing by Case Topic (Alphabetical)

Listing by Case Number

CASE NO.	TOPIC	CASE PAGE
1	Anterior Shoulder Dislocation	24
2	Distal Radius (Colles) Fracture	34
3	Posterior Hip Dislocation	42
4	Femoral Neck Fracture	50
5	Intertrochanteric Hip Fracture	60
6	Periprosthetic Hip Fracture	68
7	Patellar Tendon Rupture	78
8	Tibial Plateau Fracture	86
9	Open Tibia Fracture	95
10	Proximal Humerus Fracture	102
11	Clavicle Fracture	112
12	Ankle Fracture	120
13	Acute Compartment Syndrome	130
14	Pediatric Both Bone Forearm Fracture	141
15	Supracondylar Humerus Fracture	148
16	Child Abuse	156
17	Slipped Capital Femoral Epiphysis	165
18	Developmental Dysplasia of the Hip	172
19	Septic Knee	180
20	Osteomyelitis	189
21	Rotator Cuff Injury	198
22	Anterior Cruciate Ligament Reconstruction	208
23	Meniscal Tears	220
24	Ulnar Collateral Ligament Injury of the Elbow	228
25	Herniated Nucleus Pulposus of the Cervical Spine	236
26	Cauda Equina Syndrome	244
27	Lumbar Burst Fracture	252
28	Adolescent Idiopathic Scoliosis	260
29	Carpal Tunnel Syndrome	268
30	Cubital Tunnel Syndrome	276
31	Dupuytren Disease	284
32	Trigger Finger	292
33	Lateral Epicondylitis	298
34	Achilles Tendon Rupture	306
35	Adult Acquired Flatfoot Deformity	314
36	Lisfranc Injury	324
37	Calcaneus Fracture	335
38	Osteosarcoma	346
39	Total Knee Arthroplasty	354

40	Hip Osteoarthritis	364
41	Shoulder Arthroplasty	372
42	Gout	382
43	Rheumatoid Arthritis	390
44	Rickets	398
45	Osteoporosis	406

Listing by Case Topic (Alphabetical)

CASE NO.	TOPIC	CASE PAGE
34	Achilles Tendon Rupture	306
13	Acute Compartment Syndrome	130
28	Adolescent Idiopathic Scoliosis	260
35	Adult Acquired Flatfoot Deformity	314
12	Ankle Fracture	120
22	Anterior Cruciate Ligament Reconstruction	208
1	Anterior Shoulder Dislocation	24
37	Calcaneus Fracture	335
29	Carpal Tunnel Syndrome	268
26	Cauda Equina Syndrome	244
16	Child Abuse	156
11	Clavicle Fracture	112
30	Cubital Tunnel Syndrome	276
18	Developmental Dysplasia of the Hip	172
2	Distal Radius (Colles) Fracture	34
31	Dupuytren Disease	284
4	Femoral Neck Fracture	50
42	Gout	382
25	Herniated Nucleus Pulposus of the Cervical Spine	236
40	Hip Osteoarthritis	364
5	Intertrochanteric Hip Fracture	60
33	Lateral Epicondylitis	298
36	Lisfranc Injury	324
27	Lumbar Burst Fracture	252
23	Meniscal Tears	220
9	Open Tibia Fracture	95
20	Osteomyelitis	189
45	Osteoporosis	406
38	Osteosarcoma	346
7	Patellar Tendon Rupture	78

14	Pediatric Both Bone Forearm Fracture	141
6	Periprosthetic Hip Fracture	68
3	Posterior Hip Dislocation	42
10	Proximal Humerus Fracture	102
43	Rheumatoid Arthritis	390
44	Rickets	398
21	Rotator Cuff Injury	198
19	Septic Knee	180
41	Shoulder Arthroplasty	372
17	Slipped Capital Femoral Epiphysis	165
15	Supracondylar Humerus Fracture	148
8	Tibial Plateau Fracture	86
39	Total Knee Arthroplasty	354
32	Trigger Finger	292
24	Ulnar Collateral Ligament Injury of the Elbow	228

INDEX

Note: Page numbers followed by a t or f indicate that the entry is included in a table or figure.

A

AAFD. *See* Adult acquired flatfoot deformity (AAFD)
ACDF (anterior cervical discectomy and fusion), 239
Acetaminophen, for cervical radiculopathy, 239
Achilles tendon rupture, 305-311
  analysis of, 306
  clinical pearls for, 311
  comprehension questions for, 310-311
  definitions related to, 307, 307*f*
  etiology of, 308
  imaging of, 308-309, 309*f*
  pathoanatomy and, 308
  physical exam for, 308
  treatment of, 309-310
Acromioclavicular joint, 113
Adolescent(s), slipped capital femoral epiphysis in. *See* Slipped capital femoral epiphysis (SCFE)
Adolescent idiopathic scoliosis (AIS), 259-265
  analysis of, 260-261
  clinical pearls for, 265
  clinical presentation of, 262
  complications of, 263-264
  comprehension questions for, 264-265
  definitions related to, 261
  etiology of, 262
  treatment of, 262-264, 263*f*
Adrenocorticotropic hormone, for gout, 385
Adult acquired flatfoot deformity (AAFD), 313-321
  analysis of, 314, 315*f*, 316*f*
  clinical pearls for, 321
  clinical presentation of, 318
  comprehension questions for, 319-320
  definitions related to, 317
  diagnosis of, 318
  etiology of, 317-318
  treatment of, 318-319
Advanced Trauma Life Support (ATLS) protocol, 2
Age of patient, 2
AIN (anterior interosseous nerve), injury to, supracondylar fractures and, 148, 149, 151, 153
AIS. *See* Adolescent idiopathic scoliosis (AIS)
Allergies, 4
Allis maneuver, 43, 45, 173*f*, 173-174
Allopurinol, for gout, 385, 386
AMBRI, 29
Anabolic agents, for osteoporosis, 411
Anal wink reflex, 245, 247
Anderson classification of open fractures, 95*t*, 96
Angiofibroblastic dysplasia, 299, 300*f*. *See also* Lateral epicondylitis
Ankle fractures, 119*f*, 119-128
  analysis of, 120
  anatomy and, 121
  classification, 122-123, 124*f*-125*f*, 126
  clinical pearls for, 128
  complications of, 126
  comprehension questions for, 126-128
  definitions related to, 121
  examination of, 121
  radiographic evaluation of, 122, 123*f*
  treatment of, 126

Ankle impingement, anterior, following calcaneus fractures, 340
Anterior cervical discectomy and fusion (ACDF), 239
Anterior cruciate ligament injury, 207-216
 analysis of, 208
 anatomy and biomechanics and, 209-211, 210*f*
 clinical pearls for, 216
 complications of, 214
 comprehension questions for, 215-216
 definitions related to, 209
 differential diagnosis of, 211
 epidemiology of, 209
 imaging of, 211, 212*f*
 nonoperative treatment of, 213
 physical exam in, 211
 reconstruction for
  postoperative care and rehabilitation for, 214-215
  rationale for, 213
Anterior drawer test, 209, 211
Anterior humeral line, 149, 150
Anterior interosseous nerve (AIN), injury to, supracondylar fractures and, 148, 149, 151, 153
Anterior talofibular ligament, 121
Antibiotics
 for open tibia fractures, 95, 96, 96*t*, 99
 for osteomyelitis, 192
Anti-cyclic citrullinated peptide (CCP), in rheumatoid arthritis, 390, 391, 392
Antiresorptive agents, for osteoporosis, 411
Apley test, 221, 221*f*, 222
Appearance, general, 4
Arizona brace, 317
Arm casts, 11
Arthritis
 calcaneocuboid, following calcaneus fractures, 340
 osteoarthritis. *See* Hip osteoarthritis; Knee osteoarthritis; Osteoarthritis (OA)
 posttraumatic, of knee, 356
 rheumatoid. *See* Rheumatoid arthritis (RA)
 septic, 181-182, 184
 subtalar, following calcaneus fractures, 339
 types of, 366
Arthrocentesis, 181
Arthrography, in rotator cuff injury, 206
Arthropathies. *See also specific arthropathies*
 crystal-induced. *See* Gout
 inflammatory, clinical presentation of, 356
 rotator cuff, 200
Arthroplasty, 13, 356
 disc, for cervical radiculopathy, 240
 for femoral neck fractures, 55
 hemiarthroplasty
  definition of, 52
  shoulder, 373, 376
 of hip, hip fracture following. *See* Hip fractures, periprosthetic
 for osteoarthritis of the knee, 357-358
 prosthetic joint lifetime and, 357
 shoulder. *See* Shoulder arthroplasty
Arthroscopy, 13
 for osteoarthritis of the knee, 357
ATLS (Advanced Trauma Life Support) protocol, 2
 with posterior hip dislocations, 42, 45
Avascular necrosis (AVN)
 definition of, 43, 52
 following femoral neck fractures, 56
 of knee, 356
 following proximal humerus fractures, 103, 107, 108
Avascular osteonecrosis. *See* Avascular necrosis (AVN)

B
Backfire fracture, 35
Bankart lesions, 25, 26
  bony, 25, 26
  operative treatment of, 29
Barlow sign, 174-175, 178
Barton fractures, 35
Baseball pitch, phases of, 228
Bauman angle, 39
BBFFs. *See* Pediatric both bone forearm fractures (BBFFs)
Biofilms, 190
Biologic DMARDs, 391, 393
Bisphosphonates, for osteoporosis, 411, 413
Bladder dysfunction, neurogenic, in cauda equina syndrome, 246
Bledsoe bracing, 12
Blumensaat line, 79, 80, 80*f*
Bohler angle, 336, 337, 337*f*
Brachial plexus, major cervical roots to, 6, 7*t*
Bracing, 12
Bruising, in children, evaluation of, 159
Bulbocavernosus reflex, 247, 254
Burst fractures, 253
  lumbar. *See* Lumbar burst fractures

C
Caffey disease, 159
Calcaneal osteotomy, medializing, 317
Calcaneocuboid arthritis, following calcaneus fractures, 340
Calcaneus fractures, 333*f*, 333-342, 334*f*
  analysis of, 335-336
  classification of, 337
  clinical pearls for, 342
  complications of, 339-341
  comprehension questions for, 341-342
  definitions related to, 336
  diagnosis of, 337, 337*f*
  etiology of, 337
  extraarticular, 336
  intraarticular, 336
  treatment of, 338-341
    nonoperative, 338
    open-reduction internal fixation, 338-339
Calcar femorale, definition of, 52
Calcium
  recommended intake of, 413
  rickets and, 399
Calcium phosphate cement, for tibial plateau fractures, 89
Calcium pyrophosphate dehydrate crystals, 383, 387
Carpal tunnel, 269
Carpal tunnel syndrome (CTS), 267-273
  analysis of, 268-269
  anatomy relevant to, 269-270
  clinical pearls for, 273
  comprehension questions for, 271-272
  definitions related to, 269
  diagnosis of, 270
  treatment of, 270-271
Cartilage, damage to, bacteria causing, 182
Casting, 11-12
  spica, for developmental hip dysplasia, 176
Cauda equina, 253
Cauda equina syndrome (CES), 243-249
  analysis of, 244-245
  anatomy and pathophysiology of, 246-247
  clinical pearls for, 249
  comprehension questions for, 247-249
  definitions related to, 245-246
  outcomes in, 247
  radiographic evaluation of, 247
  treatment of, 247
Cellular atypia, diffuse, with osteosarcoma, 348
Cephalomedullary nails
  definition of, 62
  for intertrochanteric fractures, 64

Cervical nerve roots to brachial and lumbar plexuses, 6, 7*t*
Cervical radiculopathy, 235-242
  analysis of, 236-237
  anatomy and pathophysiology of, 237-238
  clinical pearls for, 242
  complications of, 240
  comprehension questions for, 240-241
  definitions related to, 237
  differential diagnosis of, 238
  history and physical exam of, 238
  imaging of, 239
  treatment of
    nonoperative, 239
    surgical, 239-240
Cervical spine, clearing, 6-7
CES. *See* Cauda equina syndrome (CES)
Chance fractures, 253-254
Chauffeur fractures, 35
Chief complaint, 2
Child abuse, 155*f*, 155-161
  analysis of, 156
  clinical pearls for, 161
  comprehension questions for, 160-161
  definitions related to, 156-157
  differentiation diagnosis and workup of, 158-159
  management of, 159
  musculoskeletal features in, 158, 158*f*
  red flags for, 157, 157*t*
Child Abuse Prevention and Treatment Act, 157
Children. *See* Child abuse; Developmental dysplasia of the hip (DDH); Pediatric both bone forearm fractures (BBFFs); Slipped capital femoral epiphysis (SCFE); Supracondylar fractures
Children's protective services, 157
Childress test, 221*f*, 222
Chronic symptomatology, 2-3
Clavicle fracture, 111*f*, 111-117
  analysis of, 112
  anatomy and mechanism of injury and, 113
  classification of, 114
  clinical pearls for, 117
  complications of, 115
  comprehension questions for, 115-116
  definitions related to, 112-113
  radiographic evaluation of, 113-114
  treatment of, 114-115
Clostridial collagenase histolyticum, for Dupuytren disease, 287
Cobb angle, 261
Codman triangle, 347, 348, 348*f*
Colchicine, for gout, 385, 386
Collagenase injection, for Dupuytren disease, 287
Colles fractures. *See* Radius fractures, distal (Colles)
Compartment syndrome
  acute, 129-137
    analysis of, 130
    clinical approach to, 131-133, 132*t*, 133*f*, 134*f*, 135
    clinical pearls for, 137
    comprehension questions for, 135-136
    definitions related to, 131
    5 Ps in, 130, 131
  with calcaneus fractures, 342
  causes of, 131-132, 132*t*
  chronic, 135
  definition of, 131, 325
  diagnosis of, 132, 133*f*
  with Lisfranc injury, 324-325, 326
  with supracondylar fractures, 151
  surgical treatment of, 132-133, 134*f*
Complex regional pain syndrome (CRPS), following distal radius fractures, 38
Complications, 17-18. *See also under specific injuries and conditions*

Compression fractures, 253
Computed tomography (CT), 8
Concomitant injuries, 2-3
Conditions. *See also specific conditions*
complications associated with, 17-18
mechanisms of, determining, 16
risk factors for, determining, 16
Conoid ligaments, 113
Contractures, flexion, following anterior cruciate ligament reconstruction, 214
Conus medullaris, 253
Coracoclavicular ligaments, 113
Corticosteroids
for carpal tunnel syndrome, 271
for cervical radiculopathy, 239
for gout, 384-385
for rheumatoid arthritis, 396
for rotator cuff injuries, 204
Coxalgic gait, with osteoarthritis of the hip, 366-367
Crankshaft phenomenon, 264
C-reactive protein (CRP) test, 8
Critical angle of Gissane, 336
CRMTOL, 150
Cross-table lateral x-rays, definition of, 52
CRPS (complex regional pain syndrome), following distal radius fractures, 38
CRP (C-reactive protein) test, 8
Crystal-induced arthropathy. *See* Gout
CT (computed tomography), 8
CTS. *See* Carpal tunnel syndrome (CTS)
Cubital tunnel syndrome, 275-281
analysis of, 276-277
anatomy relevant to, 277-278, 278*f*
clinical pearls for, 281
comprehension questions for, 280-281
definitions related to, 277
physical exam for, 278-279
treatment of, 279-280
Cubitus varus, with supracondylar fractures, 151
Cyclops lesions, 214

D

Dashboard injuries, 43, 47
DDH. *See* Developmental dysplasia of the hip (DDH)
Deep vein thrombosis (DVT), following knee arthroplasty, 358
Deltoid ligament injury, with ankle fractures, 128
Deltoid muscle, 113, 202*t*
Developmental dysplasia of the hip (DDH), 171-178
analysis of, 172
clinical pearls for, 178
complications of, 177
comprehension questions for, 177-178
definitions related to, 173-174
diagnosis of, 174-175, 175*f*
etiology of, 174
treatment of, 176*f*, 176-177
DXA (dual-energy x-ray absorptiometry) scans, 8, 407, 408, 413
Diabetes mellitus, osteomyelitis in. *See* Osteomyelitis
Diagnosis
confirmation of, 16-17
making, 9-10
Disc arthroplasty, for cervical radiculopathy, 240
Disease-modifying antirheumatic drugs (DMARDs), 391
for rheumatoid arthritis, 393, 396
Disease severity
assessing, 10
treatment based on, 10-13
Dislocations. *See* Developmental dysplasia of the hip (DDH); Hip dislocation; Shoulder dislocation, anterior
Divergent Lisfranc injury, 325

DMARDs (disease-modifying antirheumatic drugs), 391
for rheumatoid arthritis, 393, 396
Docking technique, for ulnar collateral ligament reconstruction, 232
Drug abuse, intravenous, osteomyelitis in, 191
Dual-energy x-ray absorptiometry (DXA) scans, 8, 407, 408, 413
Dupuytren diathesis, 285
Dupuytren disease, 283-289
analysis of, 284, 285*f*
clinical pearls for, 289
clinical presentation and evaluation of, 286-287
comprehension questions for, 288-289
definitions related to, 285
etiology and anatomic features relevant to, 285-287
outcomes and complications of, 287
treatment of, 287
Durkan test, 270
DVT (deep vein thrombosis), following knee arthroplasty, 358

E

Eccentric contractions, 307
Elbow
fractures of, in children. *See* Supracondylar fractures
functional range of motion of, 279
nursemaid's, 160
tennis. *See* Lateral epicondylitis
Emboli, pulmonary, with hip or knee arthroplasty, 360
Empty can test, in rotator cuff injury, 199*t*
Enneking staging system, 346, 347, 349
Epicondylitis, lateral. *See* Lateral epicondylitis
EPL (extensor pollicis longus) tendon, rupture of, with distal radius fractures, 38
Erythrocyte sedimentation rate (ESR), 8
septic knee and, 182-183
Evans classification, of intertrochanteric fractures, 63
Extensor mechanism of knee, definition of, 79
Extensor pollicis longus (EPL) tendon, rupture of, with distal radius fractures, 38, 39
External fixation, 13

F

Family history, 2-3
Fasciotomy, for compartment syndrome, 132-133, 134*f*
Febuxostat, for gout, 385
Femoral epiphysis, capital, slipped. *See* Slipped capital femoral epiphysis (SCFE)
Femoral neck, intracapsular and extracapsular, definition of, 52
Femoral neck fractures, 49-57, 50*f*
analysis of, 51
anatomy and, 52-53
basicervical, 53
classification of, 53-54
clinical pearls for, 57
complications of, 56
comprehension questions for, 56-57
definitions related to, 52
evaluation and diagnosis of, 53
mechanisms of injury and, 53
subcapital, 53
transcervical, 53
treatment of, 54-55
for displaced fractures, 55
for nondisplaced fractures, 54-55
Femur fractures, spiral, 156
Fernandez classification, of distal radius fractures, 37

Finger, trigger. *See* Trigger finger
5 Ps, 130, 131
Fixation, loss of, with intertrochanteric fractures, 64
Flatfoot deformity, in adults. *See* Adult acquired flatfoot deformity (AAFD)
Fleck sign, with Lisfranc injury, 328
Flexion contractures, following anterior cruciate ligament reconstruction, 214
Flexor digitorum longus transfer, 317
Floating shoulder, 113, 114
Foot compartment syndrome, with calcaneus fractures, 342
Forearm fractures, both bone, in children. *See* Pediatric both bone forearm fractures (BBFFs)
Forefoot abduction, 317
Fracture(s). *See also specific fractures*
- compartment syndrome associated with, 131-132. *See also* Compartment syndrome
- fixation of, 13
  - external, 13
  - internal, with open reduction, 13
  - loss of, with intertrochanteric fractures, 64
- intramedullary nailing for, 13
- malunion of
  - following calcaneus fractures, 340-341
  - of distal radius fractures, 38
  - of proximal humerus fractures, 103, 105
- nonunion of
  - of femoral neck fractures, 56
  - of intertrochanteric fractures, 64
  - of proximal humerus fractures, 103, 105
- open, definition of, 96
- percutaneous pinning of, 13

Fragility fractures, 407
FRAX, 407
Froment sign, 277, 279
Frykman classification, of distal radius fractures, 37
Functional bracing, 12

G

Gait
- coxalgic, with osteoarthritis of the hip, 366-367
- Trendelenburg, 366-367

Galeazzi test, 173*f*, 173-174
Gap sign, positive, with Lisfranc injury, 326
Garden classification, of femoral neck fractures, 54, 54*t*
Gastrocnemius recession, 317
General appearance, 4
Genu valgum, 399
Genu varum, 399, 400
Glenohumeral joint. *See also* Shoulder *entries*
- anatomy of, 26*t*, 26-27
- biomechanics of, 373-374, 374*f*
- dislocation of
  - anteroinferior. See Shoulder dislocation, anterior
  - inferior, 25, 29
  - posterior, 25, 29

Gout, 381-387
- analysis of, 382-383
- clinical pearls for, 387
- comprehension questions for, 386-387
- definitions related to, 383
- differential diagnosis of, 383
- medical management of, 384-385
- natural history of, 384
- risk factors for, 383
- tophaceous, 384
- uric acid undersecretion in, 387
- workup of, 383-384

Greenstick fractures, 142
- in rickets, 400

Gunstock deformity, with supracondylar fractures, 151

Gustilo classification of open fractures, 95*t*, 96
Guyon canal, 269

H
Hand splinting, 12
Hemiarthroplasty
  definition of, 52
  shoulder, 373, 376
Hemoglobinuria, diagnosis of, 136
Hemophilia, bruising in, 159
Herniated nucleus pulposus
  cauda equina syndrome and, 249
  cervical radiculopathy due to. *See* Cervical radiculopathy
High-turnover osteoporosis, 408
Hill-Sachs lesions, 24, 25, 28
  reverse, 29
Hindfoot valgus, 317, 318
Hip arthroplasty
  hip fracture following. *See* Hip fractures, periprosthetic
  pulmonary embolism following, 360
Hip dislocation. *See also* Developmental dysplasia of the hip (DDH)
  posterior, 41*f*, 41-48
    analysis of, 42
    anatomy of hip joint and, 43
    clinical pearls for, 48
    complications of, 46
    comprehension questions for, 46-47
    definitions related to, 43
    etiology and mechanisms of injury and, 43, 44*f*
    initial management, diagnosis, and classification of, 45, 45*t*
    treatment and postreduction management of, 45-46
Hip dysplasia, developmental. *See* Developmental dysplasia of the hip (DDH)
Hip fractures, intertrochanteric, 59-66, 60*f*
  analysis of, 61
  anatomy and, 62
  classification of, 63
  clinical pearls for, 66
  complications of, 64
  comprehension questions for, 65-66
  definitions fel, 61-62
  evaluation and diagnosis of, 62-63
  mechanism of injury and, 62
  treatment of, 63-64
    nonoperative, 63
    operative, 63-64
Hip fractures, periprosthetic, 67*f*, 67-75
  analysis of, 68-69
  clinical pearls for, 75
  clinical presentation of, 70
  complications of, 72
  comprehension questions for, 73*f*, 73-74
  definitions related to, 69
  diagnosis of, 70
  etiologies of, 69-70
  treatment of, 71, 71*t*
Hip joint, anatomy of, 43, 52-53
Hip osteoarthritis, 363-369, 364*f*, 365*f*
  analysis of, 364-365
  clinical pearls for, 369
  clinical presentation of, 366-367
  comprehension questions for, 368-369
  etiology of, 366
  treatment of, 367
Hippocratic maneuver, 28
Hip precautions, definition of, 43
History taking, 2-4
Hoffman sign, 237, 238
Homolateral Lisfranc injury, 325
Horner syndrome, following anterior cervical discectomy and fusion, 240
β-Human chorionic gonadotropin test, 9
Humerus fracture, proximal, 101*f*, 101-109

analysis of, 102-103
clinical pearls for, 109
clinical presentation of, 104
complications of, 107-108
comprehension questions for, 108-109
definitions related to, 103
diagnosis of, 104-105, 106*f*
etiologies of, 103-104
parts, 103, 105, 106*f*, 107
treatment of, 105, 107
Hutchinson fracture, 35
Hyperkyphosis, 261
Hyperuricemia, gout and. *See* Gout
Hypovascularity, adult acquired flatfoot deformity and, 318

I
Immunocompromised patients, osteomyelitis in, 191
Infection
following calcaneus fractures, 339-340
following knee arthroplasty, 358
following open tibia fracture, 98
osteomyelitis and. *See* Osteomyelitis
septic arthritis and, 181-182, 184
septic knee and. *See* Knee, septic
Infraspinatus muscle, 202*t*, 375
Infraspinatus test, in rotator cuff injury, 199*t*
Injuries. *See also specific injuries*
complications associated with, 17-18
concomitant, 2-3
mechanisms of, 2-3
determining, 16
risk factors for, determining, 16
Insall-Salvati ratio, 80, 80*f*
definition of, 79
Inspection, in spine examination, 5-6
Intermedullary nailing, 13
cephalomedullary
definition of, 62
for intertrochanteric fractures, 64
Interosseous ligament, oblique, 326. *See also* Lisfranc injury
Interosseous nerve, anterior, injury to, supracondylar fractures and, 148, 149, 151
Intertrochanteric, definition of, 61
Intertrochanteric hip fractures. *See* Hip fractures, intertrochanteric
Intravenous drug abuse, osteomyelitis in, 191
Intravenous fluids, for acute compartment syndrome, 133, 136
Involucrum, 191
Ischemic necrosis, with developmental dysplasia of the hip, 177

J
Jumper's knee, 79

K
Knee
extensor mechanism of, 79
osteoarthritis of. *See* Knee osteoarthritis
septic, 170-185
analysis of, 180-181, 181*t*
clinical pearls for, 185
clinical presentation and workup for, 182-183
comprehension questions for, 183-184
definitions related to, 181
pathophysiology of, 181-182, 182*t*
treatment of, 183
Knee immobilizer, 12
Knee osteoarthritis, 353-361, 354*f*
analysis of, 355
clinical pearls for, 361
comprehension questions for, 359-360
differential diagnosis of, 356
treatment of, 357-358
arthroplasty as, 357-358

Knee osteoarthritis, treatment of (*Cont.*):
  arthroscopy and osteotomies as, 357
  complications of, 358
  nonoperative, 357
Kyphosis, 261

L
Laboratory tests, 8-9. *See also specific tests*
  inflammatory, 8
  preoperative, 8
  synovial fluid analyses, 9
  urine pregnancy test, 9
Lacey osteoid matrix production, with osteosarcoma, 348
Lachman test, 209, 211
Laminoforaminotomy, posterior, for cervical radiculopathy, 240
Lateral column lengthening, 317
Lateral epicondylitis, 297-303
  analysis of, 298-299
  classification of and diagnosis of, 299-300
  clinical pearls for, 303
  comprehension questions for, 301-302
  definitions related to, 299
  etiology of, 299, 300*f*
  treatment of, 301
Latissimus dorsi muscle, 202*t*
Lauge-Hansen classification, of ankle fractures, 123, 124*f*–125*f*, 126
Ledderhose disease, 286
Leflunomide, for rheumatoid arthritis, 393
Leg cases, 11-12
Leukemia, bruising in, 159
Levoscoliosis, 261
Li-Fraumeni syndrome, osteosarcoma and, 347
Lift-off test in rotator cuff injury, 199*t*, 205
Ligaments. *See also specific ligaments*
  definition of, 229
Limb-salvage surgery, 347
Lisfranc, Jacques, 325
Lisfranc injury, 323-330
  analysis of, 324-325
  anatomy relevant to, 326
  clinical pearls for, 330
  comprehension questions for, 329-330
  definitions related to, 325
  divergent, 325
  homolateral, 325
  mechanism of injury and, 326
  treatment of, 328
  workup and diagnosis of, 326-328, 327*f*
Lisfranc joint, 325
Lisfranc ligament, 326
Load and shift test, 27
Long arm casts, 11
Long leg casts, 12
Lower motor neuron lesions, 246
Low-turnover osteoporosis, 408
Lumbar burst fractures, 251*f*, 251-257
  analysis of, 252-253
  clinical pearls for, 257
  comprehension questions for, 256-257
  definitions related to, 253-254
  history and physical exam for, 254
  imaging of, 254-255
  treatment of, 255
Lumbar plexus, major cervical roots to, 6, 7*t*
Luxatio erecta, 25, 29

M
Magnetic resonance imaging (MRI), 8
Maisonneuve fractures, 127
Malleolus, lateral and medial, 121
Malunion
  following calcaneus fractures, 340-341
  of distal radius fractures, 38
  of proximal humerus fractures, 103, 105
Maudsley test, 299, 300
McCash technique, for Dupuytren disease, 287

McMurray test, 221, 221*f*, 222, 225
Mechanism of injury, 2-3
determining, 16
Medial clear space, 122, 123*f*
Medializing calcaneal osteotomy, 317
Medial plantar ecchymosis, with Lisfranc injury, 324, 328
Median nerve
in carpal tunnel syndrome, 272
function of, with pediatric both bone forearm fractures, evaluation of, 142
Median nerve compression syndrome, 269
Medical history, past, 2-3
Medications. *See* Pharmacologic therapy
Meniscal tears, 219-225
analysis of, 220-221
clinical pearls for, 225
complications of, 223
comprehension questions for, 224-225
definitions related to, 221
diagnosis of, 222, 223*f*
etiology of, 222
treatment of, 222-223
Menisci, definition of, 221
Methotrexate, for rheumatoid arthritis, 391, 393, 396
Milking maneuver, 229, 230*f*
Modified Jobe technique, for ulnar collateral ligament reconstruction, 232
Monosodium urate crystals, 383
Mortise, 121
Mortise view, 122, 123*f*
Motor vehicle collisions (MVCs), hip dislocation caused by. *See* Hip dislocation, posterior
Moving valgus tress test, 229, 231, 231*f*
MRI (magnetic resonance imaging), 8
MSTS (Musculoskeletal Tumor Society Staging System), 346, 347, 349
Musculoskeletal examination, of extremities, basic approach to, 4-5
Musculoskeletal Tumor Society Staging System (MSTS), 346, 347, 349
MVCs (motor vehicle collisions), hip dislocation caused by. *See* Hip dislocation, posterior
Myofibroblasts, Dupuytren disease and, 286
Myoglobulinemia
with compartment syndrome, 133
diagnosis of, 136

N

Necrosis. *See also* Osteonecrosis
avascular
definition of, 43, 52
following femoral neck fractures, 56
of knee, 356
following proximal humerus fractures, 103, 107, 108
ischemic, with developmental dysplasia of the hip, 177
Neer classification of proximal humerus fractures, 103, 105
Neurogenic bladder dysfunction, in cauda equina syndrome, 246
Neuromuscular scoliosis, 261
Neuropathy, osteomyelitis and, 189
Neurovascular exam
with anterior shoulder dislocation, 24
in musculoskeletal examination of extremities, 5
in spine examination, 6, 7*t*
with supracondylar fractures, 150
Nonnutritional rickets, 399-400, 401*f*
Nonsteroidal anti-inflammatory drugs (NSAIDs)
for cervical radiculopathy, 239
for gout, 384
for rheumatoid arthritis, 393, 396

Nonunion
  of clavicle fractures, 116
  of femoral neck fractures, 56
  of intertrochanteric fractures, 64
  of proximal humerus fractures, 103, 105
NSAIDs (nonsteroidal anti-inflammatory drugs)
  for cervical radiculopathy, 239
  for gout, 384
  for rheumatoid arthritis, 393, 396
Nuclear medicine scans, 8
Nucleus pulposus, herniated
  cauda equina syndrome and, 249
  cervical radiculopathy due to. *See* Cervical radiculopathy
Nursemaid's elbow, 160
Nutritional rickets, 399-400, 401*f*

O

OA (osteoarthritis)
  following distal radius fractures, 38
  of hip. *See* Hip osteoarthritis
  of knee. *See* Knee osteoarthritis
  primary and secondary, 392
Oblique interosseous ligament, 326. *See also* Lisfranc injury
OI (osteogenesis imperfecta), 159, 160, 161
Open fractures, definition of, 96
Open reduction internal fixation (ORIF), 13
Operative treatments, 13
ORIF (open reduction internal fixation), 13
Ortolani sign, 174-175, 178
Ossification centers, of elbow, order of ossification for, 150, 153
Osteoarthritis (OA)
  following distal radius fractures, 38
  of hip. *See* Hip osteoarthritis
  of knee. *See* Knee osteoarthritis
  primary and secondary, 392
Osteogenesis imperfecta (OI), 159, 160, 161
Osteomalacia, 399
Osteomyelitis, 181, 187-195, 188*f*
  acute, 190
  analysis of, 189-190
  chronic, 190
  clinical pearls for, 195
  complications of, 192-193
  comprehension questions for, 193-194
  definitions related to, 190-191
  diagnosis of, 191
  pathophysiology of, 191
  radiographic evaluation of, 191-192
  in sickle cell disease, 194
  treatment of, 192-193
Osteonecrosis, 166, 356
  definition of, 43
  following posterior hip dislocation, 46
  with slipped capital femoral epiphysis, 168
Osteopenia, 399
Osteoporosis, 405-414
  analysis of, 406-407
  clinical pearls for, 414
  comprehension questions for, 411-413
  definition of, 103
  definitions related to, 407
  high-turnover, 408
  low-turnover, 408
  pathophysiology of, 407-409
  patient evaluation in, 408-409, 409*t*
  primary, 407
  secondary, 407, 408*t*
  treatment of, 409-411
    nonpharmacologic, 409-410, 410*f*
    pharmacologic, 410-411
Osteosarcoma, 345*f*, 345-350
  analysis of, 346
  clinical approach to, 347-349, 348*f*
  clinical pearls for, 350
  comprehension questions for, 349-350
  definitions related to, 347

Osteotomies
calcaneal, medializing, 317
for osteoarthritis of the knee, 357
Ottawa Ankle Criteria, 122, 123*f*

P

Palpation
in musculoskeletal examination of extremities, 5
in spine examination, 6
Patellar tendon rupture, 77-83
analysis of, 77
clinical pearls for, 83
complications of, 81
comprehension questions for, 81-82
definitions related to, 79
etiology of, 79
physical examination of, 80
radiographic diagnosis of, 80*f*, 80-81
treatment of, 81
Pauwel classification of femoral neck fractures, 54
Pavlik harness, 176, 176*f*
PE (pulmonary emboli), with hip or knee arthroplasty, 360
Peak growth velocity, 261, 262
Pectoralis major muscle, 113, 202*t*
Pediatric both bone forearm fractures (BBFFs), 139-145, 140*f*
analysis of, 141
classification of, 142
clinical pearls for, 145
complications of, 143-144
comprehension questions for, 144-145
definitions related to, 141-142
mechanism of injury and, 142
treatment of, 143
workup for, 142
Pediatric patients. *See* Child abuse; Developmental dysplasia of the hip (DDH); Pediatric both bone forearm fractures (BBFFs); Slipped capital femoral epiphysis (SCFE); Supracondylar fractures
Pegloticase, for gout, 385
Pendulum exercises, for clavicle fractures, 114
Percutaneous pinning, 13
Peroneal irritation, following calcaneus fractures, 340
Peyronie disease, 286
p53 gene, osteosarcoma and, 347
Phalen sign, 270
Pharmacologic therapy
for cervical radiculopathy, 239
for Dupuytren disease, 287
for gout, 384-385
history taking and, 4
for open tibia fractures, 95, 96, 96*t*, 99
for osteomyelitis, 192
for osteoporosis, 410-411, 413
for rheumatoid arthritis, 391, 393, 396
Phosphorus, rickets and, 399
Physical exam, 4-7
Pivot shift test, 209, 211
Plain films, 7
Pleomorphism, nuclear, with osteosarcoma, 348
PMMA (polymethylmethacrylate), 356
for osteomyelitis, 192
Podagra, 383
Polymethylmethacrylate (PMMA), 356
for osteomyelitis, 192
Positive gap sign, with Lisfranc injury, 326
Posterior drawer test, 211
Posterior fat pad sign, 149, 150
Posterior tibial tendon, 317
Posttraumatic arthritis, of knee, 356
Prednisone, for gout, 384-385
Pregnancy test, urine, 9
Probenecid, for gout, 385
Pseudogout, 383, 387
Pulley, 293, 293*f*
Pulmonary emboli (PE), with hip or knee arthroplasty, 360

R

RA. *See* Rheumatoid arthritis (RA)
Radial nerve function, with pediatric both bone forearm fractures, evaluation of, 142
Radiculopathy
  cervical. *See* Cervical radiculopathy
  definition of, 237
Radiographs, 7
  stress, of ankle, 122
Radiologic evaluation, 7-8. *See also under specific conditions and injuries*
  in suspected child abuse, 159
Radius fracture
  distal (Colles), 33*f*, 33-40
    analysis of, 34-35
    anatomy and mechanisms of injury and, 35
    carpal tunnel syndrome associated with, 272
    classification of, 37
    clinical pearls for, 40
    comprehension questions for, 39-40
    definitions related to, 35
    outcomes and complications of, 38
    radiographic evaluation of, 35, 36*f*, 37
    treatment of, 37-38
  with ulna fracture, in children. *See* Pediatric both bone forearm fractures (BBFFs)
Raloxifene, for osteoporosis, 411
Range of motion
  in musculoskeletal examination of extremities, 5
  in spine examination, 6
RB1 (retinoblastoma tumor suppressor gene), osteosarcoma and, 347
Reading, clinical problem-oriented approach to, 14-18
Reflexes
  anal wink, 245, 247
  bulbocavernosus, 247, 254
Response to treatment, 14
Retinoblastoma tumor suppressor gene (*RB1*), osteosarcoma and, 347
Retropulsion, 253
Reverse obliquity, definition of, 62
Review of systems, 4
Rhabdomyolysis, 131
  with compartment syndrome, 135
Rheumatoid arthritis (RA), 389-396, 390*f*
  analysis of, 391
  clinical pearls for, 396
  comprehension questions for, 394-396
  definitions related to, 391
  diagnosis of, 392
  differential diagnosis of, 392
  extraarticular manifestations of, 393
  prognosis of, 393-394
  radiology in, 392
  septic arthritis associated with, 184
  serologies in, 392
  treatment of, 391, 393
Rickets, 159, 397-403
  analysis of, 398
  clinical features of, 400
  clinical pearls for, 403
  comprehension questions for, 402-403
  definitions related to, 399
  etiology of, 399
  laboratory findings in, 400
  management of, 400-401
  nonnutritional, 400
  nutritional, 399-400, 401*f*
  pathophysiology of, 399
  radiologic findings in, 400
Risser sign, 261
Rotator cuff
  definition of, 200
  function and testing of muscles of, 374-375
  injury of, 197-206
    analysis of, 198, 199*f*, 199*t*, 200*f*
    classification of, 203-204
    clinical pearls for, 206

comprehension questions for, 205-206
definitions related to, 200-201
diagnosis of, 203
etiology of, 202-203
presentation of, 203
shoulder anatomy and biomechanics, 201*f*, 201-202, 202*t*
tears, 200
treatment of, 204-205
muscles of, 101*t*
Rotator cuff arthropathy, 200
Rugger jersey spine, 403

S

Sanders classification of calcaneus fractures, 337
Sarcoma. *See* Osteosarcoma
Sarmiento bracing, 12
SCFE. *See* Slipped capital femoral epiphysis (SCFE)
Schatzker classification, 87, 88*f*, 89
Sciatica, 245
Scoliosis
definition of, 261
idiopathic, adolescent. *See* Adolescent idiopathic scoliosis (AIS)
neuromuscular, 261
Segond fracture, 211
Septic arthritis, 181-182, 184
Sequestrum, 190
Serendipity view, 112, 113-114
Sex of patient, 2
Shock, spinal, 254
Short arm casts, 11
Short leg casts, 11
Shoulder. *See also* Glenohumeral joint; Rotator cuff *entries*
anatomy and biomechanics of, 201*f*, 201-202, 202*t*
anatomy of, 373-374, 374, 375*f*
floating, 113, 114
instability of, 25
anterior, 27
laxity of, 25
Shoulder arthroplasty, 371-380
analysis of, 372
clinical pearls for, 380
complications of, 377
comprehension questions for, 378-379
definitions related to, 373
hemiarthroplasty as, 376
radiographic evaluation and, 375-376
rehabilitation following, 377
rotator cuff muscle function and testing, 374-375
shoulder anatomy and normal glenohumeral biomechanics and, 373-374, 374*f*, 375*f*
total, 373, 376
reverse, 376-377
Shoulder dislocation, anterior, 23*f*, 23-31
analysis of, 24-25
clinical pearls for, 31
clinical presentation of, 27-28
comprehension questions for, 30
definitions related to, 25
epidemiology of, 25
glenohumeral joint anatomy and, 26*t*, 26-27
treatment of, 28-29
closed reduction as, 28
operative, 29
Sickle cell disease, osteomyelitis associated with, 194
Skeletal survey, in suspected child abuse, 156
Sliding hip screws
definition of, 62
for intertrochanteric fractures, 63-64
Slipped capital femoral epiphysis (SCFE), 163, 164*f*, 165-170
analysis of, 165
classification of, 167
clinical pearls for, 170
complications of, 168

Slipped capital femoral epiphysis (SCFE) (*Cont.*):
- comprehension questions for, 168-169
- definitions related to, 166
- epidemiology of, 166
- pathogenesis of, 166
- radiographic evaluation of, 167
- stable, 166
- treatment of, 167-168
- unstable, 166

Smith fractures, 35
Social history, 4
Spica cast, for developmental hip dysplasia, 176
Spinal asymmetry, 262
Spinal shock, 254
Spine
- cervical
  - clearing, 6-7
  - radiculopathy and. *See* Cervical radiculopathy
- examination of, basic approach to, 5-6
- lumbar, burst fractures of. *See* Lumbar burst fractures
- rugger jersey, 403
- scoliosis of. *See* Adolescent idiopathic scoliosis (AIS); Scoliosis

Spiral cords, 285, 286
Splinting, of hand, 12
Spring ligament, 317
Spurling sign, 237
Squat test, 221*f*, 222
Sternoclavicular muscle, 113
Sternocleidomastoid muscle, 113
Stiffness, following proximal humerus fractures, 107
Stimson technique, 28
Stress radiographs, of ankle, 122
Subacromial impingement, 200
Subscapularis muscle, 202*t*, 374-375
- lift-off test for, 199*t*

Subtalar arthritis, following calcaneus fractures, 339
Sulfasalazine, for rheumatoid arthritis, 393
Superior shoulder suspensory complex, 113
Supracondylar fractures, 147*f*, 147-153
- analysis of, 148-149
- classifications and treatment of, 150-151
- clinical pearls for, 153
- complications of, 151
- comprehension questions for, 152-153
- definitions related to, 149
- epidemiology of, 149
- history and physical examination of, 150
- mechanism of injury and anatomy relevant to, 149
- radiographic evaluation of, 150

Supraspinatus muscle, 202*t*, 375
- empty can test for, 199*t*

Surgical history, past, 2-3
Suspensory ligaments, 113
Syndesmosis, 121
Synovial fluid, from adult knee joint, classification of, 180, 181*t*
Synovial fluid analyses, 9
Syphilis, congenital, 159

T

Talocrural angle, 122, 123*f*
Tarsometatarsal (TMT) joint. *See* Lisfranc injury; Lisfranc joint
Tendinitis, 79
Tendinosis, 79
Tennis elbow. *See* Lateral epicondylitis
Tenosynovium, 293
Tensile strength, 228, 229
Teres major muscle, 202*t*
Teres minor muscle, 202*t*, 375
Teriparatide, for osteoporosis, 411
Thomas test, 367
Thompson test, 307, 307*f*
Thoracic dextroscoliosis, 261
Throwers series, 231

Tibia fractures, open, 93-100, 94*f*
  analysis of, 95*t*, 95-96, 96*t*
  clinical pearls for, 100
  comprehension questions for, 98-99
  definitions related to, 96-97
  initial assessment of, 97
  operative intervention for, 97-98
  risks and complications of, 98
  secondary surgery for, 98
Tibial plafond, 121
Tibial plateau
  definition of, 87
  fractures of, 85*f*, 85-91
    analysis of, 86
    anatomy and mechanisms of injury and, 87
    classification of, 87, 88*f*
    clinical pearls for, 91
    comprehension questions for, 89-91, 90*f*
    definitions related to, 87
    medial, 87
    outcomes and complications of, 89
    radiographic evaluation of, 88
    Schatzker classification of, 87, 88*f*, 89
    treatment of, 89
Tibial tendon, posterior, 317
Tibiofibular clear space, 122, 123*f*
Tinel test, 270, 277, 279
Tip-to-apex distance
  definition of, 62
  with intertrochanteric fractures, 64
TKA (total knee arthroplasty), 358
TMT (tarsometatarsal) joint. *See* Lisfranc injury; Lisfranc joint
TNF (tumor necrosis factor), 391
TNF (tumor necrosis factor) inhibitors, for rheumatoid arthritis, 393, 396
TNT (tarsometatarsal) joint. *See* Lisfranc injury; Lisfranc joint
Tophaceous gout, 384
Total knee arthroplasty (TKA), 358
Traction, 12
Traction-countertraction, 28
Trapezius muscle, 113
Trapezoid ligaments, 113
Trauma, acute, ATLS protocol for, 2
Treatment, determination of, 17
Treatment response, 14
Trendelenburg gait, 173, 366-367
Trigger finger, 291-296
  analysis of, 292-293
  clinical pearls for, 296
  clinical presentation of, 294-295
  comprehension questions for, 295-296
  etiology of, 294
  treatment of, 295
TUBS (traumatic, unidirectional, Bankart, surgery), 29
Tumor necrosis factor (TNF), 391
Tumor necrosis factor (TNF) inhibitors, for rheumatoid arthritis, 393, 396

U

UCL. *See* Ulnar collateral ligament (UCL)
UKA (unicompartmental knee arthroplasty), 357
Ulna fracture, with radius fracture, in children. *See* Pediatric both bone forearm fractures (BBFFs)
Ulnar collateral ligament (UCL)
  injury of, 227-233
    analysis of, 228
    clinical approach to, 229, 230*f*, 231*f*, 231-232
    comprehension questions for, 232-233
    definitions related to, 229
reconstruction of, 232
Ulnar nerve
  evaluation of function and, 142
  injury of
    with pediatric both bone forearm fractures, 151
    with ulnar collateral ligament injury, 233

Ultrasound, 8
Unicompartmental knee arthroplasty (UKA), 357
Uric acid-lowering agents, for gout, 385
Urine pregnancy test, 9

V
Vacuum-assisted wound closure (VAC), definition of, 97
Valgus, hindfoot, 317, 318
Valgus stress, 228, 229
Valgus stress test, 229, 230*f*
  moving, 229, 231, 231*f*
Vascular disease, osteomyelitis in, 191
Vascular exam. *See* Neurovascular exam
Vascular zones, 221
Velpeau axillary radiographs, 28
Vertebrae. *See also* Spine
  burst fractures of, 253
    lumbar. See Lumbar burst fractures
  columns of, 253
Vital signs, 4
Vitamin D deficiency, rickets and. *See* Rickets
Vitamin D supplementation, for rickets, 400-401

W
Wartenberg sign, 277, 279
WBC (white blood cell count), septic knee and, 182
Weber classification of ankle fractures, 122-123
White blood cell count (WBC), septic knee and, 182
Wound complications, following calcaneus fractures, 339-340
Wrinkle test, with calcaneus fractures, 338

X
Xiaflex, for Dupuytren disease, 287, 289
X-rays, 7

Z
Zanca view, 113-114
Zone of injury, definition of, 96